Advanced Therapy of
HEADACHE

Advanced Therapy of **HEADACHE**

Alan M. Rapoport, MD

Assistant Clinical Professor of Neurology
Yale University School of Medicine, New Haven, Connecticut
Director, The New England Center for Headache
Stamford, Connecticut

Fred D. Sheftell, MD

Assistant Clinical Professor, Department of Psychiatry
New York Medical College, Valhalla, New York
Director, The New England Center for Headache
Stamford, Connecticut

R. Allan Purdy, MD

Professor and Head, Division of Neurology
Dalhousie University
Chief, Neurology Service
Queen Elizabeth II Health Sciences Centre
Halifax, Nova Scotia, Canada

1999
B.C. Decker Inc.
Hamilton • London • Saint Louis

B.C. Decker Inc.

4 Hughson Street South
P.O. Box 620, L.C.D. 1
Hamilton, Ontario L8N 3K7
Tel: 905-522-7017; 1-800-568-7281
Fax: 905-522-7839
e-mail: info@bcdecker.com
Website: http://www.bcdecker.com

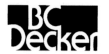

ISBN 1-55009-057-7

Printed in Canada

Sales and Distribution

United States
B.C. Decker Inc.
P.O. Box 785
Lewiston, NY 14092-0785 USA
Tel: 905-522-7017; 1-800-568-7281
Fax: 905-522-7389
e-mail: info@bcdecker.com

Canada
B.C. Decker Inc.
4 Hughson Street South
P.O. Box 620, L.C.D. 1
Hamilton, Ontario L8N 3K7
Tel: 905-522-7017; 1-800-568-7281
Fax: 905-522-7839
e-mail: info@bcdecker.com

Japan
Igaku-Shoin Ltd.
Foreign Publications Department
3-24-17 Hongo, Bunkyo-ku,
Tokyo 113-8719, Japan
Tel: 3 3817 5676
Fax: 3 3815 6776

U.K., Europe, Scandinavia, Middle East
Blackwell Science Ltd.
c/o Marston Book Services Ltd.
P.O. Box 87
Oxford OX2 0DT
England
Tel: 44-1865-79115

Australia
Blackwell Science Pty, Ltd.
54 University Street
Carlton, Victoria 3053
Australia
Tel: 03 9347 0300
Fax: 03 9349 3016

Korea
Jee Seung Publishing Company
236-15 Neung-Dong
Seung Dong P.O. Box 134
Seoul 133-600 Korea
Tel: 2-454-5463
Fax: 2-456-5058

South America
Ernesto Reichmann, Distribuidora de Livros Ltda.
Rua Coronel Marques
335-Tatuape, 03440-000
Sao Paulo-SP-Brazil
Tel/Fax: 011-218-2122

Foreign Rights
John Scott & Co.
International Publishers' Agency
P.O. Box 878
Kimberton, PA 19442
Tel: 610-827-1640
Fax: 610-827-1671

CONTRIBUTORS

STEVEN M. BASKIN, PhD
Director, New England Institute for Behavioral Medicine
Stamford, Connecticut
Neuropsychologist, Section of Neurology
Greenwich Hospital
Greenwich, Connecticut

WERNER J. BECKER, MD, FRCPC
Professor, Department of Clinical Neurosciences
University of Calgary
Director, Division of Neurology
Calgary Regional Health Authority
Calgary, Alberta, Canada

RANDALL BERLINER, MD
Assistant Professor of Neurology and Psychiatry
Albert Einstein College of Medicine
Montefiore Medical Center and Community Hospital
  at Dobbs Ferry
Bronx, New York

OSCAR BERNAL, MD
Clinical Assistant Instructor
Department of Neurology, School of Medicine
State University of New York at Stony Brook
Stony Brook, New York

VALÉRIE BIOUSSE, MD
Assistant in Neurology, Lariboisière Medical Faculty
Paris University VII
Assistant, Neurology Department
Hôpital Lariboisière
Paris, France

HARVEY J. BLUMENTHAL, MD
Clinical Professor of Neurology
University of Oklahoma College of Medicine
Neurological Associates of Tulsa
St. Francis Hospital
Tulsa, Oklahoma

NIKOLAI BOGDUK, MD, PhD, DSc
Professor of Anatomy and Musculoskeletal Medicine
University of Newcastle
Director, Newcastle Bone and Joint Medicine
Royal Newcastle Hospital
Visiting Medical Officer, Pain Management
Mater Hospital
Newcastle, Australia

MARIE-GERMAINE BOUSSER, MD
Professor of Neurology, Lariboisière Medical Faculty
University Paris VII
Head, Neurology Department
Hôpital Lariboisière
Paris, France

GENNARO BUSSONE, MD
Neurological Institute "Carlo Besta"
Head, Department of Clinical Neurology
Director of Headache and Craniofacial Pain Center
Milan, Italy

J. KEITH CAMPBELL, MD, FRCP
Emeritus Professor of Neurology
Mayo Medical School and Mayo Clinic
Rochester, Minnesota

LOUIS R. CAPLAN, MD
Department of Neurology
Beth Israel Deaconess Medical Center
Boston, Massachusetts

DAVID J. CAPOBIANCO, MD
Assistant Professor, Mayo Medical School
Consultant, Department of Neurology
Mayo Clinic Jacksonville
Jacksonville, Florida

PATRICIA K. COYLE, MD
Professor of Neurology
Department of Neurology, School of Medicine
State University of New York at Stony Brook
Stony Brook, New York

SEYMOUR DIAMOND, MD
Adjunct Professor of Clinical Pharmacology
  and Molecular Biology
Finch University of Health Sciences
Chicago Medical School
Director, Diamond Headache Clinic
Director, Inpatient Headache Unit
Columbus Hospital
Chicago, Illinois

DAVID W. DODICK, MD, FRCPC, FACP
Assistant Professor of Neurology
Department of Neurology
Mayo Clinic Scottsdale
Mayo Graduate School of Medicine
Scottsdale, Arizona

IVY M. FETTES, MD, PhD, FRCPC
Associate Professor of Medicine
University of Toronto
Staff Endocrinologist and Co-director, Mature Women's Clinic
Division of Endocrinology and Metabolism
Sunnybrook Hospital
Women's College Health Sciences Centre
Toronto, Ontario, Canada

MAREK J. GAWEL, MD
University of Toronto
Sunnybrook Health Sciences Centre
Toronto, Ontario, Canada

JACK GLADSTEIN, MD
Associate Dean for Student and Minority Affairs
Associate Professor, Pediatrics
Director, Pediatric Headache Clinic
University of Maryland Hospital
Baltimore School of Medicine
Baltimore, Maryland

PETER J. GOADSBY, MD, PhD, DSc, FRACP, FRCP
Professor of Clinical Neurology
Institute of Neurology
Consultant Neurologist
National Hospital for Neurology and Neurosurgery
London, England

JEROME GOLDSTEIN, MD
Assistant Clinical Professor of Neurology
University of California—San Francisco
Chairman, Department of Internal Medicine
St. Francis Memorial Hospital
Director, San Francisco Headache Clinic
San Francisco, California

MARK GORMAN, MD
Assistant Professor of Neurology
Department of Neurology
Wayne State University School of Medicine
Detroit, Michigan

STEPHEN B. GRAFF-RADFORD, DDS
Adjunct Associate Professor
UCLA School of Dentistry
Director, The Pain Center
Cedars Sinai Medical Center
Los Angeles, California

MARK W. GREEN, MD
Associate Clinical Professor of Neurology
New York Medical College
Mt. Kisco, New York

SHELDON G. GROSS, DDS, PC
Postgraduate Orofacial Pain Program
New York University School of Dental Medicine
New York, New York
Consultant, Pain Associates
Manchester Memorial Hospital
Manchester, Connecticut

DAVID KUDROW, MD
California Medical Clinic for Headache
Encino, California

ROBERT S. KUNKEL, MD, FACP
Clinical Assistant Professor of Medicine
Pennsylvania State College of Medicine
Staff Physician
Cleveland Clinic Headache Center
Cleveland, Ohio

RICHARD B. LIPTON, MD
Professor of Neurology, Epidemiology, and
  Social Medicine
Albert Einstein College of Medicine
Bronx, New York
CEO, Innovative Medical Research
Stamford, Connecticut

ELIZABETH LODER, MD
Instructor in Medicine
Harvard Medical School
Director, Pain and Headache Program
Spaulding Rehabilitation Hospital
Boston, Massachusetts

ANNE MAGGISANO
Research Assistant, Headache Clinic
Sunnybrook Health Science Centre
Toronto, Ontario, Canada

RUTH ANN MARRIE, MD
Resident in Neurology
McGill University
Montreal Neurological Institute
Montreal, Quebec, Canada

THOMAS J. MARRIE, MD, FRCPC, FACP
Division of Infectious Diseases
Dalhousie University
Queen Elizabeth II Health Sciences Centre
Halifax, Nova Scotia, Canada

FRANCA MOSCHIANO, MD
Department of Neurology
Neurological Institute "Carlo Besta"
Milan, Italy

NINAN T. MATHEW, MD, FRCPC
Houston Headache Clinic
Houston, Texas

STEPHEN A. MAYER, MD
Assistant Professor of Neurology
Department of Neurosurgery
Columbia University
College of Physicians and Surgeons
New York, New York

RAGUI H. MICHAEL
Clinical Research Coordinator
San Francisco Headache Clinic
San Francisco, California

ROBERT F. NELSON MD, FRCPC
Professor of Medicine
Division of Neurology
University of Ottawa
Ottawa General Hospital
Ottawa, Ontario, Canada

LAWRENCE C. NEWMAN, MD
Assistant Professor of Neurology
Albert Einstein College of Medicine
Director, The Headache Institute at St. Luke's-Roosevelt
  and Beth Israel Medical Centers
Bronx, New York

JOSEPH M. PHILLIPS, MD, PhD
Section of Neurosurgery
Dartmouth Hitchcock Medical Center
Lebanon, New Hampshire

WILLIAM PRYSE-PHILLIPS, MD
Professor of Medicine (Neurology)
Memorial University of Newfoundland
Neurologist, Health Sciences Centre
St. John's, Newfoundland, Canada

R. ALLAN PURDY, MD
Professor and Head, Division of Neurology
Dalhousie University
Chief, Neurology Service
Queen Elizabeth II Health Sciences Centre
Halifax, Nova Scotia, Canada

NABIH M. RAMADAN, MD
Associate Professor of Neurology
University of Cincinnati Medical Center
Director, Cincinnati Headache Center
Cincinnati, Ohio

ALAN M. RAPOPORT, MD
Assistant Clinical Professor of Neurology
Yale University School of Medicine
New Haven, Connecticut
Medical Director
Greenwich Hospital Inpatient Headache Unit
Greenwich, Connecticut
Co-founder and Co-director
The New England Center for Headache
Stamford, Connecticut

GORDON ROBINSON, MD, FRCPC
Clinical Associate Professor
University of British Columbia
Active Staff Neurologist
Division of Neurology, Vancouver Hospital
Vancouver, British Columbia, Canada

JOHN F. ROTHROCK, MD
Professor and Chairman of Neurology
University of South Alabama
College of Medicine
Mobile, Alabama

TODD D. ROZEN, MD
Assistant Professor in Neurology
Jefferson Headache Center
Thomas Jefferson University Hospital
Department of Neurology
Philadelphia, Pennsylvania

ROBERT E. RYAN JR., MS, MD
Assistant Clinical Professor
Department of Otolaryngology
St. Louis University School of Medicine
Director, Ryan Headache Center
Executive Director, Unity Health Research
St. Louis, Missouri

FRED D. SHEFTELL, MD
Assistant Clinical Professor
Department of Psychiatry
New York Medical College
Valhalla, New York
Co-founder and Co-director
The New England Center for Headache
Stamford, Connecticut

STEPHEN D. SILBERSTEIN, MD
Professor of Neurology
Jefferson Medical College
Director, Jefferson Headache Center
Thomas Jefferson University
Philadelphia, Pennsylvania

GLEN D. SOLOMON, MD, FACP
Associate Professor of Medicine
The Ohio State University
Department of General Internal Medicine
 and Neurology
Cleveland Clinic Foundation
Cleveland, Ohio

SEYMOUR SOLOMON, MD
Professor of Neurology
Albert Einstein College of Medicine
Director Emeritus, Headache Unit
Montefiore Medical Center
Bronx, New York

WILLIAM G. SPEED III, MD
Director Emeritus, Speed Headache Associates
Baltimore, Maryland

EGILIUS L.H. SPIERINGS, MD, PhD
Lecturer in Neurology
Harvard Medical School
Consultant in Neurology
Brigham and Women's Hospital
Wellesley Hills, Maryland

NAGANAND SRIPATHI, MD
Staff Neurologist
Department of Neurology
Henry Ford Hospital and Health Sciences Center
Detroit, Michigan

STEWART J. TEPPER, MD
Clinical Assistant Professor of Neurology
University of Washington Medical School
Polyclinic
Attending, Swedish Hospital Medical Center
Harborview Medical Center
Seattle, Washington

KATAYOUN VAHEDI, MD
Chef de Clinique
Assistant in Neurology
University Paris VII
Hôpital Lariboisière
Paris, France

NAZHIYATH VIJAYAN, MD
Professor of Neurology
U.C. Davis School of Medicine
Director, U.C. Davis Headache Clinic
Sacramento, California

THOMAS N. WARD, MD
Director, Headache Clinic
Dartmouth-Hitchcock Medical Center
Lebanon, New Hampshire

JOHN S. WARNER, MD
Professor of Neurology
Vanderbilt University Medical Center
Director, The Vanderbilt Headache Clinic
Nashville, Tennessee

RANDALL WEEKS, PhD
Neuropsychologist
Department of Neurology
Greenwich Hospital
Director, New England Institute for
 Behavioral Medicine
Stamford, Connecticut

PAUL K. WINNER, DO
Assistant Clinical Professor in Neurology
NOVA Southeastern University
Co-director, Palm Beach Headache Center
Co-director, Perieme Research Institute
St. Mary's Neuroscience Center
West Palm Beach, Florida

ANNA M. WONG, MD
Neurology Resident
Memorial University of Newfoundland
Health Sciences Centre
St. John's, Newfoundland, Canada

WILLIAM YOUNG, MD
Assistant Professor of Neurology
Jefferson Headache Center
Philadelphia, Pennsylvania

FOREWORD

THIS IS ANOTHER BOOK ABOUT HEADACHE.

When I began studying medicine almost 50 years ago, headache was rather a disreputable subject. Patients with headaches were widely perceived as being neurotic if they had migraine, weak if they had tension headache, or venal if they complained of head pain following an occupational or traffic accident. Only the demonstration of a brain tumor or a subdural hematoma would restore them to respectability. Physicians who specialized in headache were regarded by their colleagues as, at best, eccentric, and, at worst, as not being up to "real" medicine.

The advent of Harold Wolff's *Headache and Other Head Pain* changed all that. Beautifully written, it tempted students to dip their toes into the murky waters of headache. Rigorously researched, it gave reassurance that there was, after all, some science underpinning the study of headache. Many of those who contributed to this book, *Advanced Therapy of Headache*, first became interested in the subject through reading Wolff. Since then, there has been a proliferation of headache books, keeping pace with the explosion of scientifically based information on the subject. There are now over a dozen headache books on the market (many written by contributors to the present volume), and every major textbook of Internal Medicine or Neurology contains at least one chapter on headache.

Do we really need another headache book—particularly this one?

Yes. This book is different. As its title *Advanced Therapy of Headache* indicates, this book is not a general purpose text for beginners nor a bookshelf-bound reference, but, rather, a case-based compendium of advice for physicians with some background in headache, from very experienced colleagues, on the management of headache disorders that are complex or difficult. This does not necessarily mean that these disorders are rare. Indeed, most of them are common but are rendered difficult either (as in the case of migraine) by the dizzying proliferation of new medications or (as with chronic daily headache) by a lack of understanding of the etiology and a paucity of effective treatments.

The case-based format of this book is appropriate to its relatively experienced audience. In our early stages of development, we learn mostly from standard texts. Later on, we read these texts either to pick up the latest advances or to satisfy our curiosity but most of our learning is from our own cases, and from those of our colleagues. Whether from our own "experience" or our colleagues' "mistakes" (same thing), this kind of learning sticks. We remember it, and we incorporate it readily into our own experience.

All the important headache problems are addressed in this book, and each chapter bears the often recognizable distinctly personal stamp of its author. If their opinions verge on the idiosyncratic from time to time, they are promptly counterbalanced by an editorial note.

In their preface, the editors of this book quote William Osler's statement about teaching beginning, continuing, and ending with the patient. Another of Osler's many quotations is appropriate: "To see patients without reading books is like going to sea without a chart; to read books without seeing patients is to never go to sea at all." So get on board, relax, and prepare to hoist sail with master mariners on a voyage of discovery about headache.

John Edmeads, MD

PREFACE

CLINICAL CASES ARE THE CURRENCY OF COMMUNICATION between physicians and have served the test of time as a most important way to learn clinical medicine and convey knowledge among peers. In this age of evidence-based medicine, it may seem odd to produce a text of case-based strategies on the subject of advanced therapy of headache.

In the area of headache management, however, it is important to recognize that there is much to be learned from having specialists with an interest in headache discuss their "thinking" about how they diagnose and manage the various disorders, including unique and unusual cases. Too many textbooks about headache do not deal with the nuances of therapy or the wisdom of the individual physicians in managing various headache problems.

This book presents headache in a different way. Cases, which are specific as to type or etiology are presented; then the reader is asked a few questions designed to allow reflection on the case and to stimulate some initial thoughts regarding the case presented. Thereafter, the authors comment specifically on how the case was diagnosed and managed. Management strategies of the cases have been added and explained, when appropriate. Then the author(s) may summarize the salient issues in the case and/or overview the diagnostic entity and conclude with useful references.

In this way, the reader can usually identify with similar cases in their practice, and because the knowledge imparted by the author is in the context of cases, the reader can use the case as a model for diagnosing and managing similar cases. Whenever possible, the authors use the most up-to-date knowledge and evidence-based therapies to discuss their cases. In this way, the reader has the advantage of learning both the "art and science" of headache management.

By using many case scenarios and concise editorials of the cases, it is expected that the reader will gain much valuable information in the field of advanced headache management. The idea of studying patients to learn is not new, as pointed out in the following quotation:

> In what is called the natural method of teaching, the student begins with the patient, continues with the patient, and ends his studies with the patient, using books and lectures as tools, as means to an end.
>
> Sir William Osler, *The Hospital as a College*, 1928

We hope the readers of this volume will enjoy this "tool," as Osler said, and, more importantly, will use the knowledge contained herein to help headache patients under their care.

RAP
AMR
FDS
October 1998

ACKNOWLEDGMENTS

AR would like to thank his wife, Arja, and his children, Terrence, Mark, and Sabrina, for their constant support and love.

FS would like to thank his wife, Karen, for her loving support and encouragement, and his children, Jason and Lauren.

AP would like to thank his wife, Pam, for her support throughout this project, and his children, Kerri and Mark.

AR and FS acknowledge the hard work of their office manager, Susan Lee, in the preparation of this book. AP acknowledges the able assistance of his secretary, Maureen Grandy.

AR, FS, and AP thank all contributors for their hard work and patience in completing this book, as well as the staff at BC Decker for their professional work on our behalf.

To the patients whose cases inspired this book and to all those whose care has helped to relieve their pain and suffering.

CONTENTS

PART II SECONDARY, RARE, AND UNUSUAL HEADACHE DISORDERS

Part I

Primary Headache Disorders

CHAPTER 1

THE WOMAN WITH EPISODIC HEADACHE

RANDALL BERLINER, MD

RICHARD B. LIPTON, MD

Case History

This 40-year-old woman has had occasional headaches for 10 years. Although she sometimes experiences up to six headaches per month, she can go for months without any headache. She describes the headaches as a tight, squeezing pain of mild to moderate intensity which is variously localized at the back of the head and at other times bifrontally. The headaches last up to 8 hours if untreated, although simple analgesics often lessen the pain within 1 hour. Sometimes the headaches recur later the same day, or upon awakening the following morning. The headaches do not awaken her from sleep. She denies associated visual, motor, or sensory disturbances, nausea, vomiting, and photophobia. She reports that loud noise exacerbates the headache. The headaches are not triggered by food or her menses and they are more frequent and severe during periods of work or personal stress.

Over the last 3 months the headaches have become more frequent. For the last month, she has had an average of two headaches per week, and the attacks have lasted up to 24 hours. The pattern of the pain is unchanged; only the frequency and severity have increased. She requires 4 to 8 ibuprofen tablets (200 mg) 2 days per week. She decided to consult a doctor because she was worried about the increasing frequency of her pain and analgesic use.

The patient has been married for 14 years and has two children, aged 10 and 7 years. She works in an office and reports that her job is sometimes stressful. Though she enjoys her work, her supervisor has become more erratic and demanding recently. She reports that she never knows quite what to expect at work and has on several occasions considered resigning. She has not resigned because she hopes that the situation will improve. "Besides," she says, "we need the money."

Recently she has felt a little blue, though not all the time. She reports that she usually sleeps soundly but she sometimes has difficulty getting to sleep because she worries. Her appetite is mildly diminished; she reports a 10-pound weight loss over the last 3 months which she attributes to stress. She denies a change in libido. Her temper flares a little more easily than usual, and this bothers her. Worries over the last few months have sometimes affected her ability to concentrate at work but she denies that the quality of her work has slipped, either at work or around the house. She reports that her main stressors are her job and the household finances. She states that her relationship with her husband is good, and that he is a source of support.

She drinks a glass or two of wine about twice a week, does not smoke, and does not use illegal drugs. Her alcohol use has not altered recently. She denies other medical problems and has never sought a consultation with a mental-health professional.

Her general medical examination was normal. Her blood pressure was 130/80, and her pulse was 82 beats per minute and regular. Her mental status examination was significant for a "tired"-appearing woman who was well balanced, though somewhat anxious. She appeared mildly dysphoric. Her neurologic examination was normal except for some mild tenderness over the temples and the cervical paraspinal muscles.

Questions about This Case

- What is your differential diagnosis of this woman's headache problem and her other symptoms?
- What is the relationship between her emotional stress and her headaches?
- What further diagnostic evaluation would you consider (if any)?
- How would you manage this patient's headaches?
- What consultations or ancillary services might you employ in evaluating and managing this patient?

Case Discussion

This patient illustrates some of the typical features of episodic tension-type headaches (ETTH). She reports bilateral episodes of mild to moderate pain without associated features other than phonophobia; her headaches meet the IHS criteria for ETTH (Table 1–1). Like most people with ETTH, she did not seek medical attention despite many years of headache. Until recently, she had managed her headaches using over-the-counter analgesics. The recent exacerbation of her headaches and her increasing medication use led her to seek medical care. Roughly 40% of the population meet IHS criteria for ETTH; most people do not see a doctor unless the headaches become frequent, disabling, or refractory to nonprescription treatment.

She does not have the nausea or vomiting, the aura (visual, sensory, or motor disturbances), or the food or hormonal triggers which often typify migraine. The headaches lack the unilateral location, the ipsilateral autonomic disturbances, and the cyclical timing of cluster headaches. Indeed, the headaches themselves are rather nondescript. As is typical of tension-type headaches, this patient's pain changes location from attack to attack. The major trigger seems to be stress. She reports phonophobia, in that noise tends to exacerbate her headache, but denies photophobia. Although photophobia and phonophobia are characteristic of migraine, either one or

TABLE 1–1. IHS Criteria for Episodic Tension-Type Headache

A. At least 10 previous headache episodes fulfilling criteria B–D listed below
   Number of days with such headache < 180/year (< 15/month)
B. Headache lasting from 30 minutes to 7 days
C. At least 2 of the following pain characteristics:
   - Pressing/tightening (nonpulsating) quality
   - Mild or moderate intensity (may inhibit, but does not prohibit activity)
   - Bilateral location
   - No aggravation through climbing stairs or similar routine physical activity
D. Both of the following:
   - No nausea or vomiting (anorexia may still occur)
   - Photophobia and phonophobia are absent, or one but not the other is present.
E. At least one of the following:
   - History, physical, and neurologic examinations do not suggest one of the disorders listed in groups 5–11.
   - History and/or physical and/or neurologic examinations do suggest such a disorder but it is ruled out by appropriate investigations.
   - Such a disorder is present, but tension-type headache attacks do not occur for the first time in close temporal relation to the disorder.

the other but not both may occur in ETTH. Tension-type headache is therefore both a diagnosis of inclusion, in that specific combinations of pain features are required, and a diagnosis of exclusion, because the presence of aura, nausea or vomiting, or the combinations of photophobia and phonophobia preclude the diagnosis.

Does the patient require additional investigation to exclude secondary causes of headache? The fact that the character of the headaches themselves has not changed is reassuring. The normal neurologic and general medical exams do not suggest the presence of a more serious disorder. However, the increased frequency and severity of attacks is one of the "headache alarms." Primary and metastatic brain tumors most often produce headaches that resemble progressive ETTH. Given the normal neurologic exam, a mass lesion, if present, would most likely be in a "silent area," a brain region that produces relatively little in the way of focal neurologic findings. Examples of silent areas include the extra-axial space (meningioma or subdural hematoma), the right frontal or temporal regions, the intrahemispheric fissures, and the cerebellum. Though a mass lesion is unlikely, a computed tomography (CT) scan or magnetic resonance imaging (MRI) is justified by the progressive nature of the headache over the last 2 months. The normal MRI reassured both the patient and the physician. It also had therapeutic value in managing this somewhat anxious patient.

The relationship between the headaches and the patient's recent stress is complex. Stress can exacerbate ETTH, migraine, and a range of other medical disorders. This patient also has several features that suggest the possibility of major depression. To diagnose depression, the Diagnostic and Statistical Manual, fourth edition, of the American Psychiatric Association (DSM-IV) requires five out of nine symptoms which meet a certain severity threshold and, in most cases, have been present for at least 2 weeks. Our patient reports feeling "blue," and that she has disturbances of sleep, appetite, and concentration. This constellation of symptoms should alert the evaluating physician that a more serious psychiatric disorder may be present. The pervasiveness of the dysphoria and the possible presence of other vegetative signs or suicidal ideation should be assessed. Headache is a common somatic presentation of depression. If the presence of a major depression is suspected, a psychiatric consultation may be in order. If depression is present, successful treatment of the headache disorder may require treatment of the depression. Furthermore, a serious major depression may, itself, be disabling or even life threatening, should the patient become suicidal.

On further assessment, this patient had a mood disturbance which was intermittent and short lived. Suicidal ideation was absent. The sleep and appetite disturbances are most probably symptoms of the patient's stress and worrying about her life situation. This would be referred to in the DSM-IV as an "adjustment disorder." Adjustment disorders usually do not require the use of antidepressant medications. Short-term anxiolytic and/or hypnotic therapy, though useful in some cases, were judged not to be necessary here. Counseling, biofeedback therapy, or the practice of relaxation techniques are often helpful strategies for managing stress. This patient wanted to learn relaxation techniques and was given instructions and an audio tape for home use.

The medical management of this patient's headaches could include prophylactic headache therapy, i.e., medication taken daily to prevent headache. Preventive medications are usually used in patients with 3 or more days of headache-related disability per month. If the patient had a major depression, the use of a tricyclic, such as nortriptyline or amitriptyline, or a serotonin reuptake inhibitor, such as paroxetine, fluoxetine, fluvoxamine, or sertraline, would have been good choices. Because the patient's headaches are not disabling and because stress is a prominent trigger, we elected to manage her pain with abortive measures in association with attempts to reduce the triggering and exacerbating factors such as stress. Although ibuprofen was effective as an abortive treatment, we elected to switch her to naproxen sodium, 375 mg every 8 hours as needed, because we hoped that its longer half-life would help prevent recurrences of her headache later in the day. With relaxation training, reassurance, and more effective acute treatment, the frequency and intensity of her headaches diminished, avoiding the need for prophylactic medication. Three months after consultation, she was having one or two headaches per month, which were well controlled with naproxen sodium. Her sleep disturbance, appetite, and concentration problems were also reduced.

Management Strategies

- Establish the correct diagnosis.
- Rule out concomitant medical, neurologic, or psychiatric disorders.
- Help the patient learn to better manage the stress in her life, possibly with referral to a therapist trained in biofeedback and/or relaxation techniques.
- Consider the use of prophylactic agents if the headaches are impairing the patient's lifestyle or are leading to frequent analgesic use.
- Initiate a program of effective acute treatment.

Case Summary

- This patient has episodic tension-type headaches which have recently become more severe and frequent, perhaps as a result of increased stress in her life.

- Care must be taken not to miss comorbid major depression.
- Discussion with the patient will allow the treating physician to determine whether a trial of prophylactic medications should be started, or whether biofeedback/relaxation training would be sufficient.
- Reassurance that her headaches are not due to a more serious problem may also reduce her stress.

Overview of Episodic Tension-Type Headache

Introduction

Having discussed a typical patient with ETTH, we will now examine the features of this disorder in greater detail. First, we will discuss the classification and diagnosis of ETTH, followed by a discussion of its epidemiology. Then we will consider the management of ETTH beginning with general principles and then reviewing acute, preventive, and nonpharmacologic treatment.

Classification and Diagnosis of ETTH

The IHS criteria differentiate two main types of tension-type headache primarily based on the frequency of the attacks. In ETTH, attacks occur on fewer than 15 days per month and on fewer than 180 days per year. Otherwise similar patients with 180 or more headache-days per year have chronic tension-type headache. Headaches can last from 30 minutes to 7 days. Diagnosis requires at least 10 attacks during the patient's life span. The headaches are often characterized by bilateral pressure pain of mild to moderate intensity. Because only 2 out of 4 IHS-defining pain features are required, the pain may be unilateral. Photophobia or phonophobia are usually entirely absent, though one or the other is compatible with the diagnosis. Nausea or vomiting exclude a diagnosis of ETTH, though anorexia is permissible.

Unlike migraine, ETTH has few trigger factors. Foods do not seem to cause the headaches, and, indeed, the only common trigger is emotional stress. Whereas migraine sufferers often need to stop their daily activities and rest in a dark, quiet room, people with episodic tension-type headache usually do not find this necessary.

The IHS also classifies episodic tension-type headache into groups with and without pericranial muscle tenderness. It further classifies tension-type headache into purported etiologic categories, such as oromandibular dysfunction, psychosocial stress, depression, anxiety, analgesic overuse (rebound), muscular stress, and delusional (psychogenic) headache. Although scientific evidence is lacking, this classification may stimulate research to evaluate these associations more rigorously.

It is important to exclude secondary headache disorders before making a diagnosis of ETTH. In particular, disorders due to increased intracranial pressure such as mass lesions or pseudotumor cerebri may produce a headache which resembles ETTH (Forsyth and Posner, 1993). The presence of new onset headache, a new type of headache, or a substantial change in headache pattern should alert the physician to the possibility of a secondary headache syndrome.

Headaches due to brain tumor often resemble ETTH, with a dull ache or pressure pain of bifrontal location (Forsyth and Posner,1993); brain tumor headaches are sometimes worse on the side of the tumor. Headaches due to idiopathic intracranial hypertension (pseudotumor cerebri) may also resemble ETTH. They may be holocranial or unilateral. Many patients with benign intracranial hypertension experience transient visual obscurations, expansion of the blind spot, and later a constriction of peripheral vision. Risk factors include being female, being obese, and having had exposure to certain vitamins and drugs. A diagnosis is suspected with an appropriate headache history and the presence of papilledema, and is confirmed by a normal neuroimaging procedure and elevated cerebrospinal fluid pressure (greater than 200 mL of water) on lumbar puncture.

Giant cell or temporal arteritis (GCA) enters into the differential diagnosis of headache beginning after the age of 50 years. Though the headache is classically temporal in location, headache patterns are quite variable. When GCA is suspected, an elevated Westergren erythrocyte sedimentation rate should be followed by a diagnostic temporal artery biopsy.

TABLE 1–2. Acute Treatments for Episodic Tension-Type Headache

Agent	Dosage
Simple analgesics	
Acetylsalicylic acid	650–1000 mg q4–6h
Choline magnesium trisalicylate	1500 mg b.i.d.
Acetaminophen	650–1000 mg q4–6h
Nonsteroidal anti-inflammatory agents	
Naproxen sodium	250–550 mg q4–6h (maximum 1100 mg/d)
Ibuprofen	400–800 mg q4–6h
Ketoprofen	50–75 mg q4–6h
Ketorolac	60 mg load in, then 30 mg q6h
	10 mg PO t.i.d., maximum 3 d
Oxaprozin	1200 mg/d
Nabumetone	1000–1500 mg/d
Other agents and combination analgesics	
Acetylsalicylic acid + acetaminophen + caffeine	2 tablets q6h
Isometheptene + acetaminophen + dichloralphenazone	2 tablets at onset, then 1 qh up to 5/d
Butalbital + caffeine + acetaminophen/ acetylsalicylic acid	1–2 tablets q4h
Tramadol	50–100 mg q4–6h
Opioids	
Codeine	15–60 mg q4–6h
Oxycodone + acetaminophen/ acetylsalicylic acid	1–2 tablets q4–6h

Check Physicians' Desk Reference (U.S. reference) for full prescribing information.

TABLE 1–3. Antidepressants Used in the Treatment of Episodic Tension-Type Headache

Drug Name	Dosage
Cyclic antidepressants	
Nortriptyline	10–150 mg/d
Amitriptyline	10–150 mg/d
Desipramine	25–200 mg/d
Imipramine	75–150 mg/d
Doxepin	10–150 mg/d
Selective serotonin reuptake inhibitors	
Fluoxetine	10–80 mg/d
Fluvoxamine	50–300 mg/d (in divided doses above 100 mg)
Sertraline	25–200 mg/d
Paroxetine	10–50 mg/d
Other antidepressants	
Venlafaxine	25–375 mg/d (in divided doses)
Nefazodone	75–600 mg/d (in divided doses)
Mirtazapine	15–45 mg/d (can be very sedating)

Epidemiology of ETTH and Its Relationship to Migraine

Although about 90% of the population has headache at one time or another, about 40% of the population meet IHS criteria for ETTH (Schwartz et al., 1998). In contrast with the striking female preponderance of migraine, episodic tension-type headache has only a slight female preponderance. Where migraine prevalence is inversely related to socioeconomic status (it is most common in groups with low income and low levels of education), the prevalence of ETTH is directly related to socioeconomic status. That is, the prevalence of ETTH rises with increasing education.

These epidemiologic contrasts suggest that migraine and episodic tension-type headache are distinct disorders. Although IHS criteria clearly distinguish the two disorders, many headache specialists view them as polar ends on a continuum of severity. This continuum is sometimes referred to as the tension-vascular headache spectrum; migraine with aura (classic migraine) is the most severe end of the spectrum while episodic tension-type headache is at the least severe end of the spectrum. We believe that the IHS criteria are correct in distinguishing tension-type headache and migraine.

Principles of Management

Pharmacotherapy for episodic tension-type headache is divided into acute treatment and prophylactic treatment. Acute treatment is given as needed to relieve individual attacks. Prophylactic treatment is given on a daily basis, whether or not headache is present, to prevent headaches. Tension-type headache in the population rarely requires daily prophylactic medication. We usually reserve prophylactic treatment for patients with at least 3 headache days per month that are severe enough to have an adverse impact on the patient's ability to function. Most patients do not have sufficiently frequent or severe attacks to justify prophylaxis. Prophylactic treatment should also be considered in patients with an accelerating frequency of attacks, lack of response, as well as contraindications or side effects to acute treatment. Prophylactic therapy may be useful to treat or prevent analgesic-rebound headaches.

Acute Pharmacotherapy of ETTH

The mainstay of managing episodic tension-type headaches is the occasional use of analgesic medication, and there are several classes that are commonly used (Table 1–2). These include nonsteroidal anti-inflammatory drugs (NSAIDs), acetaminophen, salicylates, muscle relaxants, and combination agents. Rarely is it necessary to use opioids to control this type of headache. The commonly used NSAIDs include naproxen sodium, ibuprofen, and ketoprofen. In addition, there are several newer and longer-acting agents such as oxaprozin and nabumetone. These may be particularly helpful for patients with prolonged headaches or those who tend to require repeated dosing during the day. Aspirin or acetaminophen is often combined with caffeine and sometimes a barbiturate such as butalbital or an opioid such as codeine. Combination agents can be very effective but their over-use must be avoided. The barbiturate and opioid may be very sedating, however, and the disability secondary to this effect may outweigh the benefit achieved in breaking the less severe headaches. Furthermore, these agents can be habit forming and are frequent causes of the rebound headache when overused. Isometheptene, a sympathomimetic amine which may act as a vasoconstrictor in the head, has been combined with dichloralphenazone (a mild sedative) and acetaminophen. This combination is somewhat less sedating and may be particularly effective in some patients, though the combination of isometheptene with dichloralphenazone and acetaminophen has not been shown to be more effective than isometheptene alone.

If there is a significant anxiety component in the headaches, adjunctive benzodiazepines may be used on rare occasions in carefully selected patients. These may help relax the patient, potentiating the benefit of an analgesic. Tolerance and psychologic as well as physiologic dependence may develop with these agents so careful patient selection and monitoring is essential. In patients unable to tolerate NSAIDs, muscle relaxants are sometimes used.

Linkage of their efficacy to the presence or absence of pericranial muscle tenderness has not been established. [*Editors' note: Butalbital-containing medications may help to relieve anxiety and are sometimes overused for this reason.*]

Prophylactic Management of ETTH

At times patients with ETTH may require prophylactic treatment. Several classes of agents are used in the prophylaxis of ETTH including antidepressants (Table 1–3), beta-blockers, calcium channel blockers, and antiepileptic medications. The choice of agent may depend upon the comorbid conditions. For example, the patient who suffers from a major depression or sleep disorder may be given an antidepressant or the hypertensive patient may be given a beta-blocker or calcium channel blocker. In particularly refractory cases, several different agents may be combined. Antidepressants are sometimes used in combination with a calcium channel blocker or a beta-blocker.

Nonpharmacologic Management of ETTH

Behavioral therapies are useful adjuncts in the management of episodic tension-type headaches; these include relaxation techniques, biofeedback training, and stress management. Studies have shown that these behavioral therapies can produce an overall reduction in tension-type headaches. If the treating physician or therapist believes that high levels of stress are interfering with a patient's ability to benefit from relaxation or biofeedback, cognitive behavior therapy may be employed to assist the patient in modifying his or her lifestyle and reducing stress to a more manageable level. Cognitive behavior therapy appears to provide an additional benefit when used in combination with biofeedback or relaxation training. Excessive distress or anxiety may be a sign of a more serious psychiatric disorder and failure to respond to the above approaches may indicate the need for psychiatric evaluation.

If an oromandibular dysfunction (OMD) appears to be exacerbating a patient's headache, a dental consultation may be indicated. The IHS criteria for OMD require three or more of the following characteristics:

- Temporomandibular joint noise when the jaw is moved
- Limited or jerky jaw movements
- Pain on jaw function
- Locking of jaw on opening
- Clenching of teeth
- Gnashing (grinding) of teeth
- Other oral parafunction (tongue, lips, or cheek biting or pressing)

Therapy may include behavioral modification, stretching and strengthening exercises, and sometimes splinting. Also used are trigger point injections and analgesic medications. In some cases, particularly when conservative management has failed, surgery may be indicated.

In summary, management of the patient with tension-type headache requires a comprehensive assessment to determine which, if any, comorbid conditions may be exacerbating the headaches. Then therapies may be targeted against these conditions as an adjunct to the analgesic medications that the patient may require during the acute headache.

Selected Readings

Couch JR, Micieli G. Prophylactic pharmacotherapy. In: Olesen J, Tfelt-Hansen P, Welch KMA, editors. The headaches. New York: Raven Press; 1993. p. 537–42.

Forsyth PA, Posner JB. Headaches in patients with brain tumors: a study of 111 patients. Neurology 1993;43: 1678–83.

Graff-Radford SB, Forssel H. Oromandibular treatment. In: Olesen J, Tfelt-Hansen P, Welch KMA, editors. The headaches. New York: Raven Press; 1993. p. 527–30.

Holroyd K. Psychological and behavioral techniques. In: Olesen J, Tfelt-Hansen P, Welch KMA, editors. The headaches. New York: Raven Press; 1993. p. 515–20.

Jensen R, Olesen J. Oromandibular dysfunction. In: Olesen J, Tfelt-Hansen P, Welch KMA, editors. The headaches. New York: Raven Press; 1993. p. 479–82.

Jensen R, Paiva T. Episodic tension-type headache. In: Olesen J, Tfelt-Hansen P, Welch KMA, editors. The headaches. New York: Raven Press; 1993. p. 497–502.

Mathew N. Acute pharmacotherapy. In: Olesen J, Tfelt-Hansen P, Welch KMA, editors. The headaches. New York: Raven Press; 1993. p. 531–6.

Olesen J. Tension-type headache: an introduction. In: Olesen J, Tfelt-Hansen P, Welch KMA, editors. The headaches. New York: Raven Press; 1993. p. 437–8.

Saper JR, Silberstein SD, Gordon CD, Hamel RL. Handbook of headache management: a practical guide to diagnosis and treatment of head, neck, and facial pain. Baltimore: Williams and Wilkins; 1993.

Schoenen J, Wang W. Tension-type headache. In: Goadsby PJ, Silberstein SD, editors. Headache. Boston: Butterworth-Heinemann; 1997. p. 177–201.

Schwartz B, Stewart WF, Simon D, Lipton RB. Epidemiology of tension-type headache. JAMA 1998;279:381–3.

Silberstein SD, Lipton RB, Goadsby PJ. Headache in clinical practice. Oxford, UK: Isis Medical Media; 1998. p. 91–101.

Stewart WF, Lipton RB, Celentino DD, et al. Prevalence of migraine headache in the United States: relation to age, income, race and other socioeconomic factors. JAMA 1992;267.

Editorial Comments

Despite attempts made to differentiate episodic tension-type headache from migraine without aura, all clinicians recognize many similarities between these headache disorders. Ultimately, all primary headache disorders lie on a spectrum, although with these two types, management principles can be similar and effective. Drs. Berliner and Lipton guide us through their case of ETTH, its diagnosis, and differential considerations with clarity and ease. Thoughtful comments on investigation are made and the spectrum of potential therapies is reviewed, even though treatment is somewhat similar to that of migraine therapy.

CHAPTER 2

THE PATIENT WITH VISUAL SYMPTOMS AND HEADACHE

ROBERT E. RYAN JR., MS, MD

Case History

This 25-year-old woman has suffered from headaches since the age of 17 years. They originally occurred quite sporadically, approximately once every 6 to 8 weeks. Over the past 3 years, she has been averaging about three headaches per month.

The pain is unilateral and throbbing and often begins in the back of the neck. It ultimately involves the entire left side of her head, being most pronounced around the left eye. It is almost always accompanied by nausea and only rarely by vomiting. There is always some degree of irritation of the gastrointestinal tract. During a headache she is usually quite sensitive to light, to the degree that on the few occasions that she came to the office during a headache, she was wearing sunglasses. During a headache attack, she is often quite sensitive to noise.

Occasionally, the headaches are associated with her menstrual period but obviously some occur where there is no hormonal relationship. One other precipitating factor for her headaches is stress. She was likely to have more frequent headaches during exam times in college, and that has carried over into her business life, with headaches often being associated with stressful times at work.

Her typical headache will last 2 days. Occasionally she is bedridden with the headache but there are days when she can complete the work day and then return home and go to bed. In the early days of her headaches, they lasted less than a day but for the past 2 to 3 years her current pattern has been in place.

Approximately once a month, or one out of every three headaches, she has an unusual set of visual experiences. Approximately an hour before the headache begins, she has a sudden development of wavy lines before her eyes. This visual disturbance lasts about 15 minutes. There is usually a period of 30 to 45 minutes when she is symptom free. At that point her headache begins and develops as described.

Her past medical history is relatively unremarkable. She is not on the birth control pill. She does not smoke and drinks only socially. She does not suffer from allergies.

During the first few years of her headaches she merely used over-the-counter medications for her headaches, without any significant relief. At the age of 20 years, she had her first visual aura. At that time she consulted her family physician and he did an evaluation which consisted of a computed tomography (CT) scan with contrast as well as an electroencephalogram.

These tests were all normal. She was seen by an ophthalmologist who did a complete eye exam which was normal. She was treated initially with analgesic-barbiturates for over a year and these provided very little relief. They never totally eradicated a headache, more often merely dulling the pain, only to have it worsen when the medication wore off. She was then prescribed isometheptene mucate which would occasionally relieve her headache, but only if she caught it early. She has had to resort to going to the emergency room for the relief of her headaches on average four times a year.

When we saw this woman, her physical exam was normal. Her blood pressure was 126/76, and her pulse was 70 and regular. Her neurologic exam was completely normal. At that time she had no headache.

Questions about This Case

- What is the diagnosis in this case?
- How would you manage this case?
- What long-term management strategies would you suggest for the patient?
- What agent would you use for abortive therapy?
- Would you place her on a prophylactic agent?

Case Discussion

It is apparent that this patient suffers from two different headache patterns. Some of her headaches are preceded by a visual aura whereas the majority of her headaches begin without the aura. The first type of headache would be classified as migraine with aura, denoting the syndrome of headache associated with characteristic premonitory sensory, motor, or visual symptoms. This has been referred to in the past as "classic migraine." The second type of headache described would be migraine without aura, which has been previously described as "common migraine." It is important to recognize, first of all, that this is a straightforward example of a patient who suffers from both migraine with and without aura. Unfortunately, not all cases of migraine are as straightforward as this. For example, while the majority of all migraines are unilateral, the pain can also be bilateral. This patient is typical in that she tries to function with her headaches but often has to give in to it and go to bed. When I hear patients tell me that they are disabled by their headaches, the first diagnosis I consider is migraine. This patient's headaches are a perfect example of how the pattern of migraines may change throughout life. It is not unusual for migraines to start off occurring infrequently and to increase in frequency as time passes.

It is a well-known fact that approximately 75% of all patients who have migraines are women. Many women experience their headaches only during menstruation while others have headaches during menstruation and ovulation. It has been studied and determined that this is caused by the sudden changes in estrogen at those times of the month. It is also well known that migraines can stop occurring during pregnancy, only to recur once the pregnancy has terminated. Fortunately for many women, their migraines stop entirely after they have completed menopause; however, many women are currently being placed on estrogen replacement therapy to prevent osteoporosis, and this often causes the migraines to continue after menopause. If a woman needs to be placed on estrogen following menopause, then the lowest dose of estrogen possible is the best choice. We find that the estrogen patch is the least likely form of replacement therapy to exacerbate a woman's migraines. Unfortunately, it is often not strong enough to overcome the postmenopausal symptoms of the patient.

In this patient, the initial concern is the visual aura that accompanies her headaches. It is important to determine the etiology of the aura, and to rule out any organic pathology that could be precipitating the neurologic symptoms. If this patient had not already had a CT scan or magnetic resonance imaging (MRI) with contrast of the head, these tests would have to be performed. If the scan was done more than 2 years previously, one would have to consider repeating the test. This would be especially important if the characteristics of the headaches had changed, or more importantly, if the visual aura had changed in any way. In rare situations, a cerebral angiography may be warranted.

It is interesting that the patients who suffer from migraine with aura describe their visual disturbance in a variety of ways, e.g., some describe it as flashing lights while others describe it as wavy lines. There are numerous descriptions in literature of patients' experiences.

The typical aura precedes the headache and lasts anywhere from a few minutes to half an hour. This is usually followed by a symptom-free period of up to an hour, which is followed by the migraine. If the visual aura lasts more than an hour, I would be very concerned about ruling out any pathologic cause for the patient's headaches.

Investigations in humans as to the pathophysiology of this aura phenomenon have been done but we are far from being able to draw clear conclusions. Most investigations have been limited to the measurement of blood flow, facilitated in migraine patients by noninvasive imaging techniques. Cerebral blood flow falls, but only to oligemic values in posterior regions of the cortex, in some patients during attacks of migraine with aura. It has also been noted that the regional hypoperfusion develops before and outlasts the focal symptoms. For the most part these cerebral blood flow changes have been demonstrated in patients with migraine with aura and not in those with migraine without aura.

A recent positron emission tomography study measured by means of O^{15} labeled water done on a patient who, by chance, had a migraine while in the machine, supports the theory of decreased neuronal function. It demonstrated that there is bilateral hypoperfusion, starting in the occipital lobes and spreading anteriorly during a migraine headache.

The most common symptoms reported in the aura phase are visual, arising from the dysfunction of occipital lobe neurons according to some authors. Scotomas may appear in the central portion of the visual field. A characteristic pattern develops in about 10% of patients; the aura begins as a small paracentral scotoma which slowly expands into a "C" shape. Luminous angles appear at the enlarging outer edge, becoming colored as the scotoma expands toward the periphery of the involved half of the visual field. It eventually disappears over the horizon of peripheral vision, with the entire process lasting less than half an hour. This often occurs during the period of time before the headache and infrequently during the headache. This set of circumstances is not usually associated with a cerebral structural anomaly.

Management Strategies

The first and most important thing to do for a patient with headaches is to make an accurate diagnosis. After all, it is difficult to render the appropriate care if we have not made the proper diagnosis. In this case, the diagnosis is straightforward. This patient has two types of headache, but both are migraines. She has migraine without aura as her most frequent type of headache but she also has

migraine with aura a smaller percent of the time. If this patient was presenting to me for the first time, I would probably order an MRI if she had not had one done in the last few years. While I am quite comfortable with the diagnosis according to her history, when neurologic symptoms other than headache become involved, some physicians might feel more comfortable with an imaging scan.

This patient is looking for abortive therapy, in other words, something to get rid of the pain. It is important to keep in mind that while we are dealing with migraine headaches, we are dealing with two different types of migraine. It is my strong opinion that the best types of abortive therapy for migraines of these types are the ergotamines and the triptans. It is very important to keep one fact in mind when dealing with migraine with aura, and that is that the triptans may not work when the headache is in the aura stage, while the ergotamines will sometimes abort the entire process, occasionally preventing the onset of the headache itself.

For this patient we have two options. We could prescribe an ergotamine for both types of headache and instruct her to take it immediately at the onset of her symptoms, whether they are the headache itself, or the visual aura. The second option would be to prescribe a triptan and instruct her to take the medication immediately upon recognition of the headache. Keep in mind that with the use of the triptans we have different formulations available and we need to individualize the prescription for each patient. Some patients may even require two different formulations for different headaches. Some patients awaken with a severe pain and at that point they will benefit more from a subcutaneous form of therapy or perhaps an intranasal spray. I prefer, for my own patients, the use of a sumatriptan nasal spray as the initial form of therapy in patients who do not require a subcutaneous injection. The reason for this is the drug's rapid onset of action and its relatively high degree of efficacy.

The other consideration for this patient is whether or not to place her on some form of preventive therapy. There is no specific therapy in the prophylactic area for migraine with aura. The same drugs that work in migraine without aura could be used in this case. I would consider the use of a prophylactic agent for the headaches that are hormone related. The drugs most commonly used for this purpose are the nonsteroidal anti-inflammatory agents (naproxen sodium), diuretics, and acetazolamide. These drugs are best used if the woman has a pattern with her headaches coming at a specific time during her cycle. The drug can be given a few days before the headache is likely to begin and taken for the next several days. Sometimes there is no specific pattern; therefore, these drugs need to be used for the entire month.

For the patient we have described in this case, the use of a prophylactic drug is questionable. If she averages three headaches per month and we can find her an abortive agent that can rid her of her headache within an hour, it is likely that she would not accept the idea of using a drug on a daily basis, especially when we have finished discussing the possible side effects of any of the prophylactic agents, and have also answered her questions about the likelihood of success with these drugs.

Selected Readings

Lashley K. Patterns of cerebral integration indicated by the scotomas of migraine. Arch Neurol Psychol 1941;46:333–9.

Lauritzen M. Links between cortical spreading depression and migraine: clinical and experimental aspects. In: Olesen J, editor. Migraine and other headaches: the vascular mechanism. Vol 1. New York: Raven Press; 1991. p. 143–51.

Lauritzen M. Pathophysiology of the migraine aura: the spreading depression theory. Brain 1994;117:199.

Lauritzen M, Olsen TS, et al. The role of spreading depression in acute brain disorders. Ann Neurol 1983;14:569–72.

McLachlan RS, Girvin JP. Spreading depression of Leão in rodent and human cortex. Brain Res 1994;666:133.

Olesen J. Cerebral and extracranial circulatory disturbances in migraine: pathophysiological implications. Cerebrovasc Brain Metab Rev 1991;3:1.

Olesen J, Larsen B, Lauritzen M, et al. Focal hyperemia followed by spreading oligemia and impaired activation of RCBF in classical migraine. Ann Neurol 1981;9:3344–52.

Raskin N. Migraine. Syllabus from The Scottsdale Headache Symposium, Nov 14–16, 1997 [handout]. The American Association for the Study of Headache (AASH); 1997.

Welch KMA. The migraine aura. Syllabus from The Scottsdale Headache Symposium, Nov. 14–16, 1997 [handout]. The American Association for the Study of Headache (AASH); 1997.

Woods RP, Iacoboni M, Mazziotta JC, et al. Brief report: bilateral spreading cerebral hypoperfusion during spontaneous migraine headache. N Engl J Med 1994;331:1689–92.

Editorial Comments

Migraine varies between patients and within each patient's history and lifetime. This case by Dr. Ryan illustrates these diagnostic variations and the importance of accurate diagnosis. His approach is reasonable, yet some would defer investigations, while others would select other abortive agents or formulations. Some might include metoclopramide and ASA during the aura. Preventive strategies may include one 80-mg dose of ASA per day and/or verapamil, 80 mg t.i.d., for migraine with aura.

Since the time of this writing, several other triptans have become available including zolmitriptan, naratriptan, and rizatriptan, and could be considered for this patient, depending on the type and severity of the migraine.

Nevertheless, Dr. Ryan clearly illustrates what the "thinking" is behind the decisions of the skilled clinician caring for the headache patient with variable migraine.

THE PATIENT WITH RECURRENT HEADACHES SINCE CHILDHOOD

ROBERT S. KUNKEL, MD, FACP

Case History

This 31-year-old woman has had recurring headaches since childhood. During her teens and twenties, the headaches occurred around the time of her menstrual period. In the year or so prior to her presentation, her headaches had increased in frequency and were occurring four to six times a month, although the character and symptoms of the headaches had not changed. When she was younger, she believed that the headache and nausea that she frequently experienced at the time of her menstrual period were episodes of the flu.

In addition to the headache, she has had years of gastrointestinal (GI) symptoms. These GI symptoms consisted mainly of indigestion and heartburn, along with bloating and excessive gas. She could not correlate these GI symptoms with her headache. These symptoms had been extensively evaluated by radiography, as well as upper GI endoscopy, and an ultrasound examination of the gallbladder. The results of these studies were normal, and she was diagnosed as having irritable bowel syndrome and was told that her headache and GI symptoms were due to her being nervous.

Her headache was described as being a throbbing pain in the temples. The pain could be on either the right or left side, or at times occur bilaterally. There was also discomfort across the bridge of the nose and behind her eyes. The headache could occur upon awakening but did not wake her during the night. She always had her worst headache associated with her menses. She also noted that if she slept late in the morning she would probably get a headache.

The day before her headache, she would feel tired and weak and stated that her head "felt heavy." She had no visual symptoms prior to or during her headache, and she had no neurologic symptoms prior to or during her headache.

The headache was accompanied by sensitivity to light and noise, dizziness, weakness, and nausea with frequent vomiting. Interestingly enough, she found that the pain in her head seemed to ease with vomiting as well as with sleep. She also would become constipated when she had a headache. Her headaches would generally last 1 to 2 days.

A review of her history revealed that there was no family history of migraine. She rarely drank alcohol and had stopped smoking 7 years prior to her visit. She drank four cans of cola per day. She admitted to being tense and anxious; however, she denied having any significant psychologic problems. She had had two pregnancies and she noted that her headache was less frequent during the pregnancies.

She was taking ibuprofen and aspirin as medication for her headaches. Other medications included metoclopramide, lorazepam, and sucralfate. She was using suppositories of trimethobenzamide for nausea. Past medications had included cimetidine, ranitidine, cisapride, and thiethylperazine, all of which were given for her stomach symptoms, but none of which gave her any relief from them.

On physical examination she weighed 127 lb. and her blood pressure was 98/70. The results of the physical examination itself lay entirely within normal limits, except for some mild tenderness in the midabdomen.

She underwent a psychophysiologic evaluation in the biofeedback department. She was found to have a high autonomic nervous system arousal which is manifested by low skin temperatures in her hands. It was felt that she had stress at work but had no major psychopathology. It was felt that she would be a good candidate to benefit from further behavioral therapy.

Questions about This Case

- What is the most likely diagnosis for this 31-year-old woman?
- Are any further diagnostic studies necessary? Would they help in the diagnosis?
- In regard to treatment, does she need daily medication as prophylaxis, as well as an abortive agent which would be taken at the onset of an attack? What specific agents would you suggest?
- She has suffered from chronic upper GI symptoms. These do not necessarily occur at the same time as her headache attacks. She has had extensive evaluation and has been unresponsive to many medications. Is there a correlation with her headache?

Case Discussion

This patient has had recurrent headaches since childhood. She has never been diagnosed as suffering from migraine and has been told that her symptoms are due to nerves. She has had a lot of GI symptoms in recent years, and has had extensive GI studies. Since all of the GI studies have been negative, she was diagnosed as having functional GI stress or irritable bowel syndrome, and her headache was felt to be due to tension. She admits to being a tense person, a worrier, and somewhat compulsive. A psychologic assessment did not demonstrate any major psychopathology.

Unfortunately, many patients who suffer from migraine without aura, i.e., without a well-defined focal deficit which precedes the headache, are not diagnosed as such. Many physicians still think of migraine as that sick headache which is associated with an aura. About 80% of patients with migraine have migraine without aura. The diagnosis of migraine has become easier with the introduction of the International Headache Society classification in 1988. Diagnostic criteria are given for the primary headache syndromes. This patient has had recurring headaches with nausea and dizziness associated with her menstrual cycle since childhood, and yet no physician has ever diagnosed her as having migraine. She was labeled as having premenstrual syndrome (PMS) and being tense and nervous.

This patient has had recurrent retro-orbital and temporal throbbing headache. It can be unilateral but also is bilateral at times and may shift from side to side. She is aware of tightness in her neck which accompanies the throbbing pain in her temples. Many of the headaches are present upon awakening but do not awaken her earlier than usual. She has many associated symptoms with her headache. Quite typical are GI symptoms including nausea, vomiting, and anorexia. Gastrointestinal symptoms are second only to the head pain as the most frequent symptoms of migraine. This woman not only had nausea and vomiting, but also had severe constipation for the duration of her headaches. Other typical migraine symptoms that she suffered were sonophobia, photophobia, dizziness, and generalized weakness.

She was able to identify very few trigger factors. She was unable to determine which foods would set off a headache. She always had 2 to 3 days of headaches with her menstrual periods, and, like many women with menstruation-related migraine, she had very few headaches during her two pregnancies. Sleeping late would often be associated with a headache attack. Most people with migraine will have fewer headaches if they keep to a regular schedule of eating and avoid skipping meals. The headaches that occur when patients sleep late are probably due to prolonged hours of fasting and delay in eating breakfast at their normal time.

Stress may well be an important factor in increasing the frequency of migraine attacks. This patient has had trouble at work, feeling that she was not appreciated. She did miss a fair amount of work due to her headaches, and this caused conflict with her supervisor. She has since quit this job and has found other employment.

A biofeedback assessment showed that she would probably benefit from learning some relaxation techniques and behavioral therapy. Unfortunately, as often happens, her insurance did not cover biofeedback therapy and she never returned for further sessions.

Her GI symptoms consisted of nausea, heartburn, and epigastric pains, as well as frequent constipation. She had a lot of nausea with her headache but she could not correlate the epigastric pains with her headache. These nonheadache symptoms are felt to be secondary to the same underlying pathophysiology that causes migraine headaches. It is of interest that in the past 4 years, since undergoing treatment for her headache, this patient has seen marked improvement in her GI symptoms while on prophylactic medication for migraine. Several medications used for upper GI symptoms had been ineffective in controlling her discomfort.

As far as treatment is concerned, in this case, one needs to consider daily preventive medication because of the frequency of her attacks. Because this patient has no contraindications to the use of beta-blockers, and because beta-blockers are effective prophylactic drugs for migraine, she was started on nadolol. Her low blood pressure (98/70) was of some concern, but usually the use of either beta-blockers or calcium channel blockers has little effect on normal or low blood pressure. She has done quite well on nadolol. She was initially started on 20 mg per day, and this has been increased over 4 years so that she has now been on 200 mg per day for the past 2 years. When she felt that nadolol was losing its effect, she was prescribed verapamil but she had increased headache, nausea, and vomiting. Diltiazem was also tried, but this had no effect on the frequency and the severity of her headaches. Nadolol was reinstituted, and the dose increased to the current level of 200 mg daily.

Other preventive medications in controlling migraine without aura include the tricyclic antidepressants. This might be a good choice for her because of her anxiety but these tend to be very sedating and she had no difficulty sleeping. The tricyclic antidepressants are an excellent choice for preventive therapy for those patients who are having trouble sleeping. Nonsteroidal drugs are often beneficial in the preventive treatment of migraine but they were avoided in this case because of the patient's significant GI symptoms. Recently valproic acid has been approved for migraine prophylaxis. Nausea, however, is a side effect of this drug, and it is not as effective as the beta-blockers or calcium channel blockers.

Regarding abortive therapy, I usually start with isometheptene mucate. This is usually combined with a sedative and acetaminophen. This agent is well tolerated and is often effective. Patients must use it early in the attack and they must use a sufficient amount. Usually two capsules are used at once followed by one or two capsules in an hour. More effective abortive agents such as ergotamine tartrate and sumatriptan have more side effects. This patient has done very well on isometheptene mucate and only needs to take one capsule followed by another capsule in an hour. Her headache is usually well controlled in about 4 hours. She did try oral sumatriptan tablets but had a recurrence of her headache in 12 hours. Isometheptene mucate, sumatriptan, and ergotamine tartrate are all vasoconstrictive agents.

Another group of medications that is often helpful for the acute treatment of migraine is the rapid-acting anti-inflammatory drugs. Meclofenamate, ibuprofen, and naproxen sodium are the ones used most often. They need to be taken in a fairly large dose at the onset of migraine.

This patient has found the use of metoclopramide to be very helpful. She doses herself with this agent prior to taking her isometheptene mucate. Metoclopramide is often helpful in controlling nausea and also enhances the absorption of any of the abortive agents. Migraineurs, in general, have decreased intestinal absorption predominantly due to gastric stasis.

This patient is very pleased with the control of her headaches on the regimen of nadolol 200 mg per day and the use of metoclopramide and isometheptene mucate for the acute attacks. She still has about three attacks per month, the worst of which occurs with her menstrual period.

Management Strategies

- Make the diagnosis of migraine without aura. Any recurrent headache accompanied by a wide variety of other symptoms is likely to be migraine. The more severe attacks usually occur with the menstrual period.
- One needs to decide whether to use daily prophylactic medications as well as abortive agents, or only abortive agents. Consider prophylactic medication when the patient has three or more attacks per month or when the attacks last for a very long time.
- Help the patient to identify various trigger factors such as foods, stress, erratic eating, and sleeping habits. Other factors that seem to play a role in migraine are the menstrual cycle and weather changes. One cannot do much about the weather changes, and hormone therapy has not been very satisfactory for migraine sufferers.
- Consider nonpharmacologic therapies such as biofeedback, relaxation techniques, and physical therapy. Physical therapy is helpful when there is much neck and shoulder tightness accompanying the headache.
- Patients such as this one need to be followed, and the medications need to be adjusted or even changed depending on their effectiveness and their side effects. Prophylactic medication should be increased to the point where headaches are well controlled or until there are uncomfortable side effects. Migraineurs often require higher doses of calcium channel blockers and beta-blockers than are used to treat hypertension, and they often require lower doses of tricyclic antidepressants than are needed to treat depression.
- The long duration of symptoms and a normal computed tomography scan done 2 months before the patient's visit make further lab and imaging studies unnecessary. Her headaches had not changed over the years other than in their increased frequency. A common cause of increased frequency and severity of migraine is mild hypertension, but her blood pressure was normal.

Case Summary

- This patient has migraine without aura and probably migrainous GI symptoms.

- Even though this patient has a typical history of migraine without aura, she was not previously diagnosed as such and suffered from years of headache and GI symptoms, which had been diagnosed as being due to stress and tension. Migraine without aura remains underdiagnosed by the medical profession.
- This patient has done very well on nadolol, although the dosage has needed to be increased. Beta-blockers remain the drugs of choice for migraine prophylaxis if there is no contraindication. Other medications that are useful for the prevention of migraine include the calcium channel blockers (usually verapamil), tricyclic antidepressants, valproic acid, and the nonsteroidal anti-inflammatory drugs.
- Abortive agents useful in the treatment of migraine include isometheptene mucate (combined with dichloralphenazone and acetaminophen), ergotamine tartrate, sumatriptan, and the short-acting nonsteroidal anti-inflammatory drugs. The use of metoclopramide prior to any of these abortive agents is often very useful in controlling nausea and potentiating the effects of the abortive agents.

Overview of Migraine without Aura

It is felt that about 80% of all migraine sufferers have migraine without aura. Epidemiologic studies are difficult, however, because many patients with migraine will have both migraine without aura and migraine with aura. Most patients who do not have an aura will never have an aura; whereas, people who have migraine with aura will often have some typical migraine headaches that are not preceded by an aura. Therefore, at any one time one might make a different diagnosis.

In spite of all that has been written about headaches and migraine, it is remarkable how many physicians still do not diagnose migraine unless the patient describes a typical aura. The fact that migraine with or without aura very frequently starts in childhood is also not well recognized. It has been demonstrated that about 50% of patients with migraine have had their first headache by the age of 15. The International Headache Society (IHS) classification of headache, which was published in 1988, provides diagnostic criteria for the various types of primary headache syndromes. Many headache physicians do not use this classification in their daily clinical practice and rely only on the history that the patient presents, and on their own diagnostic expertise as to whether the headache is of a migrainous type. The IHS classification has been very useful in research studies where all headache patients can be classified according to the IHS criteria.

There is much debate as to whether migraine with aura and migraine without aura have the same basic pathophysiology. Some studies have demonstrated differences in the circulation and metabolism of the brain prior to the two types of migraine whereas other studies have not demonstrated any significant differences. The fact that many patients who suffer primarily from migraine with aura will also have some migraine attacks without aura leads me to believe that they are manifestations of the same basic pathophysiology. There are also patients who have migraine without aura and have never had migraine with aura who develop aura symptoms without headache in their later years.

Many patients suffering from migraine without aura will have prodromal symptoms. A migraine aura is a focal visual or neurologic symptom, which lasts less than 1 hour and is followed by a headache within 1 hour of the end of the symptoms. Prodromal symptoms are generalized and vague and last hours to days prior to the onset of the migraine attack. Such symptoms as depression, irritability, fatigue, and hunger are common prodromal symptoms. Patients or spouses and family can come to recognize that a headache will be coming on within a day or two because of some of these prodromal symptoms. Prodromal symptoms, which are manifestations of cerebral dysfunction, are further evidence that migraine starts in the brain, with the blood vessels reacting secondarily to neurologic dysfunction.

The migraine attack has been divided by Blau into five phases. Not all patients have these five phases, and they may overlap in some patients. The first phase is a prodromal phase, which is a change in mood or behavior, and, as mentioned, occurs for hours or days before the headache begins. The second phase, which is the aura when it does occur, is a well-defined focal deficit lasting less than an hour.

The third phase is the headache phase, with the pain and other associated symptoms. The termination phase, which is the fourth phase, is the lessening of pain, and the fifth phase, which Blau calls the postdrome, consists of residual symptoms such as fatigue that occur after the pain has ceased.

The onset of most attacks of migraine is in the morning. It is unusual for the headache to actually awaken the patient but frequently the headache is present when the patient awakens. Headaches that are present upon awakening often are more difficult to control because patients do not take their abortive therapy as early in the attack as they would have had they recognized the onset of the headache. Although migraine without aura is usually a unilateral throbbing or pulsatile pain, many patients do have bilateral pain. Nausea and vomiting are the second most common symptoms. A symptom that I find very helpful in differentiating migraine without aura from other types of headache, such as tension-type headache, is that migraine is usually aggravated by any physical activity. Patients with migraine will want to go to a dark room and be very quiet. Photophobia and phonophobia as well as osmophobia are all commonly associated symptoms of the migraine attack. In addition to nausea, vomiting, and anorexia, other GI symptoms such as diarrhea or constipation are not uncommon.

Generalized fatigue may occur as a prodromal symptom but is very common in the postdrome phase after the headache pain has ceased. Chills and sweats also may occur. Migraine without aura is truly a generalized condition with systemic manifestations. The typical attack of migraine without aura lasts between 4 and 72 hours. Any migraine lasting longer than 72 hours fits the criteria for status migrainosus and usually has to be dealt with differently.

The diagnosis of migraine without aura is based solely on the history of the patients. We have found it useful to send out a questionnaire to patients prior to their initial visit so that they can spend some time thinking about some of the aspects of their headache. It is very difficult for patients to remember details of the onset of their headache and various associated symptoms when presenting to the doctor's office for the first time. Often they will consult with parents and then present some history of having had migrainous symptoms at a much earlier age than they had suspected. The complete history of all other symptoms will often unfold as one sees a patient over several visits.

Patients often request that the physician do imaging studies to exclude disease in the head. Scans are not usually necessary for anyone who has had a recurring headache for many years. It is helpful to remember that patients who have headache due to an organic disease usually also have neurologic symptoms and abnormalities on physical examination. Indications for considering imaging patients include a recent onset of headache or a change in the pattern or frequency of their headache. Certainly the development of any neurologic symptoms warrants close scrutiny with examination and probably scanning. If the headache frequency or pattern changes, it is good practice to do some laboratory studies as well. Anemia, electrolyte disturbances, thyroid disorders, or other endocrine disorders may have developed and may be a factor in a changing migraine pattern.

Migraine without aura, like migraine with aura, is an inherited condition. It is, therefore, very important to tell the patient up front that at present there is no cure for their headaches, and that successful treatment will consist of trying to reduce the frequency and severity of their attacks and to abort the attacks quickly when they occur. Many patients have unreasonable expectations that the headache can be cured and completely eliminated with some of the new drugs that they have heard about. Successful treatment of migraine involves a close partnership of the patient with the treating physician.

Management of migraine without aura includes both pharmacologic and nonpharmacologic modalities. Patients should be advised to keep regular living patterns and to avoid erratic sleep patterns and eating patterns. Skipping meals is a common trigger of a migraine attack. Excessive tiredness or excessive sleeping, which result in patients not eating for long periods of time, can aggravate migraine. Perhaps 10 to 15% of patients can identify certain foods which may trigger an attack. Patients who have migraine without aura may find substances triggering attacks at one time, but not always. This is very frustrating for patients, but it seems that above a certain threshold, and when there are multiple factors present, any one substance may act as a trigger. Women with migraine are much more prone to have a headache at the time of menses. If the weather is changeable and they ingest some chocolate or alcohol, they may find the alcohol provokes a headache. At other times of the month, alcohol may not induce a headache. Keeping a diet diary and writing down all of the foods they ingested within 24 hours prior to the onset of headache will often help patients identify a food or substance which may act as a trigger.

Stress, as well as depression, may play a role in the frequency and severity of migraine attacks. Biofeedback training along with other means of relaxation may help reduce the severity and frequency of attacks. In patients who have a significant amount of muscle tension in the neck and shoulders, physical therapy and exercise on a regular daily basis may help as well.

Although some of these nonpharmacologic techniques are helpful in reducing the frequency and severity of migraine, the mainstay of treatment is pharmacologic. The decision whether or not to use daily prophylactic medication is based on consultation and discussion with the patient. Some patients who have very frequent attacks just do not want to take daily medication. Other patients who may only have one attack a month are so fearful of the attack that they want to take something daily in the hope that the attack will not occur or will be less intense. In general, however, daily preventive treatment should be considered for patients having three or more attacks per month. [*Editors' note: Some headache specialists would consider that preventive treatment is needed for a patient who gets six attacks or more per month and who gets long-lasting relief without side effects from a triptan.*] In the United States, the only preventive agents approved by the Food and Drug Administration (FDA) for migraine are the beta-blockers propranolol and timolol, methysergide, and divalproex sodium. Other beta-blockers are useful as well, and the calcium channel blockers, particularly verapamil, have been found to be fairly effective. Numerous studies have demonstrated the effectiveness of tricyclic antidepressants in the management of migraine as well. The nonsteroidal anti-inflammatory drugs can be quite beneficial in migraine prophylaxis. Their long-term use, however, needs to be closely monitored, and GI symptoms are frequent side effects. The patient may have other medical problems, which would contraindicate the use of these medications.

The best approach to the use of these preventive medications is to start with a fairly low dose and gradually increase the amount used depending on the patient's response or side effects. In many instances these agents are not used long enough. Frustration on the part of both the physician and the patient leads to frequent changing to other medications. Some of these preventive agents, particularly verapamil and divalproex sodium, may take 6 to 8 weeks before one sees a significant reduction of headache frequency and severity. Often patients have their drugs changed every couple of weeks and never give the medication an adequate trial.

Whether the patient is put on preventive medication, all patients with migraine need abortive therapy, i.e., something to take at the time of the acute attack. Ergotamine tartrate, which is usually combined with caffeine, has been very effective for many years. Unfortunately this agent makes many people nauseated. Isometheptene, which is combined with dichloralphenazone and acetaminophen, is not as effective but it certainly is better tolerated and often will be helpful. It is important to use enough of these abortive agents and to use them early in the attack. The rapid-acting anti-inflammatory drugs such as meclofenamate, ibuprofen, and naproxen sodium, when used in large amounts early in the headache attack, are often very effective.

A newer agent, sumatriptan, is effective in about 60 to 65% of patients and is available as an oral medication, as a nasal spray, or in self-injectable form. Our studies have shown that about 40% of responders do so to 25 mg in the oral form. Another 40% need 50 mg and about 20% need 100 mg or more. The dose seems to be quite variable, probably because of the variation in absorption during a GI attack. Zolmitriptan, naratriptan, and rizatriptan are new abortive agents available as oral tablets.

Summary

In summary, migraine without aura is the most common type of migraine, but is often not diagnosed. Helping the patient to recognize the factors that trigger their headache will help reduce the frequency of attacks. Good prophylactic and abortive medication is available, so that most patients with migraine without aura can control their attacks.

Selected Readings

Blau JN. Adult migraine: the patient observed. In: Blau JN, editor. Migraine, clinic and research aspects. Baltimore: Johns Hopkins University Press; 1987. p. 3–30.

Blau JN. Migraine with aura and migraine without aura are not different entities. Cephalalgia 1995;15:186–90.

Diamond S. Medical management of recurrent migraine. In: Tollison CD, Kunkel RS, editors. Headache diagnosis and management. Baltimore: Williams and Wilkins; 1993. p. 89–106.

Headache Classification Committee of the International Headache Society. Classification and diagnostic criteria for headache disorders, cranial neuralgias and facial pain. Cephalalgia 1988;Suppl VII:1–96.

Kunkel RS. Medical management of acute migraine episodes. In: Tollison CD, Kunkel RS, editors. Headache diagnosis and management. Baltimore: Williams and Wilkins; 1993. p. 85–8.

Lewis TA, Solomon GD. Advances in migraine management. Cleve Clin J Med 1995;62:148–55.

Lipton RB, Rapoport AM. Migraine with and without aura. In: Sammuels MA, Feske S, editors. Office practice of neurology. New York: Churchill Livingstone; 1996. p. 1105–11.

Rasmussen BK. Migraine with aura and migraine without aura are two different entities. Cephalalgia 1995;15:183–5.

Silberstein SD. Preventive treatment of migraine—an overview. Cephalalgia 1996;17:67–72.

Tietjen GE. Migraine with aura and migraine without aura: one entity or two or more? Cephalalgia 1995;15:182–3.

Editorial Comments

Migraine is more than headache, with many varied presentations, some stereotypical, and many systemic symptoms and manifestations. This case by Dr. Kunkel explores the nature of migraine symptoms and the importance of associated gastrointestinal symptomology. The case is rich in description, and his management suggestions and strategies are sound and reflect the experience of a seasoned clinician. When neurologic aura does not accompany migraine, diagnosis can be more difficult. The fine line between repetitive usage of abortive agents, such as the triptans, and institution of preventive agents will become more defined in the future. In the meantime, approaches to therapy as outlined in this case are most welcome.

CHAPTER 4

THE YOUNG GIRL WITH INCAPACITATING HEADACHES

PAUL K. WINNER, DO

Case History

A 12-year-old girl presents with a 6-month history of incapacitating headaches. These headaches occur on average two times a month. These headaches begin gradually in the bifrontal region and intensify over the course of 1 to 2 hours to incapacitating, throbbing headaches that are worsened with activity. She notes nausea and photophobia but denies suffering from prominent vomiting or phonophobia. The patient indicates that the headaches have slightly intensified over the course of the last 6 months. She notes that these headaches are often precipitated by skipping meals or eating hot dogs. She denies having had any head trauma or any recent episodes of meningitis or encephalitis.

The patient denies having any sensorial changes, motor or sensory weaknesses, any visual changes, lightheadedness, or dizziness associated with the above episodes. She describes these episodes as lasting on average 3 hours but occasionally lasting slightly longer. She has at this point, with the help of her parents, attempted to treat her headaches with over-the-counter medicines, primarily acetaminophen and ibuprofen, with minimal benefit.

Her past medical history is unremarkable except for asthma which is presently stable. There is a family history of migraine on the maternal side. The patient denies having any gastrointestinal symptomatology. The patient is not on any standard medications. She says that she has had no exposure to any environmental toxins or to alcohol, smoking, or illicit drugs.

Both the patient and her parents express a desire to control these headaches since the patient is missing on average 1 to 2 days of school a month. They are also concerned about the intensity of the headache which has increased over the past few months.

Her general examination is within normal limits. Her blood pressure is 100/66. Her pulse is 76 beats per minute and regular. A neurologic examination reveals some diffuse discomfort in the cervical region. Motor, sensory, and cognitive examinations are normal, as is an examination of the cranial nerves.

Questions about This Case

- What is your diagnosis in this case?
- Why do you think the headaches may be intensifying?
- Is there any other information that you would like to know regarding this case?
- How would you manage this patient's headaches?
- What specific therapies would you initially suggest and, if they are ineffective, what would be alternative therapies?
- What is your long-term suggestion for comprehensive care and the future outlook for this patient?

Case Discussion

This 12-year-old girl presents with a history that is consistent with the International Headache Society (IHS) criteria for migraine. This patient has a history described as 6 months of intermittent headaches that last on average 2 to 3 hours. The IHS criteria does make an adjustment for children, specifically under the age of 15, for headache duration being 2 to 48 hours. It has been noted by many researchers that children will often experience headaches of a duration shorter than that of adults. The patient also presents with a bifrontal headache symptomatology which is often seen in children, especially in the younger age group. It has been the author's experience when following these children into adulthood that their headaches often become of longer duration and often become unilateral. The patient does have incapacitating, throbbing headache that is one of the necessary criteria for migraine according to the IHS. The patient also describes having nausea without prominent vomiting. Children often will experience vomiting very early in the headache symptomatology, although this individual did not. Children often experience photophobia without phonophobia or the reverse.

This patient has described having headache for roughly 6 months with slight intensification. The possibility of a prominent central nervous system (CNS) lesion, specifically a brain tumor, is a concern when physicians see individuals who have had a headache for fewer than 4 months and who are under the age of 12 years, and even more so when they are under the age of 7 years. This individual, however, has had 6 months of headaches and on further questioning it appears that they have only moderately increased and there has not been a prominent progression of the incapacitation of the headaches, nor has there been a prominent progression of the duration. She has not been awakened by headache, a characteristic which might suggest a CNS neoplastic lesion.

Children in this age group and younger have a higher incidence of posterior fossa lesions. Whenever there is a history of more prominent occipital headache symptoms, especially with intensification and a short headache history such as 4 months, it is important to rule out a posterior fossa neoplasm.

In review, there is a family history of migraine in this individual. This child did not have prominent aura symptomatology. It is important to note that often in children there is the initial presentation of the various subclasses of migraine with aura and some of the migraine variants that are often diagnosed later in life. This is not the case with our present patient.

This patient attempted to treat these headaches unsuccessfully with over-the-counter medication. With a headache of short duration it still may be possible to use other medications such as analgesics to control this patient's headache. A butalbital-containing compound may be used in limited amounts with proper education of both the patient and the family to avoid potential overuse. Butalbital-containing compounds with acetaminophen may prove extremely effective in this individual, especially with the shorter duration of headache. Over-the-counter nonsteroidal anti-inflammatory drugs (NSAIDs) may prove beneficial. In my experience, sometimes prescription NSAIDs have proved more efficacious. Ibuprofen in appropriate dosages per weight can often be helpful for young children. This individual, however, did not respond to acetaminophen or to over-the-counter ibuprofen. Nausea is present but not prominent vomiting.

Sometimes these individuals, especially as they progress from childhood through adolescence, will benefit greatly from the use of a serotonin (5-HT-1) agonist. There are presently published studies with the use of 5-HT-1 agonists, specifically sumatriptan, naratriptan, and dihydroergotamine, and ongoing studies are presently evaluating zolmitriptan, rizatriptan, and eletriptan. This patient may benefit significantly from the use of a sumatriptan 25 mg-tablet that can relieve headache symptoms within 1 to 2 hours. Other delivery systems (e.g. SQ, nasal) of sumatriptan may also prove beneficial with a quicker onset of action to relieve this patient's symptoms or those of individuals with a similar symptomatology. Dihydroergotamine is also an option and, again, various delivery systems may be considered.

This individual has on average one to two migraines without aura per month. At this point, I would continue to use abortive approaches but should this individual's headaches intensify or should this individual have headaches lasting several days or continue not to respond to abortive therapy, preventive therapy may be considered. This patient has asthma and, as such, beta-blockers are not an appropriate choice, although there are studies to show that in patients without asthma, this would be a consideration. This individual may benefit from the use of cyproheptadine hydrochloride, which can be given in divided doses from 4 to 12 mg daily.

Other preventive therapies such as tricyclic antidepressants can be used with caution because of the potential cardiac side effects. Unfortunately, the most effective of the calcium channel blockers, flunarizine, is not available in the United States but there is published data regarding its efficacy in children and it is used widely in other countries.

The long-term outlook for remission in children is good. In discussion with both the patients and their parents, I feel that it is important not only to outline our knowledge of the pathophysiology of migraine as well as the various medications, but also to suggest a comprehensive approach including addressing this patient's triggers such as dietary issues, a proper schedule for meals, exercise, proper sleep hygiene, and the use of a headache diary for future assistance in the management of this patient's headaches. Roughly 30 to 40% of individuals in this age group with migraine will have remission of their migraines for years to decades and sometimes completely.

Management Strategies

Establishing the correct diagnosis is paramount. If you feel uncomfortable with the evaluation and treatment of children or adolescents, it is recommended that you refer this individual to a specialist in this field such as a pediatric neurologist, a neurologist, a pediatrician, or a primary care physician who is very comfortable with these patients.

For individuals who have had headaches for less than 4 months, where there has been an increase in frequency and severity of the headaches and where there has been a reported neurologic sign or symptom, it is imperative that these patients be evaluated appropriately and considered for a work-up to rule out a structural lesion or other disorders.

For individuals who do not respond to the initial abortive and symptomatic therapies such as simple analgesics or NSAIDs, there are various medications such as 5-HT-1 agonists which have been tested, and under testing at this time, which may prove beneficial. The use of opioids at this age can be undertaken safely but it is important to discuss the long-term consequences of excessive use, including rebound issues to avoid overuse of analgesics. It is important to tell these individuals that should their headaches worsen or change, they need to be re-evaluated by their health care professional.

Case Summary

This child has migraine without aura. Her headaches may go into remission for many decades or for the rest of her life. There is also the possibility that these headaches will fluctuate significantly with increased severity and intensity, especially around the time of menstruation.

The majority of these patients can be managed successfully with the use of an abortive or symptomatic medication. For the majority of individuals whose headaches do intensify in frequency and severity, who are evaluated appropriately, and are known to still maintain a migraine with or without aura, preventive therapies can be appropriately and successfully used.

It is important to approach children and adolescents with a comprehensive headache management profile with an emphasis on diet, exercise, sleep hygiene, biofeedback where appropriate (over the age of 9 years), and the appropriate use of abortive/symptomatic and, when necessary, preventive therapy.

Overview of Migraine in Children

Parents usually seek medical attention for their children and adolescents with severe headaches in an effort to obtain reassurance that the underlying cause is not a brain tumor or other serious illness. Many parents do not realize that it is common for migraine headaches to begin in childhood. Migraine is found in 4 to 5% of school-age children. Among adults with headaches, 20% report that the symptoms began before the age of 10 years and more than 45% report the onset of their severe headaches before the age of 20 years. The prevalence of migraine is equal in young boys and girls. However, after puberty, the ratio of women to men increases to three to one.

The IHS provides explicit criteria for the diagnosis of migraine. However, the IHS criteria do not characterize headaches in children separately and lack sensitivity in this age group. Therefore, a revised criteria for children has been proposed and is being tested.

Both the IHS criteria and the proposed criteria for children require multiple attacks for diagnosis because the first migaine attack cannot always be distinguished from a secondary headache. Secondary headaches may result from infection, concussion, or neoplasm.

In children, headaches may last as little as 1 hour and they are often bifrontal or bi-temporal. Headaches in the occipital region are less common and may have an underlying organic cause.

Associated symptoms are an integral part of migraine and are essential for diagnosis; these include photophobia, phonophobia, nausea, and vomiting. Most migraineurs, whether children or adults, experience nausea. All age groups also report vomiting but it may occur earlier in the headache episodes in children. Adults often experience both photophobia and phonophobia, whereas children may be more likely to experience one or the other.

A diagnosis of migraine with aura requires the presence of one or more fully reversible neurologic symptoms: visual, motor, or sensory. This finding helps distinguish migraine from a progressive organic disorder, which requires further diagnostic assessment. Aura develops gradually over at least 4 minutes and usually lasts 20 to 30 minutes, but may be as long as 60 munutes. An aura that is rapid in onset and short in duration may be caused by a paroxysmal event.

Nonspecific electroencephalographic abnormalities have been reported in migraineurs. Some of these findings are believed to be normal variants.

Practitioners may encounter several varied presentations of migraine in children, as outlined below.

Hemiplegic migraine is a type of migraine that may occur in young children. Usually the headache follows a hemiparesis which lasts for hours to days. Attacks are infrequent and may be accompanied by dysarthria, aphasia, and altered levels of consciousness that often involve visual symptomatology.

A familial form of hemiplegic migraine requires identical attacks in a first-degree relative to establish a diagnosis. This is the first form of migraine to be linked to a genetic cause, a point mutation on chromosome 19, which is found in roughly 55% of families experiencing this clinical symptomatology. Recently, a mutation in chromosome 1 has been reported to affect 15% of families with this clinical symptomatology.

Basilar migraine often occurs in adolescent girls with a positive family history of migraine. Brainstem symptomatology, including blurred vision, tinnitus, vertigo, and ataxia, is common. About half of the patients experience bilateral weakness and paresthesias, which may be very frightening to the patient.

Benign paroxysmal vertigo, a periodic syndrome of childhood according to the IHS criteria, usually occurs monthly and resolves as the child becomes older. The presentation may be rather abrupt with the child becoming suddenly pale, seemingly frightened, and grabbing on to any item nearby for stability. Nausea and vomiting often accompany the episode and nystagmus may be noted. The attacks are very short, usually lasting 1 to 2 minutes, without loss of consciousness. If the attacks have no residual deficit, abate quickly, and follow the presentation as noted, follow-up is all that is necessary; should the attacks vary from the above, a complete work-up is recommended. Patients experiencing benign paroxysmal vertigo in childhood have a positive family history of migraine.

Cyclic vomiting has its onset usually between the ages of 4 and 8 years. Episodes occur at regular intervals, usually about every 4 to 5 weeks. Headache may or may not be associated. Cyclic vomiting is not progressive. If the condition becomes worse, a thorough examination is suggested, including a complete gastrointestinal work-up and magnetic resonance imaging (MRI) of the brain.

Once the diagnosis of migrane has been made, the practitioner should take the opportunity to review the causative mechanisms with both the patient and his or her parents. The treatment of acute migraines in children and adolescents often requires modifications of the adult approach. A comprehensive approach using both pharmacologic and nonpharmacologic methods is often helpful in children.

Nonpharmacologic methods include the elimination of known triggers and training in biofeedback and stress management techniques. Several studies have reported the beneficial effects for biofeedback and relaxation training in children.

In children under the age of 6 years, limited amounts of acetaminophen are effective and cause few problems since headaches are usually short lived and resolve with sleep. In older children, acetaminophen, nonsteroidal anti-inflammatory agents, and butalbital-containing analgesic compounds may be useful in the absence of significant nausea. A brief discussion with parents and patients about the potential for analgesic-induced rebound headache is recommended as a precaution against long-term misuse. In children under the age of 15 years, aspirin must be avoided because of the continued concerns for Reye's syndrome.

Opioids such as meperidine hydrochloride and codeine can usually be used in children over the age of 6 years, if caution and supervision are exercised and physician monitoring is provided.

The use of 5-HT-1 agonists has proved to be effective in the treatment of acute moderate to severe migraine in children and adolescents. The parenteral use of both dihydroergotamine mesylate and sumatriptan has been found to be effective in patients aged 6 years and older. Recently, patients aged 12 years and older have been shown to respond to oral sumatriptan, 25 mg, with pain relief noted within 4 hours accompanied by relief of disability. At present these medications have not been formally approved by the Food and Drug Administration (FDA) for use in children and adolescents but studies toward this end are ongoing. Other 5-HT-1 agonist medications (naratriptan, zolmitriptan, rizatriptan, and eletriptan) for the treatment of children and adolescents are under evaluation in several delivery systems (SQ, nasal, and tablets).

Antiemetics, both in suppository and oral forms, are useful in children with acute migraines accompanied by nausea and vomiting. The 25-mg suppository form of promethazine hydrochloride is often effective in young children, while the 50 mg formulation may be necessary in older children. Prochlorperazine should be used with caution in children because of the potential extrapyramidal side effects.

Preventive therapy should be considered in children who miss excessive amounts of school or do not respond to abortive therapies. Age plays a role in the selection of prophylactic agents, and often dosages need to be tailored to individual children and adolescents. Beta-blockers have proved to be beneficial migraine preventive agents in both adults and children. We have had excellent results with the use of beta-blockers, specifically propanolol. In children, we start with a dosage of 1 mg per kilogram, not to exceed 10 mg twice a day in a young child, and the dosage is gradually increased until a therapeutic response is achieved or side effects prohibit further increase. Often, a clinical response is not seen for several weeks. We caution patients, physicians, and parents to monitor for the potential precipitation of depression when this medication is used in adolescents.

Antihistamines, specifically cyproheptadine hydrochloride, are often used as a preventive agent in young children. The dosage ranges from 4 to 12 mg and is to be given in divided doses or at bedtime as a single dose. The most common side effects are drowsiness and weight gain.

The antimigraine effects of tricyclic antidepressants seem to be independent of their antidepressant effects. Amitriptyline and nortriptyline have proved to be effective. No controlled studies of these agents in children have been reported and the side-effect profile, especially cardiac, limits their usefulness as a first-line agent in young children.

Calcium channel blockers have been shown to be helpful in double-blind, placebo-controlled studies using nimodipine for the prevention of migraine in children aged 7 through 18 years. Flunarizine has also been proved to be effective but it is not available in the United States.

The anticonvulsant sodium valproate has been shown in recent double-blind, controlled studies to be effective in the prevention of migraine in adults. This agent must be considered with caution especially in children under the age of 10 years for the potential side effects of hepatotoxicity and pancreatitis. The effectiveness of phenobarbital, phenytoin, and carbamazepine have been demonstrated in older studies. Whether the patients included in the study population had comorbid seizures as well as migraine is not known. However, anticonvulsants can be used effectively in children whose condition is refractive to other prophylactic agents.

Migraine often presents for the first time during childhood and adolescence. Patients require an appropriate evaluation and follow-up. The management of migraines should include a discussion of therapeutic goals with both the patients and their parents. Appropriate medications are limited in younger children, but in older children and adolescents, more options are becoming available especially with the addition of 5-HT-1 agonists. Preventive therapy should be discussed with both patients and parents so that they fully understand the options available regarding headache management.

Selected Readings

Allen K, Shriver M. Enhanced performance feedback to strengthen biofeedback treatment outcome with childhood migraine. Headache 1997;37:169–73.

Battistella P, Ruffilli R, Moro R, et al. A placebo-controlled crossover trial of nimodipine in pediatric migraine. Headache 1990;30:264–8.

Bille B. Migraine in school children. Acta Paediatr Scand 1961; 51 Suppl 136:1–151.

Congdon PJ, Forsythe WI. Migraine in childhood: a study of 300 children. Dev Med Child Neurol 1979;21:209–16.

Duckro P, Cantwell-Simmons E. A review of studies evaluating biofeedback and relaxation training in the management of pediatric headache. Headache 1989;29:428.

Gladstein J, Holden EW, Peralta L, Raven M. Diagnosis and symptom patterns in children presenting to a pediatric headache clinic. Headache 1993;33:497–500.

Headache Classification Committee of the International Headache Society. Classification and diagnostic criteria for headache disorders, cranial neuralgia, and facial pain. Cephalalgia 1988;8 Suppl 7:1–96.

Hering R, Kuritzky A. Sodium valproate in the prophylactic treatment of migraine: a double-blind study versus placebo. Cephalalgia 1992;12:81–4.

Kudrow L. Cluster headache: mechanisms and management. Oxford: Oxford University Press; 1980.

Lewis DW. Migraine and migraine variants in children and adolescents. Semin Pediatr Neurol 1995;2(2):127–43.

Linder S. Treatment of childhood headache with dihydroergotamine mesylate. Headache 1994;34:578–80.

Linder S. Subcutaneous sumatriptan in the clinical setting: the first 50 consecutive patients with acute migraine in a pediatric neurology office practice. Headache 1996;36:419–22.

Raskin NH. Migraine: clinical aspects. In: Headache. 2nd ed. New York: Churchill-Livingston; 1988. p. 41.

Rothner D. Miscellaneous headache syndromes in children and adolescents. Semin Pediatr Neurol 1995;2(2):159–64.

Scheller JM. The history, epidemiology, and classification of headache in children. Semin Pediatr Neurol 1995;2(2): 102–8.

Seshia SS, Wolstein JR, Adams C, et al. International Headache Society criteria and childhood headache. Dev Med Child Neurol 1994;36:419–28.

Singer HS. Migraine headaches in children. Pediatr Rev 1994; 15(3):94–100.

Solomon GD. Pharmacology and use of headache medications. Cleve Clin J Med 1990;57:627–35.

Swaiman KF, Frank Y. Seizure headache in children. Dev Med Child Neurol 1978;20:580.

Winner P, Martinez W, Mate L, Bello L. Classification of pediatric migraine: proposed revision of the IHS criteria. Headache 1995;35:407–10.

Winner P, Prensky A, Linder S, et al. Efficacy and safety of oral sumatriptan in adolescent migraines. Presented at the American Association for the study of Headache Scientific Meeting. San Diego, CA, May 1996.

Young GB, Blume WT. Painful epileptic seizures. Brain 1983;106:537.

Editorial Comments

Headache in children has always been regarded as quite different from adult headache disorders. There are significantly different diagnostic categories in children and some clinical differences, however, when it comes to migraine there are many similarities. Pediatric migraine headache is probably under-recognized and treated, but as Dr. Winner points out, such disorders can be incapacitating in children. Careful explanation and education of the children and their parents, along with the judicious use of appropriate medications and behavioral techniques, including biofeedback, are warranted. This, in fact, is a good formula for the management of all headache patients.

CHAPTER 5

THE WOMAN WHO COULD NOT DECIDE WHICH MEDICATION TO TAKE

R. ALLAN PURDY, MD, FRCPC

FRED D. SHEFTELL, MD

ALAN M. RAPOPORT, MD

STEWART J. TEPPER, MD

Case History

This 35-year-old female patient presented with a long history of headache, which had begun since childhood. Since the age of 22, she had had attacks about eight to twelve times a year. In the past year, she has had attacks three or more times a month, and the headache would last 4 to 6 hours.

The headaches were located on the side of her head, usually on the left but occasionally on the right, and were throbbing in nature. Frequently, just prior to each headache she would have visual symptoms consisting of "zigzag lines" in her right visual field, which would slowly move across her vision from right to left and be followed by a black blank area in her vision. On other occasions, she noticed that her headaches were preceded by numbness in her right tongue, then in her face and arm. She has noted trouble with her speech on occasion, in that she would have difficulty finding the right word. These headaches were usually associated with nausea and, if severe, with vomiting. She found that her headaches were worse if she moved her head or if she was exposed to bright lights, sounds, or perfumes.

Interestingly, but not surprisingly, she has occasional tension-type headaches, which can occur after a "migraine" or independent of her "migraine headaches." There is a family history of migraine in her mother and sister, and a maternal uncle died of a "brain tumor."

The patient is an accountant who finds that her migraine headaches are interfering with her work and her family activities. She finds it hard to care for her two children, work, and carry on with her personal life. She wants to find a way to reduce the number of headaches she is having and is very interested in all forms of therapy for migraine. She was worried about a "tumor" originally but recognizes that such a concern is "irrational." She does not like taking too many medications and wants to avoid side effects. Her expectation is that the "doctor" will manage her headaches. She has had and continues to have great difficulty deciding which treatment or medication she should take for her headaches. She had tried various medications without success.

Her neurologic and general examinations were completely within normal limits.

Questions about This Case

- What are your initial impressions of this case?
- What would you recommend in terms of investigations and why?

- What would you recommend in terms of treatment and management of her case?
- If she decides to take a triptan medication, then which one should she take and why?

Case Discussion

This is a case of migraine with aura, fitting the usual International Headache Society (IHS) criteria. The aura consists of the usual visual symptoms but on some occasions, she has more speech and sensory symptoms, suggesting a more anterior localization of her neurologic dysfunction during some of her auras, which in her case precede her headaches. She has a typical "sensory march," which is analogous to the classical jacksonian motor and sensory marches seen in epilepsy but is much slower in onset and increased in duration.

This case does indicate that migraine has variability in each patient. It is not unusual for migraine patients to have different auras on occasion, and many have different intensities of headache as well. She also has some of her migraine headaches without aura.

This patient had a normal examination, which is what one would expect in a patient not having a migraine attack during an office visit, unlike someone in severe pain in the emergency room (ER). It is important that the patient is between migraine attacks since if she was in the ER having an attack, she would look ill, and usually in such situations, it is difficult to get a precise history. Thus, the ER is not the place to start a therapeutic relationship with a migraine patient in severe pain. Treat the pain and have the patient return to your office to get a more detailed account of the headache, its triggers, and other medical information pertinent to the case.

It is interesting in this case to consider the mechanisms of migraine headache, the difference between various subtypes of migraine headache, the idea of aura, trigger factors, and prodromal symptoms. The patient did have some migraine headaches in childhood, and her migraine headaches were worse when she used oral contraceptives.

She has occasional "tension-type headaches" that can occur after a migraine or independent of her migraine headaches. This is not at all uncommon in migraine patients.

It is now accepted that neither computed tomography (CT) nor magnetic resonance imaging (MRI) are necessary in adult patients whose headaches fit a broad definition of recurrent migraine and who do not demonstrate any change in headache pattern, a history of seizures, or the presence of focal neurologic signs. In this case, one would be justified in not doing a neuroimaging procedure. However, all good clinicians would temper this decision, based on the patient's concerns and family history, which in this case did not appear relevant. Sometimes CT or MRI can be "therapeutic" or help the patient and their physician get "beyond" the worry about an organic etiology.

The patient had tried simple analgesics, ergotamine, NSAIDs, as well as a dihydroergotamine (DHE) nasal spray. She did not feel the analgesics helped at all, and the NSAIDs only helped if her migraine was mild. She did not prefer nasal DHE because of nasal congestion and the device needed to administer the spray although it did seem to help but took a long time. She had tried oral sumatriptan at a dose of 100 mg but had experienced chest symptoms that she did not like; however, she did feel that it helped her more moderate and severe headaches within a couple of hours. She also noted that several times after oral sumatriptan, she would get a recurrence of her headaches or that it did not work for every migraine, and she did not wish to take any more.

In terms of future management, her case represents the typical dilemma faced by clinicians and patients. Although guidelines are available for acute and prophylactic treatment of migraine, they do not specify which agent to use but suggest that treatment be based on severity. This makes sense to the physician as well as the patient but with the development in recent years of more migraine-specific medications for abortive therapy, it could become increasingly more difficult to give advice on which medication to use and when.

She should certainly explore all the nonpharmacologic therapies and look at the management of migraine triggers, all of which have been dealt with in other cases in this book. However, when it comes to managing her severe migraine headaches, she will have to decide which of the new triptans to use, as they appear to have the greatest efficacy, best side-effect profile, and safety. The discussion of all the current triptans available will follow but for now, her therapeutic options include the following management strategies.

Management Strategies

- Consider using an ergot preparation including a suppository.
- Use oral sumatriptan at a dose of 50 mg or less, which could help many of her moderate and some of her severe headaches, with fewer side effects than with an ergot.
- Use nasal sumatriptan, 20 mg, which could reduce her chest symptoms and give fast onset of relief as well as, if not better than, oral sumatriptan.
- Use naratriptan in a dose of 2.5 mg for her moderate migraines and recognize that the onset of relief may be slower, up to 4 hours, but recurrence is less frequent and side effects are negligible in most patients.
- Use oral zolmitriptan, which may be more consistent in response than sumatriptan. The optimal dose is 2.5 mg and is at least as effective as sumatriptan, 50 mg, with similar side effects and a slightly longer duration of action.
- Consider rizatriptan fast tablets or melt tablets, which may induce less nausea than sumatriptan, although perhaps more drowsiness. The 10 mg dose is the most effective but the 5 mg dose works well in many patients and has fewer side effects, so it could be used for moderate migraine. The effectiveness of 10 mg rizatriptan and 50 mg sumatriptan is indistinguishable at 2 hours but rizatriptan has a shorter duration of action.

She decided, after discussion, to try sumatriptan, 50 mg, and found it helpful, with few problems, but not as good as the higher dosage. She did have a very good response to nasal sumatriptan and was very thankful that she had no chest symptoms, so she decided to stay with that medication for now. With one headache per month she was not a candidate for prophylaxis. As you can see from the above and the following discussion, she has many options for the future management of her migraine headaches.

Case Summary

- This patient has migraine with aura and without aura, which is variable in severity.
- She has both visual and sensory auras.
- She does not require investigation based on current knowledge but this is always a matter of clinical judgement in an individual patient.
- She represents what will become an increasing problem for patients and physicians managing migraine in the future, with respect to what medication to use for acute treatment. Her case also raises the question of what prophylactic treatment actually means, when there are so many new effective abortive agents available.

Overview of How to Pick a Triptan or Ergot for Your Patient

The patient in this case has a varying, but rather typical, migraine picture. She has migraine with aura and migraine without aura. She has moderate migraine, and she has severe migraine. When she has severe attacks, she is disabled from work, and she is unable to take oral medication. The frequency of migraine is low enough to suggest that daily preventive therapy may not be necessary if acute treatment is available to reliably restore her to normal function. So the question for the treating physician is how to craft an acute migraine strategy given all her clinical variables?

Two concepts may prove helpful, **stratifying** her care and **staging** her attacks. Stratifying her care means figuring out how high the treatment needs are for the patient.

There are several ways to do this. One can take a history of peak intensity of the migraine, time to peak intensity, disability, and time to disability, e.g., nausea, vomiting, and those associated symptoms that would prevent the patient from functioning normally. Or one could use a validated, simple disability scale, such as the Migraine Disability Assessment Scale (MIDAS), which allows one to stratify the patient's disability in terms of work and social losses over the previous 3 months. Either way, this patient would stratify to a high level of disability with high treatment needs because of the intensity of the pain and the time lost due to illness. High treatment needs dictate the use of migraine-specific medications such as the triptans and, to a lesser extent, the ergots.

Clearly not every attack that this patient has requires injectable triptan or ergot use, so this is an opportunity for the doctor to allow the patient to stage her attacks, giving her several medication options to use, depending on the severity and speed of development of the attack. Lower-level attacks might be treated with oral mixed analgesics such as aspirin/acetaminophen/caffeine combinations, anti-headache compounds, containing isometheptene or butalbital, and/or antinauseants such as metoclopramide. The concern in staging with low-level medication is that overuse of these medications can lead to analgesic rebound or transformed migraine, with increased overall frequency of headache and decreasing response to all medications. And if the patient guesses wrong, and the attack becomes severe, she must have a higher-level medication to stage up to, to restore normal function.

For the more severe attacks, use of an ergot or triptan is indicated. Ergots are the old standby but they are difficult to use and, to a great extent, have been superseded by the triptans. **Ergotamine tartrate** is available in the United States in oral-tablet, sublingual, and suppository forms. However, the oral form is poorly absorbed, and all forms usually produce nausea. Ergotamine is also habituating, with a low threshold for triggering rebound. Finally, peripheral vasoconstriction can be a problem with its use.

If the patient is distressed by the occasional aura, she might wish to use an ergotamine suppository at the beginning of the aura since ergots, but not triptans, have been shown to shorten the aura and the attack that follows. She would need to try out the suppository in advance and titrate her dose by cutting it with a razor blade to find the highest non-nauseating dose up to a full suppository to use at the onset of aura. The starting dose is no more than one-quarter of a suppository (0.5 mg).

Dihydroergotamine mesylate (DHE) is used both parenterally and intranasally. It is less nauseating and less habituating than ergotamine. The nasal spray is somewhat cumbersome to use, as it requires considerable patient preparation but it achieves headache relief in about 60% of patients in 2 hours. It has a long duration of action, with a low recurrence rate, which makes it reasonable for longer menstrual migraines, especially if the patient wakes up too nauseated to take a tablet. Adverse effects of DHE are few, consisting primarily of nausea, leg cramps, gastrointestinal problems, and local intranasal problems with the spray.

Sumatriptan is available as a tablet, as a nasal spray, and as a subcutaneous 6 mg injection with autoinjector. Both the tablet and the spray yield a headache response of 60 to 65% in 2 hours but the spray works faster for some patients. The optimal dose is 50 mg for the tablet and 20 mg for the spray. The injection gives 50% of patients pain relief in 30 minutes and 80 to 90% in 2 hours.

Sumatriptan offers this patient some unique advantages since patients are advised that switching between ergots and triptans or among different triptans in the same day is contraindicated. So, if this patient takes one nonsumatriptan orally and it does not work, she cannot rescue herself with injectable DHE or sumatriptan in the same 24 hours. However, it is acceptable to switch forms of sumatriptan, so if she takes the pill and then the migraine worsens and she proceeds to prostration, she can use the injection. So, providing her with multiple sumatriptan forms will allow her to stage her headache and virtually guarantee her ability to restore herself to normal function.

Maximum amounts per 24 hours are 200 mg of sumatriptan tablets, two injections, two sprays, or combinations of a 100 mg tablet plus one injection or spray, or one injection plus one spray. All doses should be separated by 2 hours.

Zolmitriptan has the best headache response at 2 hours for an oral triptan (67.1% for 2.5 mg versus 63.8% for 50 mg sumatriptan) and the highest consistency reported in open-label studies over a year (95% of attacks aborted with one to two doses). The optimal dose is 2.5 mg, and the maximum total dose is 10 mg per 24 hours. If a 2.5 mg dose is not effective, a 5 mg dose often is.

Naratriptan is the most unusual of the available triptans in that it has a different profile for use. It is slow in its onset of activity with 48% of patients showing pain relief at 2 hours and 66% at 4 hours. However, it has a very gentle adverse-event profile, with side effects comparable to placebo. It has a long duration of action, with half the recurrence rate seen with sumatriptan or rizatriptan.

Naratriptan can thus be used in a number of specific situations. It can be used for moderate migraine, especially if the lower-level, nonspecific medications have failed. It can be used in a prolonged migraine, in place of DHE, if the patient can take an oral tablet. Recurrence is least likely if the naratriptan is taken in the first 90 minutes of the attack. It can also be used in depressed patients as a monoamine oxidase (MAO) inhibitor as it is the only currently available triptan that is not metabolized by MAO. Finally, in patients who are sensitive to the adverse effects of these medications, naratriptan is the "gentle triptan."

Rizatriptan is an oral triptan available in both conventional oral-tablet and orally dissolvable-tablet or melt form. The optimal dose is 10 mg but patients who are on propranolol need to be given the 5 mg dose. The 2-hour headache relief resulting from the 10 mg dose is indistinguishable from that obtained with the 50 mg sumatriptan dose.

The melt has a mint taste, dissolves rapidly in saliva, and is swallowed without water. It is not absorbed through the oral mucosa but is absorbed like any other tablet in the gut. The rate of onset of effect and the overall headache response is identical for the tablet and melt forms.

This patient could use the melt in a number of circumstances. If getting to water was difficult (i.e., at a movie or while driving) or embarrassing (i.e., in a corporate board room making a presentation), dropping a mint-like tablet on the tongue would be both convenient and discreet.

So, to summarize, if a patient has migraine that varies widely in speed and intensity, the use of sumatriptan allows for switching forms in the same day. The injection sets the standard for speed of onset and overall efficacy. The nasal spray is usually faster than any tablet and bypasses the gut in a nauseated patient. The tablet has identical efficacy to rizatriptan.

If the patient desires the most effective tablet at 2 hours, with the highest consistency, and never needs a spray or injection, zolmitriptan is the correct choice. When the patient needs discretion, cannot get to water, or does not like to drink liquid when having a migraine, the rizatriptan melt can be used.

If the patient wants to shorten the aura and the migraine that follows, an ergot should be used. If a patient needs to bypass the gut in a long menstrual migraine, a DHE nasal spray can be used. Finally, for moderate migraine, for prolonged migraine, or in patients who are sensitive to side effects or on MAO inhibitors, naratriptan is optimal.

Allowing multiple options to stage the headache empowers the patient and furthers the therapeutic alliance. Stratifying the patient to low-, moderate-, or high-treatment needs matches the treatment to the patient to maximize the likelihood of success.

Selected Readings

Ahrens SP, Visser WH, Jiang K, Reines SA and the Rizatriptan RPD Study Group. Rizatriptan RPD for the acute treatment of migraine. [poster]. Eur Neurol 1998;5(Suppl 3):S52.

Dahlof C, Hogenhuis L, Olesen J, et al. Early clinical experience with subcutaneous naratriptan in the acute treatment of migraine; a dose ranging study. Eur Neurol 1998;5:469–77.

Gallagher RM. Acute treatment of migraine with dihydroergotamine nasal spray. Arch Neurol 1996;53:1285–91.

Gallagher RM, Tepper SJ. Maximizing treatment response to acute migraine therapy. Presented at the American Association for the Study of Headache meeting; 1998 June 27; San Francisco CA.

Klassen A, Elkind A, Asgharnejad M, et al, on behalf of the Naratriptan S2WA3001 Study Group. Naratriptan is effective and well tolerated in the acute treatment of migraine. Results of a double-blind, placebo-controlled, parallel group study. Headache 1997;37:640–5.

Mathew NT, Mahnaz A, Peykamian M, Laurenza A, on behalf the Naratriptan S2WA3003 Study Group. Naratriptan is effective and well tolerated in the acute treatment of migraine: results of a double-blind, placebo-controlled, crossover study. Neurology 1997;49:1485–90.

Meyler WJ. Side effects of ergotamine. Cephalalgia 1996;16:5–10.

Norman BA, Block GA, Jiang K, Ahrens S. Two-period crossover comparison of rizatriptan 5 mg and 10 mg to sumatriptan 25 mg and 50 mg for the acute treatment of migraine. Neurology 1998;50:A341 (presented at the American Academy of Neurology meeting; 1998 Apr; Minneapolis MN).

Pffaffenrath V, Cunin G, Sjonell G, Prendergast S. Efficacy and safety of sumatriptan tablets (25 mg, 50 mg, and 100 mg) in the acute treatment of migraine: defining the optimum doses of oral sumatriptan. Headache 1998;38:184–90.

Ryan R, Elkind A, Baker CC, et al. Sumatriptan nasal spray for the acute treatment of migraine. Neurology. 1997;49:1225–30.

Sawyer J, Lipton RB, et al. Clinical utility of a new instrument assessing migraine disability: the migraine disability assessment (MIDAS) questionnaire. Neurology 1998;50:A433–4.

Sheftell FD, Weeks RE, Rapoport AM, et al. Subcutaneous sumatriptan in a clinical setting: the first 100 consecutive patients with acute migraine in a tertiary care center. Headache 1994;34:67–72.

Sheftell F, Watson C, Pait DG, O'Quinn S. Low headache recurrence with naratriptan: clinical parameters related to recurrence. Headache 1998;38:405.

Subcutaneous Sumatriptan International Study Group. Treatment of headache attacks with sumatriptan. NEJM 1992;12:214–20.

Tepper SJ. Selection of new triptan or ergot for your patient. Seminars in Headache Management. 3:10–4.

Editorial Comments

Undoubtedly, one of the major problems for patients and their physicians in the foreseeable future will be in deciding which is the best acute care agent for their migraine attacks. It may be that with all of the new triptan medications available at present and in the future, the choice will be much easier but one does not necessarily expect that this will be the case.

Physicians make choices based on the best knowledge and experience; patients make choices for similar reasons but on other occasions make entirely separate choices regarding therapies, some of which make no sense to clinicians at all.

This will then be the challenge, which we as editors offer to the reader in this case, with the excellent assistance of Dr. Tepper, and that is that patients and their doctors must sit down together, discuss what they know and do not know, and agree on a mutually acceptable management strategy. Now, that sounds like good medicine and must be seen as in the best interests of our patients.

The knowledge and science behind the triptans has markedly increased the awareness of migraine and its unique neurobiology. One of the outcomes, however, may never have been expected in the laboratories where these compounds are made, and that is that patients and doctors will have to start "talking" again, suggesting to us that the art of migraine management is still very much alive. Advanced headache therapy will require advanced communication skills!

CHAPTER 6

THE WOMAN WITH MONTHLY HEADACHE

ELIZABETH LODER, MD

Case History

This patient is a 28-year-old woman who has experienced severe headaches since menarche at the age of 12 years. Initially, the headaches occurred several days before her menstrual period began and lasted 1 to 2 days at a time. She recalls that these headaches were generalized, throbbing, and associated with nausea and vomiting. She generally missed at least a day of school each month and recalls lying in a dark room and using ibuprofen at the recommendation of her family doctor. She had only occasional headaches at other times of the month, and those were generally less severe than the headaches associated with her menstrual period.

Over the years, her headaches have waxed and waned. There have been times when she has had no headaches for several months, and then at other times, she has seemed to have almost daily headache. For the past few months, she reports that she has had on average one or two severe headaches a month, with more frequent, milder headaches three to four times a month. She has not kept formal records but is quite certain that the severe headaches correlate with her menstrual period and ovulation. In addition to the headaches associated with her menstrual periods, she reports mood swings, fluid retention, and sleep difficulties, which she refers to as premenstrual syndrome (PMS). She does not report neurologic signs or symptoms prior to headache but says she can tell when a headache is coming because she experiences emotional lability and increased appetite.

She has been treating her headaches with over-the-counter ibuprofen, which helps "a little" but is not useful when she is vomiting. She has also been given a combination acetylsalicylic acid-caffeine-butalbital medication. It makes her drowsy and she cannot function well when she takes it. However, she says that the drowsiness is "better than having a headache" and asks to have the prescription refilled.

Her mother and grandmother had similar headaches. Her mother's headaches "went away" after menopause. She has been told that she cannot use oral contraceptives because of her headache problem. Her general and neurologic examination is normal.

Questions about This Case

- What are your diagnostic considerations?
- What treatment options are available for the patient?
- What advice would you give her about the use of oral contraceptives?
- What effect are pregnancy, breast-feeding, menopause, and estrogen replacement therapy (ERT) likely to have on her headaches?

Case Discussion

This case is a composite of issues commonly encountered in the treatment of women with headache. There is no doubt that the normal hormonal milestones of a woman's life (menarche, the monthly menstrual cycle, pregnancy, lactation, and menopause) can have a significant influence on the course of migraine. These milestones are imbued with a great deal of social significance. All of the attention paid to these occurrences makes it important to distinguish real effects from those of attribution, in which headaches which would have occurred anyway are attributed to the hormonal event near which they (presumably randomly) occurred. There is no better way to sort this out than by asking a woman to keep a careful diary of her headaches, menstrual periods, and other symptoms. Then, an accurate understanding of the true contribution of hormonal events can inform subsequent treatment.

The patient's description of her headaches meets the International Headache Society (IHS) criteria for migraine without aura. She reports a link between the headaches and her menstrual cycle, as do 60 to 70% of women who have migraine. When headache occurs in relation to the menstrual cycle, it generally begins 1 to 2 days prior to the menstrual flow itself, presumably reflecting the drop in estrogen levels and the consequent changes in central nervous system sensitivity to endogenous opioids, increases in circulating levels of prostaglandins, and many other complex events.

Most women whose migraines correlate with their menstrual periods also have similar headaches at other times of the month. As with this patient, they frequently report that the headaches occurring in relation to the menstrual period are longer, more difficult to treat, and more debilitating than those which occur at other times of the month. The headaches which occur around the time of menses in these women are termed "menstruation-associated migraine," and it is estimated that around 50% of women with migraine fall into this category. This is distinguished from true "menstrual migraine," in which migraine occurs exclusively with menstrual periods, and which affects 7 to 14% of women with migraine. In this situation, the headache by definition must occur between days −1 and +2 of the cycle.

Headaches occurring with ovulation are less common, and it is said that menstruation-associated migraine is almost exclusively migraine without aura. Patients with menstruation-associated headaches

often worry that there is something abnormal about their hormone levels or cycles, and may request "tests of my hormone levels" to rule this out. There is no evidence, though, that abnormal or aberrant hormonal levels play a role in these headaches. Rather, it is the central nervous system response to normal hormonal cycles which is the problem. For women who have inherited a vulnerability to migraine, the normal ebb and flow of hormones may be an important trigger which increases susceptibility to migraine.

To determine whether the relationship between menstrual periods and headache is real or perceived, it is helpful to ask the patient to keep a log of all headache attacks and menstrual periods for several months; the statement that headaches are, in fact, linked with menstrual periods should be supported by several months of carefully kept headache calendars. If it becomes clear that headaches are only erratically associated with menstrual periods, or if the menstrual periods are very irregular, it is unlikely that treatment aimed specifically at menstruation-associated headaches will be fruitful. In that case, standard migraine treatment should be employed.

If, however, the headache diary reveals that headaches are predictably associated with the menstrual period, and that the menstrual periods are regular, specific treatment strategies aimed at the menstruation-associated headaches can be attempted. Often a perimenstrual course of scheduled nonsteroidal anti-inflammatory drugs (NSAIDs) will be very helpful, e.g., ibuprofen, 400 mg three times a day. Although any of the NSAIDs can be used, compliance is enhanced with those which need to be taken fewer times a day. General practice is to begin the NSAID 1 to 2 days prior to the expected headache. (While the headache most often begins a day or two before the actual menstrual flow, individual headache patterns vary, and attention to the headache diaries kept previously will be useful in judging when to begin treatment.) Treatment should be continued for a total of 4 to 5 days and headache logs should be kept. These can be compared to the headache logs obtained before treatment to judge its effectiveness and whether to adjust treatment.

Studies are ongoing to determine if this kind of perimenstrual use of other drugs, such as the triptans, might be useful in menstrual migraine. One small open trial showed good results from sumatriptan, 25 mg orally taken three times a day, perimenstrually. Zolmitriptan may also prove efficacious; a clinical trial is under way to test this hypothesis.

The scheduled perimenstrual use of other agents such as ergotamine preparations can be helpful in some patients but care must be taken to ensure that these drugs are not overused for other headaches during the month, in order to avoid drug-induced rebound headaches. It should be remembered, too, that in women who are already on a daily drug for migraine prophylaxis the dose can be increased perimenstrually. Occasionally, the typical prophylactic drugs (beta-blockers, tricyclic antidepressants, etc.) are used only perimenstrually but there are no trials to support this.

Recognition that menstruation-associated migraine is probably triggered by a fall in estrogen levels has led to interest in hormonal treatments for the headaches. Perimenstrual use of estrogen, most often in the form of an estrogen patch, is helpful in some cases, presumably by blunting the fall in estrogen levels. For example, a 0.05 or 1.0 mg estrogen patch can be applied 1 to 2 days before the expected headache and continued for 4 to 5 days. This is generally well tolerated. Among the potential side effects of this treatment, however, is disruption of menstrual periods and when that occurs, the unpredictability of the periods renders continued treatment difficult.

It is also possible to place the woman on oral contraceptives continuously for up to 4 months at a time (skipping the pill-free or placebo-pill week). This approach, which is similar to that employed for women with endometriosis, minimizes the number of times a woman experiences estrogen withdrawal with its attendant priming of the migraine mechanism. As long as withdrawal bleeding occurs several times a year, the risk of endometrial build-up and uterine cancer is minimal. It is probably advisable, however, to attempt this type of treatment in conjunction with a gynecologist.

More drastic attempts at hormone manipulation are sometimes employed, such as the use of danazol, 200 mg twice a day, from days 3 to 28 of the menstrual cycle; tamoxifen, bromocriptine, and luteinizing hormone–releasing hormone (LH–RH) analogues have also been used. Because of their significant side effects, these drugs should be reserved for resistant cases. Finally, there is no solid evidence that oophorectomy produces long-lasting improvement in menstruation-associated migraine. It is major surgery with all of the attendant risks, and a woman then faces the question of estrogen replacement therapy, which can also affect migraine.

The availability of pharmacologic treatment for migraine should not distract attention from non-pharmacologic treatment methods. These are a cornerstone of treatment for any patient with significant headaches and are especially important for those whose headaches are refractory to treatment. Such precautions as obtaining adequate rest, not skipping meals, avoiding dietary triggers for migraine, and establishing a regular aerobic exercise program benefit all patients. There is solid evidence that relaxation training and biofeedback are helpful as well. Patients who know they are more likely to get headaches in certain situations, such as around the menstrual period, can practice "avoidance therapy," in which they are especially careful to avoid lifestyle triggers for migraine at a vulnerable time, whereas at other times of the month they may be able to relax proscriptions about alcohol or lack of sleep.

Whereas, in many cases, the headaches associated with menstrual periods are the major problem and the focus of attention for both patient and doctor, in other cases, headache is but one of a number of troubling symptoms occurring in conjunction with menstrual periods. The association of emotional lability, fluid retention, headache, and other symptoms with the luteal phase of the menstrual cycle has long been referred to as PMS. Since mild versions of these complaints are part of the normal physiology of the menstrual cycle, these symptoms must be severe enough to disrupt normal functioning in order to be considered abnormal. The fourth edition of the *Diagnostic and Statistical Manual of Psychiatric Disorders* refers to this as "late luteal phase dysphoric disorder." Little research has been done to characterize the headaches which are said to occur in conjunction with this syndrome, and it is far from clear that they are migrainous. In contrast to non-PMS menstruation-associated headaches, which occur on the first or second day of the flow, PMS headaches tend to occur just prior to onset of the menstrual flow.

Recent studies have suggested that various of the serotonin reuptake inhibitors, such as fluoxetine and sertraline, can be helpful with many of these premenstrual symptoms; these drugs have not been shown to be useful in the treatment of migraine. Nonetheless, there is often an overlap between menstruation-associated headaches and other symptoms, as in this case. Carefully kept symptom diaries can help distinguish reality from perception. If the two problems coexist, both may merit treatment. Progesterone has not been shown to be of value in the treatment of PMS.

The use of oral contraceptives (OCs) in patients with migraine is the subject of controversy. Although popular wisdom is that "the pill" will make migraine worse, that is not invariably so. In fact, one study of migraine patients who took OCs showed that one-third reported improvement in headache, one-third reported worsening of headache, and one-third reported no change in pre-existing headache. The perceived association may reflect the high background incidence of migraine in the age group of women who are likely to begin the oral contraceptive, and certainly in patients genetically predisposed to develop migraine, use of oral contraceptives may hasten its appearance. It seems likely that most of them would have developed migraine anyway at a later point. The apparent association also almost certainly reflects the fact that patients whose headaches worsen while on the pill are likely to return to their doctor and complain of this; those whose headaches are unchanged or improved are less likely to report back to their physician, and the consequence is that the physician, relying on his or her experience, will overestimate the likelihood that oral contraceptives worsen migraine.

A more realistic concern is that use of oral contraceptives may increase the risk of ischemic stroke in women who have migraine. Older studies which attempted to clarify the link between stroke and migraine suffered from methodologic problems. A more recent review by Backer (1997) and a carefully done study by Tzourio et al. (1995) give good reasons to believe that while migraine is a risk factor for stroke, the increased risk is quite small in women who have migraine without aura and who do not have other risk factors for stroke.

The use of oral contraceptives is, however, one of those risk factors, and it seems prudent that migraine patients who smoke, are obese, have poorly controlled hypertension, or other attributes which raise the risk of stroke, should use oral contraceptives with caution, if at all. The risk of stroke is higher in patients who have migraine with aura, for reasons that are not yet understood, and those patients should weigh the risks and benefits of OC use carefully. If a migraine patient does decide to use OCs, her headache pattern should be monitored. If her headaches worsen, if she develops neurologic prodromes with her headache that did not occur prior to OC use, or if a pre-existing aura lengthens or becomes more complicated, OCs should be discontinued. The lowest possible dose of estrogen should be used.

In deciding whether or not to prescribe OCs for a migraine patient, it should be borne in mind that unintended pregnancy can have important health consequences and that OCs are currently the most effective contraceptive method available. In addition, other contraceptive methods such as medroxy progesterone acetate suspension and levonorgestrol implants are also reputed to worsen or trigger migraine in susceptible women. For an individual patient, the benefits of OC use may outweigh the risks. Discussion of the risks and benefits of OC use, including stroke risk, is important.

Migraine affects an estimated 20% of the female population and its prevalence is greatest during the childbearing years; for this reason careful consideration must be given to the likelihood of pregnancy in patients and the best way in which to manage migraine during this time. It is fortunate that 60 to 70% of women who have migraine without aura will experience significant improvement or even cessation of migraine attacks during pregnancy. This improvement is most pronounced in the second and third trimesters of pregnancy, and seems to be most likely in women whose prepregnancy headaches were closely linked to menstrual periods. Their demonstrated tendency to develop headache in response to normal decreases in estrogen levels means that the stable estrogen levels of pregnancy will most probably remove one of their most important trigger factors. Women who have migraine with aura are less likely to note improvement, and a small but not insignificant percentage of women will have worsening of headache during pregnancy.

Many women with migraine who are considering pregnancy worry about what they will do if their headaches continue when they are pregnant, knowing that it is best to avoid medication use if possible. In clinical practice, it is the periconceptional period that can be most difficult. When a woman is attempting to become pregnant, it is especially important to try to avoid exposure to unnecessary medications. This puts many women in a difficult position; they must often decide whether or not to stop prophylactic medications that have been useful to them and suffer worsening headaches until they become pregnant. In addition, the use of acute medication for headache becomes problematic as well when they develop their usual headaches at a time when they might be pregnant but pregnancy has not been confirmed.

Some of these problems can be avoided by planning ahead. Certain broad principles apply to the pharmacologic treatment of headache in the periconceptional and pregnancy periods. Nonpharmacologic treatment of migraine, such as biofeedback training, exercise, and adequate sleep and nutrition should be emphasized. If pharmacologic prophylaxis must be continued, accumulated experience suggests the use of beta-blockers or tricyclic antidepressants, both of which belong to classes of medication which have long been used to treat other conditions during pregnancy, and which appear devoid of major teratogenic effects.

With regard to acute treatment, it is important to avoid the use of obviously problematic medications such as ergotamine compounds. All of the triptans are also contraindicated during pregnancy. A sumatriptan pregnancy registry maintained by Glaxo Wellcome has so far shown no evidence of teratogenic effects with in utero exposure to sumatriptan; however, case numbers are limited and these results, while encouraging, must be interpreted with caution. It is surprising how often barbiturate-containing medications are used to treat headaches during pregnancy. Recent evidence of potential cognitive effects from exposure to barbiturates during pregnancy suggests that these agents be avoided. Given long-term experience with acetaminophen and opi-

oid medications during pregnancy, combination compounds such as acetaminophen and oxycodone may be appropriate for use in small and carefully monitored quantities, although they are far from being ideal agents for many obvious reasons.

The sudden drop in estrogen levels occurring after delivery can trigger headache in some migraine patients, as can the resumption of normal menstrual cycles which follows weaning. Although it is not approved by the Food and Drug Administration for use by lactating women, the short half-life of sumatriptan (2 hours) has made many clinicians feel comfortable in allowing breast-feeding women to use sumatriptan, provided they pump and discard their breast milk for 6 to 8 hours after use.

Many migraine patients look forward to menopause as a time when their headaches will improve. It is commonly supposed that migraine will disappear at menopause and many patients will recount stories of women they know whose headaches did just that. However, carefully done epidemiologic studies suggest that for many women, migraine worsens in the perimenopausal period, when hormonal fluctuations can be unpredictable. With the cessation of menses and the monthly cycle, some women do experience improvement in migraine, but a sizable number of migraine sufferers note no change or even worsening in their headaches. As mentioned previously, women whose headaches before menopause correlated closely with menstrual cycles are most likely to experience improvement in migraine after menopause.

In addition, evidence is accumulating as to the benefits for many women of taking ERT after menopause. The modern practice of continuous estrogen and progesterone treatment (for women with an intact uterus) and continuous estrogen alone (for women without a uterus) is less likely than older, interrupted dosing regimens to trigger or aggravate migraine. In those women who do note worsening of migraine with ERT, a change from natural to synthetic estrogen, reduction of the estrogen dose, or use of the patch or gel instead of oral estrogen are all anecdotally reputed to be strategies worth trying.

In summary, the normal physiologic hormone fluctuations of a woman's life (menarche, the menstrual cycle, pregnancy, lactation, and menopause) often have an important effect on the frequency, severity, and timing of migraine. In some women, hormone fluctuations will be the most important and obvious etiologic agent of migraine. For most women, however, hormone fluctuations are *one element among many others* which influence the course of migraine. For this reason, it is important to take a balanced view of the role hormonal factors play in an individual woman's migraine experience. It is rarely appropriate to focus on hormonal factors in migraine to the exclusion of other factors which influence the course of the disorder.

Management Strategies

- Try to put hormonal factors in perspective among other important triggers for each patient by keeping a diary of headaches and other symptoms.
- The problem with hormonally influenced migraine is enhanced sensitivity of the central nervous system to normal physiologic events. Therefore, tests of hormone levels will not be fruitful.
- Most women whose headaches correlate with menstrual periods will have other headaches throughout the month. These should not be ignored in the rush to treat the menstruation-associated headaches.
- There is limited evidence for the efficacy of most treatment strategies for menstruation-associated migraine but perimenstrual prophylaxis with NSAIDs or other agents may be useful.
- Less conventional hormone treatments should be reserved for truly refractory patients. Oophorectomy as a treatment for menstruation-associated migraine is to be discouraged.
- Oral contraceptives and ERT can be used safely by most migraine patients. They aggravate pre-existing migraine less often than is supposed.

- Migraine in women is most common in the childbearing years and the possibility of pregnancy should be kept in mind when treating female patients.
- Careful planning and judicious use of medication can improve the management of migraine in pregnancy and puerperium.

Selected Readings

Becker WJ. Migraine and oral contraceptives. Can J Neurol Sci 1997 Feb;24(1):16–21.

MacGregor EA. Menstruation, sex hormones and migraine. In: Mathew NT, editor. Neurologic clinics: advances in headache. Philadelphia: WB Saunders; 1997. p. 125–41.

Somerville BW. The role of estradiol withdrawal in the etiology of menstrual migraine. Neurology 1972;22:355–65.

Tzourio C, Tehindrazanorivelo A, Iglesias S, et al. Case-control study of migraine and risk of ischaemic stroke in young women. BMJ 1995;310:830–3.

Welch KMA. Migraine and ovarian steroid hormones. Cephalalgia 1997 Dec;17(Suppl 20):12–6.

Editorial Comments

The management of menstruation-associated migraine can be difficult for some women. The use of NSAIDs and other nonspecific abortive agents may simply be inadequate for severe migraine. Dr. Loder overviews this important area with insightful discussion based on clinical experience and recent trial data. This case and its discussion provide another balanced view of the treatment of such patients, similar to Dr. Fettes' approach (see Chapter 8). An added feature of the excellent discussion is the commentary on all estrogen-related headache disorders in pregnancy, menopause, and with the use of oral contraceptive agents.

CHAPTER 7

THE WOMAN WITH THE NUMB HAND AND FACE

WERNER J. BECKER, MD, FRCPC

Case History

A 22-year-old woman arrived at the emergency department with numbness of the right hand and face, and difficulty expressing herself. Her symptoms had begun while at work. She had first noted tingling in her right thumb. Over about 5 minutes, the tingling and associated numbness had spread to all the fingers of the hand and up the right arm to the midforearm. The sensation then began to affect her face, with progressive involvement of the right cheek, mouth, and the right half of her tongue. Her symptoms reached their maximum anatomic involvement about 10 minutes after onset in the right thumb. She then developed some difficulty expressing herself as well, but this was short lived, lasting only 10 to 20 minutes. The numbness persisted for almost 3 hours. About 90 minutes after the numbness began, she developed a mild constant left-sided headache. This became more severe later in the evening, with moderate pain intensity and some nausea. The headache lasted 5 or 6 hours.

In the emergency department, the only positive neurologic finding was some evidence of patchy sensory loss to pinprick over the right hand and face. When seen in follow-up several days later, her examination was normal.

When questioned about her past history, she indicated that she had begun to experience episodes of numbness and tingling in the right hand 2 years previously. Since that time, she had had several of these episodes. One year ago, she had a more intense attack in which the numbness had gradually progressed to involve the right forearm. This episode had also lasted somewhat longer, perhaps a total of 30 minutes. She could not recall any significant headache with these attacks, and denied any past history of significant headache.

She had been taking oral contraceptives for 4 years, and was currently on a preparation of 30 µg of ethinyl estradiol.

Questions about This Case

- What is the most likely diagnosis, and what would be an appropriate differential diagnosis?
- If her symptoms are the result of migraine, how would you specifically classify her migraine type?
- What investigations should be done?
- Is the fact that she is taking oral contraceptives important, and if it is, why?
- What would be your advice to her with regard to the treatment and prevention of her attacks?

Case Discussion

Diagnosis

The most likely diagnosis for this patient for most of her attacks would be migraine aura without headache (category 1.2.5, using the classification of the International Headache Society [IHS]). Her most recent attack might qualify for migraine with aura (IHS 1.2), in that she did have a unilateral headache of moderate intensity with associated nausea afterwards. However, to make this diagnosis, two attacks are necessary, and she had had only one. Finally, her aura was prolonged with one symptom (numbness and tingling) lasting 3 hours, well beyond the 60-minute time limit imposed by the IHS. Therefore, if classified as migraine with aura, she would be classified as having migraine with prolonged aura (IHS 1.2.2).

At the time when she came to the emergency department, with symptoms at that point of over 2 hours' duration, one could consider whether she was developing a migrainous infarction (IHS 1.6.2). Consistent with this diagnosis, she had persistent symptoms of the kind that occurred with her usual migraine aura but to make a clinical diagnosis of migrainous infarction, the neurologic deficit must still be present to some extent 7 days later. Alternatively, the diagnosis can be made if neuroimaging demonstrates infarction in the relevant area.

The differential diagnosis would include a transient ischemic attack of the usual type secondary to an artery-to-artery embolus or an embolus of cardiac source. A third consideration would be a partial (focal) seizure, perhaps arising from a structural lesion in the left cerebral hemisphere.

For several reasons, migraine would be by far the most likely diagnosis in this patient. Her symptoms showed many features typical of the migraine aura.

- Her symptoms showed a slow progression through the anatomically involved areas, taking 10 minutes to progress from their onset in her right thumb to the time of maximal anatomic involvement of the right hand, forearm, face, and tongue.
- Her symptoms had pronounced positive components. Very considerable associated tingling was present in addition to the numbness.
- Involvement of the hand and lower face is a common form of somatosensory migraine aura. In recognition of this, auras of the type described by our patient have been called the "cheiro-oral" (hand-mouth) syndrome.

In addition, our patient had no significant cardiovascular risk factors, apart from the use of oral contraceptives (OCs), and had no signs on examination to suggest a source of embolus or a structural lesion which might cause focal seizures.

Investigation

In patients with a typical clinical presentation of migraine with aura which meets IHS diagnostic criteria, including a normal neurologic examination, laboratory and neuroimaging investigations are very likely to be fruitless and usually are not needed.

In patients with migraine aura without headache, or if the aura is atypical because it is prolonged, the situation is less clear-cut. Our patient had the typical slow march of symptoms consistent with migraine, and had a normal cardiovascular examination. Because of this, we did not do an electroencephalogram, an investigation which may be helpful if partial epilepsy is considered a significant possibility. Investigations directed at potential embolic sources, such as carotid ultrasound examinations and echocardiograms, likewise were not done. Because her focal neurologic symptoms had consistently involved the same central nervous system anatomic site, and appeared to be progressing in severity, an elective (nonurgent) brain magnetic resonance imaging (MRI) was done to exclude a focal lesion, such as an arteriovenous malformation. The MRI scan could also have shown a migrainous infarction had one occurred despite the resolution of the patient's clinical symptoms. Admittedly, the chances of an MRI scan showing a significant lesion in her case were small, and in areas of the world where medical resources are limited, it could not be justified.

Hemoglobin, white blood cell count and differential, sedimentation rate, and antinuclear antibody tests were also done, and were normal.

Management Strategies

This patient's attacks of right-sided numbness were infrequent and for the most part short lived. Like most patients with a migraine aura, she required no symptomatic treatment directed at the aura symptoms themselves.

The main management questions to be considered in her case are:

- Can the frequency of her attacks be reduced through avoidance of migraine trigger factors?
- Do her attacks place her at risk of any serious complications such as a stroke, and can this risk

be reduced? In her case, this relates most specifically to her use of oral contraceptives.

In a patient such as this, her history might reveal that the attacks tend to occur when she has missed a meal, has been exposed to bright sunlight or glare, or is under unusual stress. The patient should be made aware of migraine trigger factors so that these can be avoided if possible.

In my opinion, the main issue in her case relates to the use of OCs. Her attacks of focal neurologic symptoms began while she was on OCs, and she was experiencing progressively more severe attacks. As early as in 1975, Bickerstaff noted that some women experienced migraine attacks for the first time after starting the pill, and that others experienced a change in the pattern of their migraine headaches. For example, women who had a long history of migraine without aura, could suddenly begin to have attacks of migraine with aura after starting OCs. Admittedly, the onset of migraine is most common in young women and this is the very population that also uses OCs. The occurrence in our patient of migraine aura without headache while she was using OCs may have been purely coincidental.

Our patient was advised to stop her OCs. The main reason for doing this was because it is likely that her OCs put her at significantly increased risk of stroke, given her history of prolonged migraine aura. This area is still somewhat controversial, but evidence is accumulating from carefully done case-control studies that migraine, and in particular migraine with aura, puts patients at an increased risk of ischemic stroke. There are also many studies in the literature which indicate that OCs increase the risk of ischemic stroke. There is reason to believe that the combination of the two risk factors may result in a quite significant and unacceptable risk of stroke in some patients with migraine with aura. Although the evidence is anecdotal, this may be especially true for patients with unusual, complex, or prolonged migraine auras. Although the newer low-estrogen-dose OCs may pose less of a risk of stroke than the older contraceptives, there is at present little reason to doubt that they do contribute some risk of stroke, at least in patients with other stroke risk factors.

The whole issue of migraine, OCs, and stroke will be addressed in more detail below.

Case Summary

The patient was a 22-year-old woman who had a history of migraine aura without headache, and in addition had suffered a recent attack which was probably migraine with prolonged aura. These symptoms developed while she was taking OCs. Her symptoms were quite characteristic of migraine aura, and investigations were limited to a brain MRI and blood tests. She was given enteric-coated acetylsalicylic acid for a few weeks until investigations were completed, and was advised to stop taking her OCs. The reasons for stopping her OCs were twofold. It was likely that her focal neurologic episodes would become less frequent and/or less severe. Secondly, given her history of migraine with prolonged aura, her OCs would put her at an increased risk of ischemic stroke.

Overview of Migraine, Oral Contraceptives, and Risk of Ischemic Stroke

Migraine and Risk of Ischemic Stroke

Several case-control studies have examined the effect of migraine on the risk of ischemic stroke in women under the age of 45 years. One of the best known is that of Tzourio et al. (1995), which found a relative risk of ischemic stroke of 3.0 for patients with migraine without aura, and of 6.2 for patients with migraine with aura, compared to controls without migraine.

Similarly, Carolei et al. (1996) also found a strong association between migraine with aura and ischemic stroke. For patients with migraine with aura (their population included both men and women), they found a relative risk of ischemic stroke of 8.6 as compared to nonmigraine controls. In their study, although patients with migraine without aura had an increased risk of transient ischemic attack, they could not confirm an increased risk of stroke in this patient subgroup.

In conclusion, to date, evidence suggests a much higher risk of stroke in young adults who have migraine with aura. It must be kept in mind, however, that given the very low incidence of ischemic stroke in young adults, the risk even in patients who have migraine with aura is not very high in absolute terms. For women with migraine with aura the risk has been estimated to be approximately eight ischemic strokes per year per 100,000 women for those under the age of 35, and 22 per year per 100,000 women ages 35 to 44.

Oral Contraceptives and Risk of Ischemic Stroke

The risk of ischemic stroke posed by oral contraceptives is controversial, partly because the estrogen content of OCs has been declining gradually during the time that the various case-control studies have been carried out.

Since 1968, no fewer than 13 case-control studies have been carried out which examine the relationship between ischemic stroke and OCs. With one exception, all have shown an increased risk of stroke, with odds ratios varying from 25 and 19, in some of the older studies, to 2.1 and 3.0 in more recent studies. There is indirect evidence from a variety of sources that the risk of thromboembolism including cerebral thromboembolism is reduced as the estrogen content of OCs is reduced.

One recent study, that of Petitti et al. (1996) raises an interesting question. This was the one case-control study which did not show an increased risk of ischemic stroke from the use of OCs. While this may have been because most women in the study used low-estrogen preparations (use of OCs with more than 50 μg of estrogen was rare), other recent studies have also included large numbers of such patients. The Petitti study, however, which came from a health maintenance organization, appears to have examined a population of young women for whom the OCs were prescribed very selectively, and were probably not often given to patients with significant stroke risk factors. Only 12% of females under the age of 45 in their control population were on OCs. This contrasts many other studies, for example the study by Tzourio et al. from France in which 36% of women in the control population were current users of OCs. The Petitti study, therefore, raises the issue of whether OCs increase the risk of stroke very little in patients without risk factors, but increase it more in patients with risk factors. The Tzourio study suggests that this might be so. They found the relative risk of ischemic stroke to be 13.9 for patients who had migraine and used OCs, compared to women without migraine who did not use OCs. These results require confirmation, as they are based on a relatively small number of cases.

It must be clearly understood that the great majority of ischemic strokes which occur in patients with migraine are not due to migrainous infarction but appear due to the usual causes of stroke, including thrombosis, embolism, and arterial dissection. The same is true of patients with migraine on OCs. Why patients with migraine, and especially those with migraine with aura, should have an increased risk of stroke is not clear. What role, for example, any migraine-related vasoconstriction might play is purely speculative. The majority of strokes occurring in migraine sufferers in the various case-control studies have occurred outside of the time period of an actual migraine headache. Documented alterations in platelet activity in migraine sufferers may be significant.

With regard to OCs, changes in blood coagulation and blood coagulation factor levels have been demonstrated. Fortunately, at least for low-dose preparations containing 20 μg and 30 μg of estrogen, the changes in the levels of the various procoagulant and anticoagulant factors appear to be balanced, with stimulation of both procoagulant and fibrinolytic activity. It is of interest that changes in the levels of some coagulation factors begin within 4 days of starting OCs, and these may progressively increase over 6 months of use. Surprisingly, once OCs are stopped, the levels of the various coagulation factors may return to baseline very quickly, i.e., within 14 days. The concern is that in some women, particularly those who may have some undetected abnormality in their coagulation or fibrinolytic systems, OCs may shift the balance significantly in favour of procoagulant effects. This has already been shown in some women with genetic mutations leading to clotting abnormalities.

Recommendations

In general, when women with migraine request OCs, the risks, as much as are known, should be discussed with them. If it is decided that OCs are the best option for the patient, she should be carefully monitored for a significant change in migraine frequency, severity, and pattern. This applies particularly if patients already have migraine with aura, or if they develop migraine with aura while on OCs.

Recommendations for specific situations are as follows:

- Women with migraine without aura can probably use OCs safely, unless other major risk factors for stroke (e.g., hypertension) are present.
- Women who have migraine with aura are often advised not to use OCs. However, if OC use is important to the patient, it would seem reasonable to consider OCs in patients with typical, relatively simple auras (i.e., typical visual auras lasting less than 60 minutes), who are young (under the age of 35), and who have no significant cardiovascular risk factors. Such patients should be carefully monitored, however, and OCs should be stopped if the aura or headache pattern changes significantly. It would seem prudent not to prescribe OCs for women with more complex or prolonged migraine auras (i.e., complete hemianopsia, hemiparesis, etc.). In other words, OCs should be avoided in women with moderate to severe neurologic events in migraine.
- Oral contraceptives should be discontinued in patients with migraine without aura who develop a migraine aura for the first time on the pill, and in patients who develop transient ischemic attacks, stroke, or ischemic vascular disease elsewhere.

Selected Readings

Becker WJ. Migraine and oral contraceptives. Can J Neurol Sci 1997;24:16–21.

Bickerstaff ER. Neurological complications of oral contraceptives. Oxford(UK): Clarendon Press; 1975.

Carolei A, Marini C, de Matteis G, et al. History of migraine and risk of cerebral ischemia in young adults. Lancet 1996;347:1503–6.

Collaborative Group for the Study of Stroke in Young Women. Oral contraceptives and stroke in young women. JAMA 1975;231:718–22.

Committee of the International Headache Society. Classification and diagnostic criteria for headache disorders, cranial neuralgias and facial pain. Cephalalgia 1988;8 Suppl 7:1–96.

Lidegaard O. Decline in cerebral thromboembolism in young women after introduction of low dose oral contraceptives: an incidence study for the period 1980–93. Contraception 1995;52:85–92.

Petitti DB, Sidney S, Bernstein A, et al. Stroke in users of low dose oral contraceptives. N Engl J Med 1996;335:8–15.

Tzourio C, Tehindrazanarivelo A, Iglesis S, et al. Case-control study of migraine and risk of ischemic stroke in young women. BMJ 1995;310:830–3.

Winkler UH, Schindler AE, Endrikat J, et al. A comparative study of the effects of the hemostatic system of two monophasic gestodene oral contraceptives containing 20 µgm and 30 µgm ethinylestradiol. Contraception 1996;53:75–84.

Editorial Comments

The area of migraine and stroke and their inter-relationships with the use of oral contraceptive agents is controversial, and demands working knowledge of the issues in order to best treat and advise migraine patients. Dr. Becker presents a most interesting case and discusses and overviews these issues in a comprehensive fashion with very reasonable recommendations. This balanced approach has great utility.

Appendix 7–1
Diagnostic Criteria of
The International Headache Society for
Selected Migraine Syndromes with Aura

The following material has been taken from the classification and diagnostic criteria for headache disorders, cranial neuralgias, and facial pain of the Headache Classification Committee of the International Headache Society, published in Cephalalgia, Volume 8, Supplement 7, 1998 by Norwegian University Press.

1.2 Migraine with Aura

DESCRIPTION

Idiopathic, recurring disorder manifesting with attacks of neurologic symptoms unequivocally localizable to cerebral cortex or brain stem, usually gradually developed over 5 to 20 minutes and usually lasting less than 60 minutes. Headache, nausea, and/or photophobia usually follow neurologic aura symptoms directly or after a free interval of less than an hour. The headache usually lasts 4 to 72 hours but may be completely absent (1.2.5).

DIAGNOSTIC CRITERIA

A. At least two attacks fulfilling B

B. At least three of the following four characteristics:
1. One or more fully reversible aura symptoms indicating focal cerebral cortical and/or brain stem dysfunction
2. At least one aura symptom develops gradually over more than 4 minutes, or two or more symptoms occur in succession.
3. No aura symptom lasts more than 60 minutes. If more than one aura symptom is present, accepted duration is proportionally increased.
4. Headache follows aura with a free interval of less than 60 minutes. (It may also begin before or simultaneously with the aura).

C. At least one of the following:
1. History, physical, and neurologic examinations do not suggest another cause for the headache.
2. History and/or physical, and/or neurologic examinations do suggest such disorder but it is ruled out by appropriate investigations.
3. Such disorder is present but migraine attacks do not occur for the first time in close temporal relation to the disorder.

1.2.1. Migraine with Typical Aura

DESCRIPTION

Migraine with an aura consisting of homonymous visual disturbances, hemisensory symptoms, hemiparesis or dysphasia, or combinations thereof. Gradual development, duration under 1 hour, and complete reversibility characterize the aura which is associated with headache.

DIAGNOSTIC CRITERIA

A. Fulfils criteria for 1.2 including all four criteria under B.

B. One or more aura symptoms of the following types:
1. Homonymous visual disturbance
2. Unilateral paresthesia and/or numbness
3. Unilateral weakness
4. Aphasia or unclassifiable speech difficulty

1.2.2 Migraine with Prolonged Aura

DESCRIPTION

Migraine with one or more aura symptoms lasting more than 60 minutes and less than a week. Neuroimaging is normal.

DIAGNOSTIC CRITERIA

A. Fulfils criteria for 1.2 but at least one symptom lasts more than 60 minutes and ≤ 7 days. If neuroimaging reveals relevant ischemic lesion, then it is classified as code 1.6.2 migrainous infarction regardless of symptom duration.

1.2.5 Migraine Aura without Headache

DESCRIPTION

Migrainous aura unaccompanied by headache

DIAGNOSTIC CRITERIA

A. Fulfils criteria for 1.2

B. No headache

COMMENT

It is common for migraine with aura that headache occasionally is absent. As patients get older, headache may disappear completely even if auras continue. It is less common to have always suffered exclusively from migraine aura without headache. When the onset occurs after the age of 40 years, and for other reasons, the distinction between this entity and thromboembolic transient ischemic attacks may be difficult and require extensive investigation. Acute onset aura without headache is not sufficiently validated.

CHAPTER 8

TWO WOMEN WITH MENOPAUSAL-RELATED HEADACHE

IVY M. FETTES, MD, PhD, FRCPC

Case 1 History: The Woman with Perimenopausal Headache

This 50-year-old woman has had migraine since menarche at the age of 13. Her headaches are characterized by a throbbing, unilateral pain and are associated with nausea, vomiting, photophobia, and phonophobia. They come monthly with the onset (day 1) of her menses. Occasionally, they occur mid-cycle with ovulation. The headaches which occur regularly with her menses are also accompanied by menstrual cramps and diarrhea.

She has had three pregnancies and was headache-free in the first two. However, during her third pregnancy, she had severe migraine attacks during the first trimester.

Her menses were regular until 1 year ago when the duration between menses increased to 3 months. She also has begun to suffer from hot flushes which disturb her sleep at night and embarass her at work during the day. Her headaches have increased in frequency from every 4 weeks to every 3 to 4 days. She uses sumatriptan and acetaminophen for pain control. She is frustrated with the exacerbation of her migraine and the hot flushes, and experiences difficulties in concentrating.

Our patient has never smoked and only occasionally drinks alcohol. Her maternal grandmother, mother, sister, and daughter have also suffered from migraines. Her mother has recently been diagnosed with osteoporosis after suffering a fracture with minimal trauma. Her father has known coronary artery disease and has had coronary artery bypass grafting and is on a cholesterol-lowering drug.

She experienced a hot flush during the interview. Subsequent physical examination revealed her to be 5'4" tall and 127 lb. in weight. Her blood pressure was 130/80 and her pulse was 80 beats per minute and regular. The remainder of the physical examination, including the neurologic examination, was normal.

Questions about Case 1

- What are your diagnostic considerations in this case?
- Why do you think her headaches have become worse?
- What is the association between menstruation and migraine?
- What usually happens to migraine during pregnancy?
- What course does migraine take as women approach menopause?
- Is there any other information you would like to know about this case?
- What benefits would hormone replacement have for this patient?
- How would you manage this patient's headaches?
- What long-term management strategies would you suggest?

Case 1 Discussion

Our patient has described a history of migraine (episodic unilateral, throbbing pain associated with nausea, vomiting, photophobia, and phonophobia) which has been related to her menstrual cycle since menarche. She suffers from migraine without aura. Since the migrainous attacks occurred exclusively with her menses and occasionally at ovulation, we would consider this "menstrual migraine."

Menstrual migraine occurs during or after the fall of estradiol levels. Estradiol levels peak prior to ovulation. They then fall off dramatically and there is a secondary peak in the luteal phase. Progesterone peaks in the midluteal phase. Both estrogen and progesterone decrease to low levels just prior to menstruation and remain low during menstruation. Since estradiol levels fall after ovulation and before menstruation, this could account for headaches at these times. As estrogen and progesterone levels decrease, the concentration of prostaglandins increases and reaches maximal concentrations at the time of menstruation. Our patient's symptoms of dysmenorrhea and diarrhea were most likely prostaglandin ($PGF_{2\alpha}$) related.

Migraine that starts at menarche often shows a menstrual periodicity and usually (60 to 70% of the time) improves with pregnancy, as it did in 2 of 3 of our patient's pregnancies. Migraine is thought to improve with pregnancy at least partly because of the noncyclic high levels of estrogen. If migraine occurs or worsens during pregnancy, it is usually during the first trimester, as was the situation with our patient. There was some improvement in the second and third trimesters, presumably because the estrogen environment stabilized. Following delivery, the migraine usually returns on the third to sixth day postpartum, after a marked fall in the estrogen level.

Our patient is experiencing a perimenopausal exacerbation of migraine. In early menopause, there are tremendous fluctuations in estrogen levels. Menopause (defined as the last menstrual period) is not a sudden event. Just prior to menopause, there is an increase in the rate of atresia of ovarian follicles. The follicles disappear and become fewer in number, the menstrual cycle becomes irregular, and the frequency of ovulatory cycles decreases. The usual orderly pattern of estrogen and progesterone secretion is lost. Transient elevations of estradiol are not usually associated with ovulation. However, it would be important to ask our patient about con-

traception and to rule out the possibility of pregnancy if she has not had a recent menstrual period.

The decline in estradiol is relatively steep in the first 12 months after the last menses. Over the following years, which may be one-third of a woman's life, estrogen levels remain low and decline only slightly with time. Levels of follicle-stimulating hormone (FSH) increase just prior to menopause and remain elevated postmenopause.

As estrogen levels are both fluctuating and falling, there may be an increase in the frequency and severity of migraine in women who experience estrogen withdrawal as a migraine trigger. Continuous hormone replacement therapy with estrogen and progesterone may be useful in stabilizing the hormonal milieu and in relieving migraine in the majority (65 to 75%) of such patients. [*Editors' note: It may worsen the situation, especially if given in a cyclical manner.*]

The average age of menopause in North America is 51. Menopause is a form of adult-onset hypogonadism and is associated with many changes. Hot flushes occur in 85% of women undergoing natural or surgical menopause and may continue for 3 to 5 years in 45% of women. Hot flushes which occur at night cause sleep disturbance and possibly insomnia. The flushes usually spread upward from the upper trunk to the shoulders, neck, and face. They may be associated with palpitations, dizziness, and headache. There is an increase in skin temperature and a decrease in core temperature during a hot flush. This vasomotor instability is thought to be due to the effects of estrogen withdrawal on catecholamines and prostaglandins in the central nervous system. Hot flushes can be relieved within 1 month of initiation of estrogen replacement in the majority of women. Other agents which may be used for the reduction of hot flushes include clonidine, NSAIDs, vitamin E, and methyldopa. High doses of medroxyprogesterone acetate can reduce hot flushes but may trigger migraine in the migraineur, especially if given cyclically.

When hot flushes interrupt sleep and cause sleep deprivation, there may be irritability, anxiety, nervousness, depression, fatigue, memory loss, and inability to concentrate. Estrogen replacement may help to restore psychological homeostasis in addition to relieving the hot flushes. Postmenopausal estrogen users may also have improved concentration and memory skills due to an estrogen-mediated improvement in cerebral blood flow. Estrogen deficiency causes urogenital atrophy and may be associated with atrophic cystitis or urethritis, urinary incontinence,and dyspareunia. The patient should be questioned about these symptoms as well as any change in libido.

Our patient has two important risk factors for osteoporosis: estrogen deficiency and a family history of osteoporosis. It is important to assess other risk factors, including physical inactivity and low calcium intake. The average intake of calcium in North American women is about 600 mg per day and 1200 to1500 mg per day is recommended for postmenopausal women. To facilitate the absorption of calcium, 400 IU of vitamin D per day are recommended. Dietary sources provide the optimal forms of calcium and vitamin D. There is also a wide variety of calcium and vitamin supplements available. Regular exercise is encouraged. Walking for 20 or 30 minutes daily or every second day is a popular choice for exercise. An objective assessment of bone density (e.g., by DEXA) is appropriate for our patient and may help her make a choice about hormone replacement therapy. Estrogen replacement is useful in both the prevention and treatment of osteoporosis. Even with established osteoporosis, hormone replacement therapy improves bone density and reduces the risk of osteoporotic fracture in the order of 50 to 60% over 5 years of use.

The likelihood of cardiovascular disease increases dramatically after menopause and is the leading cause of death in women in North America. Our patient has a family history of coronary artery disease. Her fatheris being treated for hypercholesterolemia and it is reasonable to do a lipid profile of our patient. After menopause, there is an increase in low-density lipoprotein (LDL) cholesterol and a decrease in high-density lipoprotein (HDL) cholesterol. Estrogen replacement has multiple cardioprotective effects in addition to reducing LDL cholesterol and increasing HDL cholesterol. Estrogen reduces the oxidation of LDL cholesterol and reduces atherosclerotic plaque formation. Estrogen preserves endothelial structure and function. Estrogen decreases vessel stiffness and acts as an important vasodilator, both acutely and chronically. Acutely, estrogen is thought to cause vasodilation by reducing the inactivation of nitric oxide. Chronically, estrogen can induce the synthesis of nitric oxide, increase levels of vasodilator prostaglandins, and decrease vasoconstriction by endothelin and other factors. Estrogen promotes fibrinolysis by decreasing the postmenopausal and age-related increase in fibrinogen and plasminogen activator inhibitor. Decreases in protein S, antithrombin III, and factor VII have also been reported with estrogen replacement, and may contribute to the prevention of thrombosis. Although both oral and transdermal estrogen replacement have beneficial vascular effects, oral estrogens are more effective in decreasing LDL cholesterol and increasing HDL cholesterol.

Epidemiologic studies have demonstrated that estrogen replacement reduces the incidence and mortality of cardiovascular disease by 50%. Short-term trials have not demonstrated a diminution of this benefit by the addition of progesterone. We are awaiting long-term trials in this regard. At the present time, continuous oral estrogen and progesterone appear to offer the most favorable cardiovascular profile. For severe lipid disorders, estrogen can be used in combination with other lipid-altering drugs such as the HMG-CoA reductase inhibitors (the statins). This may be a consideration for our patient if she has a marked elevation of LDL cholesterol, perhaps partly due to a genetic predisposition.

Prior to the initiation of hormone replacement therapy, a baseline mammogram should be done. The traditional contraindications to estrogen replacement include estrogen-dependent malignancies of the breast or endometrium, acute liver disease or acute vascular thrombosis, unexplained abnormal uterine bleeding, and the possibility of pregnancy.

Response to hormone replacement can be assessed at 6 and 12 weeks. During this time the patient may document hot flushes, sleep patterns, and any vaginal bleeding in her headache diary.

Continuous estrogen and progesterone replacement will cause endometrial atrophy and amenorrhea within 12 months in the majority of women. Most commonly, there is irregular bleeding within the first 6 months of therapy. Pelvic ultrasound examination and/or an endometrial biopsy may be indicated if the bleeding pattern is inappropriate, especially after 12 to 15 months, when amenorrhea would be expected. Breast tenderness may occur with estrogen replacement but tends to resolve with time. Restriction of caffeine may help to reduce the tenderness. It is important to remember that estrogen replacement provides only physiologic levels of estrogen and, thus, does not suppress ovulation. Contraception may be gainfully employed in the first year after the onset of menopause.

Management Strategies

Establish the correct diagnoses:

- Exacerbation of migraine (increase in frequency and severity)
- Perimenopausal (hot flushes, irregular menses, consider beta human chorionic gonadotropin [βhCG], check for elevated follicle-stimulating hormone [FSH])
- ? Osteopenia (positive family history, estrogen deficiency, inactivity, and low calcium intake; consider measuring bone density)
- ? Hypercholesterolemia (father has elevated cholesterol and coronary artery disease)

You may request the assistance of one or more specialists to help with the diagnoses and to cooperate with the management plans.

If there are no contraindications, continuous hormone replacement therapy (HRT) is a very reasonable option for this patient. A negative mammogram should be documented prior to the onset of HRT. If she has hypercholesterolemia, oral estrogen is preferred. Conjugated equine estrogen 0.3 mg every 12 hours, or an equivalent such as estropipate, one half tablet of 0.625 mg every 12 hours, or micronized estradiol, 0.5 mg every 12 hours, may be used. If her cholesterol status is normal, transdermal estrogen, 0.05 mg, can be used on a continuous basis. The progesterone replacement is given at bedtime as medroxyprogesterone acetate, 2.5 mg daily, or micronized progesterone, 100 mg every evening as a starting dosage.

Any acute migrainous attacks may be treated in the same way as a "nonhormonal" migraine. Acetylsalicylic acid (ASA) and nonsteroidal anti-inflammatory drugs (NSAIDs) are recommended for mild attacks. The NSAIDs (e.g., naproxen sodium or ibuprofen) may also be used for moderate attacks. Combinations of ASA or acetaminophen with codeine and caffeine may also be helpful. Our patient previously found sumatriptan to be effective. This medication could be used, as could dihydroergotamine (DHE), for either moderate or severe migraine attacks. Sumatriptan should not be given within 24 hours of administration of DHE or ergotamine. Sumatriptan is faster acting than DHE but DHE lasts longer (leads to a lower rate of recurrent headache). Dihydroergotamine, which may be given subcutaneously (SQ), intramuscularly (IM), intravenously (IV), or intranasally, is more likely to cause nausea than sumatriptan but sumatriptan, which may be given orally, nasally, or subcutaneously, may be more likely to cause chest pain. Sumatriptan is given as 50 to 100 mg by mouth and may be repeated twice within 24 hours. If the subcutaneous route is employed, 6 mg are given and the sumatriptan may be repeated only once in 24 hours. Alternatively, zolmitriptan may be given as 2.5 or 5 mg by mouth, followed by a repeat dose in 2 hours if necessary, or naratriptan, 1 or 2.5 mg by mouth, followed by a repeat dose in 4 hours if required. Dihydroergotamine, 0.5 to 1.0 mg SQ, IM, or IV, can be given initially and may be repeated at 1 hour with a recommended maximum of 3 doses within 24 hours.

Long-term management will involve headache surveillance in addition to regular breast examinations and Pap smears. For our patient, bone density and cardiovascular status must also be followed. If her migraines are not adequately controlled with HRT, other prophylactic agents can be considered. These include beta-blockers, calcium channel blockers, tricyclic analgesics, antiepileptics, serotonin receptor antagonists, and NSAIDs. However, the majority of postmenopausal women respond well to HRT and a healthy lifestyle without needing additional prophylactic medication.

Case 1 Summary

Our patient is suffering from a perimenopausal exacerbation of migraine. She has a history of menstrual migraine with freedom from migraine in 2 of 3 pregnancies. Fluctuations in estrogen and estrogen withdrawal are probably the triggers for the increase in the frequency of her migraines, in addition to causing the hot flushes.

The usual prophylactic medications are unlikely to be effective given her fluctuating estrogen status. She risks using larger amounts of analgesics and acute abortive measures with the increase in frequency and severity of her headaches.

Continuous HRT is an important consideration for her. The restoration and stabilization of estrogen levels within the physiologic range will eliminate the hot flushes and is likely to diminish the migraine significantly. The family history of osteoporosis and heart disease provide additional reasons for the consideration of HRT. Further discussion of the pros and cons of HRT is included with the next case.

Management of this patient is likely to involve the cooperation of physicians with different areas of expertise, to provide the best possible comprehensive care.

Case 2 History: The Woman with Postmenopausal Headache

This 49-year-old woman had her first migraine at the age of 20 years. The headaches are characterized by a throbbing unilateral pain, nausea, photophobia, and phonophobia. Her menses were regular every 28 days until the age of 48 when she became amenorrheal and was prescribed cyclic HRT. Prior to menopause, her migraines occurred every 3 to 4 months, although she did experience an increase in the frequency of migraines when she was transiently on an oral contraceptive.

The hormone replacement which was initiated consisted of conjugated equine estrogens, 0.9 mg per day on days 1 to 25, and medroxyprogesterone acetate, 10 mg per day on days 16 to 25. The medroxyprogesterone acetate was decreased to 5 mg because of the headaches which would develop within a day or two of the patient starting the medroxyprogesterone acetate. In addition, she had a severe migraine in the week off her hormone replacement, during the time of the withdrawal bleed (menses).

She is physically active and generally well. She does not smoke and has a glass of wine on occasion. She is well informed about the benefits of estrogen replacement but is unhappy about the exacerbation of her migraine and asked questions about other possible risks of hormone replacement, including breast cancer, blood clots, and weight gain.

Her physical examination was completely normal.

Questions about Case 2

- What are your diagnostic considerations in this case?
- What is the association between oral contraceptives and migraine?
- Are the risks of venous thromboembolism different when oral contraceptives are used compared with hormone replacement therapy?
- Why is progesterone added to estrogen replacement in postmenopausal women with a uterus?
- Is there an increase in the risk of breast cancer in women on HRT?
- Do postmenopausal women on HRT gain more weight than those who are not on HRT?
- Is there any other information you would like to know about this case?
- Why do you think her headaches have become worse?
- What is the natural history of migraine after menopause?
- How would you manage this patient's headaches?
- What long-term management strategies would you suggest?

Case 2 Discussion

The criteria for diagnosing migraine without aura include at least five attacks lasting 4 to 72 hours with two of the following characteristics: (1) unilateral, (2) pulsating, (3) moderate or severe intensity, (4) aggravated by routine physical activity, and at least one of the following symptoms: (1) nausea or vomiting, (2) photophobia and phonophobia. There should be no evidence from the history and physical examination to suggest any other cause of headache. A family history of migraine also makes the physician feel more confident about the diagnosis.

Our patient fulfils the criteria with her episodic recurrent headaches with unilateral throbbing head pain associated with nausea, photophobia, and phonophobia. Her mother also suffered from migraine.

As a younger woman, our patient experienced an accentuation of migraine shortly after starting an oral contraceptive. In the majority of women there is no change in the pattern of migraine while on an oral contraceptive. Some women (at least 10%) experience an improvement or alleviation of migraine while on the birth control pill. Sometimes there is relief while on the pill but attacks occur during the "placebo" portion or during the week off the pill, suggesting a withdrawal phenomenon. In about 20% (reports vary from 18 to 50%) of migraineurs, there is an increase in the incidence or severity of attacks while on the pill. If the migraines increase in frequency by three to four times as they did in our patient, the pill is usually discontinued. If a woman who has a history of migraine without aura suddenly develops migraine with aura after starting an oral contraceptive, the pill is typically stopped because of a possible increased risk of stroke.

There continues to be controversy about the risk of stroke in migraineurs who take oral contraceptives. Migraine itself, especially migraine with aura in young women, may be a risk for stroke. The vasoconstriction associated with aura (if it exists) may result in cerebral perfusion defects or cerebral infarction. This may be aggravated by dehydration from severe vomiting and by platelet activation. The risk of ischemic stroke while on an oral contraceptive has decreased as the dose of estrogen in oral contraceptives has decreased from 150 µg to between 20 and 35 µg. The incidence of cerebral infarction is low in young women but may be increased by the use of oral contraceptives by about 3.5 times. Additional risk factors, such as migraine with aura or smoking, will further increase the risk. The relative risk of ischemic stroke is about 10 times greater in the migraineurs who smoke than in nonmigraineurs who do not smoke. **Oral contraceptives are not advised for women with prolonged or complex migraine auras. Oral contraceptives should be discontinued if a woman develops an aura for the first time while on the pill, or if there is development of transient ischemic attacks or stroke. Smoking is not advised, particularly for migraineurs.**

An increased risk of venous thromboembolism has been associated with the concurrent use of combination oral contraceptives. The effect is primarily related to the dose of the synthetic estrogen (usually ethinyl estradiol) used in the pill and is thought to be related to changes in coagulation factors. The increase in the risk of thrombosis is about threefold for current users. Other risk factors such as immobilization, trauma, or genetic resistance to activated protein C (factor V Leiden mutation) would further increase the risk of venous thrombosis.

In oral contraceptives, pharmacologic doses of synthetic steroidal estrogens are used to inhibit ovulation. For menopause, we use low doses of naturally occurring estrogens for physiologic replacement. One milligram of micronized estradiol is equivalent to 5 µg of ethinyl estradiol. Most oral contraceptives contain 30 to 35 µg of ethinyl estradiol. The estrogenic enhancement of coagulation factors is dose related. Hormone replacement therapy is not generally believed to increase the risk of venous thromboembolism. The reported relative risks have varied from 0.7 to 3.6. The risk increases with increasing doses of estrogen and the risk may be higher in the first year of use. However, the absolute risk of venous thromboembolism (VTE) is low in women aged 45 to 64 years. If there is a small increase in the risk of VTE, this must be weighed against the benefits of the relief of menopausal symptoms and the reductions in the risk of coronary heart disease and osteoporosis.

The estrogen preparations currently available for HRT require the addition of progesterone to prevent endometrial hyperplasia and endometrial cancer. Unopposed estrogen, that is estrogen in the absence of progestin, stimulates endometrial cell division and increases the risk of endometrial cancer by 5 to 7 times. Obesity also increases the risk. The risk of endometrial cancer is decreased by an earlier age at menopause, increasing parity, oral contraceptive use, and the addition of a progestin to HRT. The incidence of endometrial cancer can be reduced even below the level observed in the control population with the addition of a progestin.

While progestins are not recommended after a hysterectomy, their use is advised if the uterus is intact. Either natural micronized progesterone or synthetic progestins such as medroxyprogesterone acetate, norethindrone, or norethindrone acetate may be employed. The progestin may be given cyclically (e.g., 12 to 14 days per month) or continuously (daily). Cyclic use of progesterone every 3 to 4 months is occasionally used for women who have side effects with the other approaches. The recommended daily doses for starting cyclical therapy are as follows: medroxyprogesterone acetate 5 mg; norethindrone 0.35 mg; natural micronized progesterone 200 mg. Higher doses, e.g., medroxyprogesterone acetate 10 mg, may be associated with more side effects such as PMS-like symptoms, headache, breast tenderness, bloating, and fluid retention in some women. The advantage of cyclic therapy, for those who can tolerate it, is the predictable monthly withdrawal bleeding which helps to eliminate concerns about endometrial dysplasia.

An increasingly popular approach to HRT, and ideal for the migraineur, is continuous combined estrogen and progestin. This results in stable hormone levels with an atrophic endometrium and amenorrhea. There may be irregular bleeding, especially in younger women, until the atrophic state is reached. Monitoring is required and an endometrial biopsy may be indicated for persistent or inappropriate bleeding.

For the postmenopausal woman, the most stable estrogen environment can be achieved with transdermal estrogen or a twice-daily administration of an oral estrogen.

Maximum serum levels of estradiol and estrone are reached within 4 to 6 hours after oral ingestion. Micronized estradiol has a shorter half-life than does conjugated equine estrogen. The daily dose of progestin, e.g., medroxyprogesterone 2.5 mg or micronized progesterone 100 mg, is given with the evening or bedtime dose of oral estrogen.

Cyclic therapy is not recommended for the migraineur who is susceptible to fluctuations in estrogen and progesterone. Within 48 hours of the last oral dose of estrogen, plasma levels may fall below the physiologic range and trigger a migraine.

Plasma estradiol levels in the low normal range can usually be achieved with 0.625 mg of conjugated equine estrogen daily. Our patient is currently on 0.9 mg daily and this could be reduced to the usual replacement of 0.625 mg daily. Splitting the dose (e.g., 0.3 mg every 12 hours) of estrogen would provide an even more stable environment. The medroxyprogesterone acetate could be decreased to 2.5 mg daily. The patient is likely to stop cycling within a few months and the migraines are likely to decrease in frequency and severity.

Breast cancer is the greatest fear associated with the use of HRT. Unlike the protective effects on the endometrium, progestins do not protect against breast cancer. It should be kept in mind that a 50-year-old woman has a 3% lifetime probability of death due to breast cancer, compared with a 31% chance of cardiovascular death. She may have already outlived the increased risk of breast cancer associated with a positive family history. Cardiovascular disease increases dramatically in the 10 to 15 years after menopause and the mortality from cardiovascular disease is 10 times greater than that from breast cancer.

The current consensus is that HRT at the usual recommended dosages, with conjugated equine estrogen of 0.625 mg per day (or equivalent), does not increase the risk of breast cancer. The risk may be increased with higher doses and with longer duration of use (>5 to 10 years). The association with increased doses is not clear, probably because doubling the dose of conjugated equine estrogen (CEE) does not double the level of unbound estradiol. The dose-response effect does not appear to be linear, at least for CEE. The most convincing association is with duration of use, with a 5 to 15% increase in risk for each 5 years of treatment. For a 50-year-old woman, a risk increase of 10% would raise the 10-year risk from 2.4% to 2.55%. The impact seems small compared to the benefits in the prevention and reduction of cardiovascular disease and osteoporosis. Screening, clinical breast examination, and mammography should be done prior to the initiation of HRT and continued thereafter on an annual basis. A healthy lifestyle with regular exercise and prevention of obesity is also recommended.

In women with known breast cancer who undergo menopause with an exacerbation of migraine, an estrogen antagonist/agonist such as tamoxifen may help decrease the frequency and severity of the migraine. Ten to 30 mg of tamoxifen are given daily. Surveillance for endometrial dysplasia must continue while the patient is on tamoxifen. Although endometrial cancer usually presents with vaginal bleeding, the majority (perhaps 80%) of such patients will not have cancer on further evaluation. With increasing age, the association of inappropriate bleeding and endometrial malignancy becomes stronger.

The incidence of obesity increases with age. Results from both clinical trials and epidemiologic studies indicate that HRT helps to reduce this age-related increase. Estrogen, with or without the addition of a progestin, appears to counteract the increase in waist and hip girth which occurs in the decade following menopause. Cigarette smoking may prevent this reduction, possibly by increasing the metabolism of estradiol and by increasing insulin resistance. After menopause, women tend to gain weight and add centimeters to their waist and hips. With estrogen replacement there is less weight gain and smaller increments in the waist and hip measurements.

With regard to further information about our patient, it would be important to know about her family history. She has a family history of migraine (mother and daughter), but not of premature heart disease, osteoporosis, breast cancer, or venous thromboembolism. She has two children and is not obese.

The headaches have probably become worse because of the cyclic withdrawal of estrogen and the dose of medroxyprogesterone. Often anything more than 5 mg of medroxyprogesterone will induce a headache in a susceptible migraineur. Using continuous low doses of estrogen and progesterone usually eliminates this problem and will provide protection against heart disease and osteoporosis.

The natural history of migraine is that it lessens with age. There may be a perimenopausal exacerbation as estrogen levels fall prior to menopause. After menopause, about 65% of women have a marked lessening or disappearance of migraine. Tension headaches tend not to improve with menopause.

Aging women who suffer from migraine with aura may notice that either the headache disappears or the aura disappears. An aura without the headache may be confused with a transient ischemic attack.

Only about 2% of migraines occur for the first time after the age of 50. In this situation, radiologic imaging (computed tomography or magnetic resonance imaging) may be prudent in helping the physician make the correct diagnosis. The other causes of headache to consider in older people include giant cell arteritis, intracranial mass lesions, ischemic cerebrovascular disease, chronic obstructive lung disease with hypercapnia sleep apnea, and drugs.

Management Strategies

Our patient has a long history of migraine, and other causes of headache are unlikely in her case. After discussing the reasons for the exacerbation of her migraine and the benefits and risks of HRT, various alternatives for continuous HRT could be offered. Estrogen may be given in the form of a patch or as oral estrogen. Since she is already on oral estrogen, the physician may choose to stay with this preparation. The progesterone may be given as medroxyprogesterone or micronized progesterone. Since she is on medroxyprogesterone, the physician can simply decrease the dose. If she continues to have headaches, the physician might try switching to micronized progesterone. Response to therapy can be assessed at 6 and 12 weeks and thereafter as required.

Surveillance of the breasts and endometrium is typically done by the primary care physician but may be done by her gynecologist. The patient should be aware of the importance of the monitoring and ensure that she is being assessed on at least an annual basis. Inappropriate vaginal bleeding, particularly after 1 year of continuous HRT, should be investigated with a pelvic ultrasound examination and/or an endometrial biopsy.

If our patient's migraines are not adequately controlled with continous HRT, the headaches and medications should be re-evaluated. Other causes of headache, including analgesic rebound can be considered. Prophylactic medications can be tried once the hormonal status has stabilized. A calcium channel blocker (e.g., verapamil 240 to 320 mg per day or flunarizine 5 to 10 mg per day) or beta-blocker (e.g., atenolol 50 to150 mg per day or nadolol 20 to 160 mg per day) may be useful. [*Editors' note: Flunarizine is not currently available in the United*

States.] Other prophylactics include the tricyclic analgesics, antiepileptics, NSAIDs, and serotonin receptor antagonists. The choice of treatment for an acute attack depends on the severity of the headache. The treatment options are as discussed in Case 1. If migraines change from mild or moderate to severe, the patient should be reviewed by a neurologist or headache specialist.

Case 2 Summary

Our patient is experiencing an exacerbation of migraine since being placed on cyclic HRT. She had a similar exacerbation several years ago when placed on an oral contraceptive. In both situations the headaches occurred in the week off the estrogen and progestin. This suggests an estrogen withdrawal phenomenon. As the estrogen falls to a certain threshold, it appears to trigger a migraine in susceptible individuals.

Her experience with cyclic HRT has led her to re-evaluate the benefits and risks of HRT. She is aware of the natural history of migraine as it affected her mother who became free of migraines after menopause. After discussion about her concerns, including cancer and weight gain, and putting them in perspective with the benefits, she decided to try continuous low-dose HRT. If she does not respond, she will be re-evaluated and other options for prophylaxis will be considered.

Selected Readings

Andrews WC. Menopause and hormonal replacement. Obstet Gynecol 1996;87:S1–53.

Colditz GA, Egan KM, Stampfer MJ. Hormone replacement therapy and risk of breast cancer: results from epidemiologic studies. Am J Obstet Gynecol 1993;168:1473–80.

Cowan BD, Seifer DB, editors. Clinical reproductive medicine. Philadelphia: Lippincott-Raven Publishers; 1997.

Edmeads J. Headaches in older people. Postgrad Med 1997; 101:91–100.

Fettes I. Menstrual migraine. Postgrad Med 1997;101:67–77.

Gambrell RD Jr. Prevention of endometrial cancer with progesterones. Maturitas 1986;8:159–68.

Lobo RA. Treatment of the postmenopausal woman. New York: Raven Press; 1994.Uknis A, Silberstein SD. Review article: migraine and pregnancy. Headache 1991;31:372–4.

O'Dea JPK, Davis EH. Tamoxifen in the treatment of menstrual migraine. Neurology 1990;40:1470–1.

Pryse-Philipps WEM, et al. Guidelines for the diagnosis and management of migraine in clinical practice. Can Med Assoc J 1997;156:1273–87.

Tzourio C, Tehindrazanarivelo A, Iglesis S, et al. Case-control study of migraine and risk of ischaemic stroke in young women. BMJ 1995;310:830–3.

Uknis A, Silberstein SD. Review article: migraine and pregnancy. Headache 1991;31:372–4.

World Health Organization Collaborative Study of Cardiovascular Disease and Steroid Hormone Contraception. Venous thromboembolic disease and combined oral contraceptives: results of an international multicentre case-control study. Lancet 1995;346:1575–82.

Editorial Comments

Perimenopausal and postmenopausal migraine headache management can be very difficult for the patient and therapist. A full understanding of the endocrinology of menopause and its relationships to migraine remains essential to the management of patients with menopausal migraine, particularly in refractory and difficult cases. Dr. Fettes guides us through the advanced management of two very representative cases with excellent practical suggestions based on the best knowledge available.

CHAPTER 9

THE PATIENT WITH HEADACHE, ARTHRITIS, AND HYPERTENSION

GLEN D. SOLOMON, MD, FACP

Case History

A 52-year-old woman was referred to the headache center for evaluation of her headaches. She noted the onset of headache at the age of 13 years. The headaches occurred once per month, usually with menses. These headaches were described as a unilateral, pounding headache, associated with nausea, vomiting, and phonophotophobia. They would last for a day and were relieved by sleep.

In her early thirties, her headaches started to become more frequent. At that time, she began having one headache every week. She was started on propranolol and her headache frequency decreased to one per month. After 6 months the propranolol was discontinued.

In her late thirties she noted symmetrical joint pain, erythema, and warmth in her fingers, wrists, and knees. She was diagnosed as having rheumatoid arthritis and was treated with nonsteroidal anti-inflammatory drugs (NSAIDs). Her condition continued to worsen, and she was eventually placed on hydroxychloroquine. Ten years later, due to continued progression of her arthritis, she was also given methotrexate. As a complication of her rheumatoid arthritis, she developed fibromyalgia, with pain particularly in the muscles of her neck and upper back. She also developed Raynaud's phenomenon.

At the age of 41 years, she was noted to have hypertension. The NSAIDs were discontinued, and she was treated with a thiazide diuretic. Her blood pressure was well controlled and she had no adverse effects with this treatment.

She did not smoke, rarely drank alcohol, and took no over-the-counter medications. She was married with two grown children, and was employed as an administrative assistant.

At the time of her headache evaluation, she was on hydroxychloroquine, methotrexate, and amitriptyline for her arthritis and associated fibromyalgia, and hydrochlorothiazide for her hypertension. For her migraines, which were again occurring once per week, she took naproxen sodium, 550 mg at onset, with a second dose 6 to 8 hours later if needed.

Her general examination was remarkable for a blood pressure of 138/90 and rheumatoid changes in her hands. She had multiple tender points on examination and increased muscle tension in her neck. Her neurologic examination was unremarkable.

Questions about This Case

- What are the appropriate strategies for the management of hypertension in the patient with migraine?
- How does the presence of Raynaud's phenomenon influence therapy choices?
- Could the patient's medications be contributing to her headaches?
- How is fibromyalgia related to headaches?
- How do you manage migraine in the presence of comorbid medical illnesses?

Case Discussion

There are several major issues that the physician must consider in evaluating and treating the headache patient with comorbid medical disorders. These include: (1) Do the headaches represent a primary headache disorder (i.e., migraine, tension-type, or cluster) or are they secondary to the patient's other medical problems? (2) Is the therapy for the comorbid condition triggering or exacerbating the headache problem? (3) Is the headache treatment likely to worsen the comorbid condition, or does the comorbid condition contraindicate certain therapies? (4) Does the presence of comorbid disease offer the opportunity to use a single drug to treat both the headache disorder and the comorbid condition?

Certain medical illnesses are more common in the headache patient. Featherstone evaluated the prevalence of concomitant medical diseases in chronic headache sufferers by reviewing 1414 life insurance applications and obtaining 200 headache cases with matched controls without chronic headaches. The average age for study patients was 45 years. The groups were equally divided by gender. Headaches were not classified by diagnosis (i.e., migraine, cluster, etc.). Six conditions were found to occur more often in the chronic headache group: hypertension, dizziness (or vertigo), gastroesophageal reflux, depression or anxiety, peptic ulcers, and irritable bowel syndrome. Three conditions were significantly more common in the nonheadache population: nephrolithiasis, alcohol abuse in men, and abdominal pain in women. Several conditions had the same prevalence in both the headache and nonheadache groups: ischemic heart disease, mitral valve prolapse, cardiovascular disease, central nervous system ischemia, cigarette smoking, emphysema, and previous surgery.

Other investigators have found associations between specific headache diagnoses and diseases. To examine the association between migraine and other conditions, Merikangas reviewed the Health and Nutrition Examination Survey (HANES I), a study of 12,200 adults aged 25 to 74 years, that was used to estimate the health of the general population of adults in the United States. Merikangas found the following conditions to be strongly associated with migraine: stroke (odds ratio 3:1); heart attack (odds ratio 2:4); bronchitis (odds ratio 2:3); colitis (odds ratio 2:3); nervous breakdown (odds ratio 2:2); urinary tract disorders (odds ratio 2:2); and ulcers (odds ratio 2:2). Migraine has also been associated with an increased prevalence of coronary vasospasm, Raynaud's phenomenon, aspirin-sensitive asthma, mitral valve prolapse, epilepsy, and hypertension.

Cluster headache is associated with a threefold increase in the prevalence of peptic ulcers. Cluster patients often have multiple risk factors for coronary artery disease. Chronic tension-type headache sufferers have an increased prevalence of depressive symptoms.

1. Do the headaches represent a primary headache disorder (i.e., migraine, tension-type, or cluster) or are they secondary to the patient's other medical problems?

In medical practice, most headaches are not caused by underlying disease. It is important to recognize, however, that headache can be the presenting symptom of several diseases. Fever, regardless of etiology, is probably the most common medical problem that causes headache. Less common causes include pheochromocytoma, chronic renal failure, hyperthyroidism, and malignant hypertension. Pheochromocytoma may present with a pounding headache associated with hypertension, diaphoresis, tachycardia, and palpitations.

Rheumatologic diseases may have headache as an early manifestation. Headache is common in systemic lupus erythematosus, polyarteritis nodosa, and giant cell arteritis. About two-thirds of patients with fibromyalgia report headache, usually tension-type headache. Many types of vasculitis can also present with headache

Headache upon awakening may be the initial symptom of sleep apnea syndrome. The headache often will improve as the day progresses. Sleep apnea is most commonly observed in obese, middle-aged males. Associated symptoms include snoring, daytime somnolence, hypertension, and arrhythmias.

In the present case, the headaches preceded the onset of comorbid rheumatoid arthritis and hypertension by at least 25 years. The age at onset and presentation were typical of migraine, and the headache quality did not change over time. In this situation, there is no reason to believe that the migraine headaches are related to the patient's other medical problems.

On the other hand, the patient does suffer from chronic neck discomfort related to her fibromyalgia. Fibromyalgia can be a primary complaint or, as in this case, associated with rheumatoid arthritis. Treatment of the underlying condition may have a direct impact on the neck pain.

2. Is the therapy for the comorbid condition triggering or exacerbating the headache problem?

Certain medications can trigger the onset of headache or exacerbate headache in patients with an underlying headache disorder. Medication-induced headache has been commonly reported with the following medications: indomethacin, nifedipine, cimetidine, atenolol, a trimethoprim-sulfamethoxazole combination, nitroglycerin, isosorbide dinitrate, ranitidine, isotretinoin, captopril, piroxicam, granisetron, epoetin, metoprolol, and diclofenac. Medications that may aggravate existing migraine include vitamin A, its retinoic-acid derivatives, and hormone therapy, such as oral contraceptives, clomiphene, and postmenopausal estrogens. Migraine and cluster headaches may be exacerbated by vasodilators such as nitrates, hydralazine, minoxidil, nifedipine, and prazosin.

Reserpine, a serotonin depleter, can cause depression, migraine, and tension-type headaches. Indomethacin, while useful in treating cluster-variant headaches, can cause a generalized headache. Frequent or chronic use of some prescription and over-the-counter medications used to treat headache, including opioids, barbiturates, caffeine, and ergots, can lead to rebound or withdrawal headaches.

A careful review of this patient's medications did not suggest that the treatment of her rheumatoid arthritis, hypertension, or fibromyalgia was complicating her headache disorder. Additionally, she avoided over-the-counter or habituating medications.

3. Is the headache treatment likely to worsen the comorbid condition, or does the comorbid condition contraindicate certain therapies?

In a patient with Raynaud's phenomenon, as well as any patient with peripheral vascular disease or coronary artery disease, any medication which can exacerbate vasoconstriction should be avoided. Therefore, we would not treat this patient with ergotamine tartrate, dihydroergotamine mesylate (DHE), isometheptene mucate, the triptans, or other 5-HT 1B/1D agonists. Beta-blockers are generally avoided in patients with vasospastic diseases like Raynaud's phenomenon or vasospastic angina.

Ergotamine tartrate, DHE, isometheptene mucate, and triptans can transiently elevate blood pressure. Patients with hypertension must have their blood pressure well controlled prior to using these drugs. As hypertension is a major risk factor for coronary artery disease, a careful appraisal of other coronary risk factors should be undertaken prior to the prescription of any of these drugs. Patients with active ischemic heart disease, or those patients likely to have occult coronary artery disease, should not be treated with ergotamine tartrate, DHE, isometheptene mucate, or triptans.

To treat this patient's migraine attacks, we chose a nonsteroidal anti-inflammatory drug (naproxen sodium). We suggested she take her initial dose at onset but if the headache persisted, she should take her second dose 1 hour later. Metoclopramide, 10 mg orally, could be added to the NSAID to improve its efficacy and to reduce nausea and vomiting.

4. Does the presence of comorbid disease offer the opportunity to use a single drug to treat both the headache disorder and the comorbid condition?

Many agents used in migraine prophylaxis have additional uses in other medical conditions. Beta-blockers and calcium channel blockers are useful in treating concomitant hypertension or ischemic heart disease. The NSAIDs are useful for many rheumatologic and musculoskeletal conditions. Divalproex sodium can be used for epilepsy.

For this patient, the calcium channel blockers offer the opportunity to use a single agent to treat three diseases. Calcium channel blockers are useful in migraine prophylaxis, and in the treatment of hypertension and Raynaud's phenomenon.

We elected not to use daily NSAIDs in this patient because she was already on disease-modifying agents for her rheumatoid arthritis, and because intermittent NSAIDs were the best choice for her acute migraine management. She was already taking a tricyclic antidepressant for the treatment of her fibromyalgia. Chronic headache is reported by over two-thirds of patients with fibromyalgia. Tricyclic antidepressant drugs may also be useful in migraine prophylaxis.

Management Strategies

- Establish the correct headache diagnosis.
- Be alert for secondary headache disorders related to the patient's comorbid diseases.
- Carefully review the current medications, including over-the-counter products. Look for drugs that may exacerbate headache or cause rebound/withdrawal headaches.
- Assess for medical problems that may have an impact on your choices of headache treatments. Screen patients for ischemic heart disease and coronary artery disease risk factors prior to prescribing ergotamine tartrate, DHE, isometheptene mucate, sumatriptan, and other 5-HT 1B/1D agonists.
- Try to select headache therapies that may also treat the patient's comorbid condition. Reducing the number of medications can improve compliance, limit adverse effects, and reduce cost.

Migraine and Cardiovascular Disease

Migraine headache and cardiovascular disease are both extremely common. This section will discuss the clinical associations between these disorders, connections in their pathophysiology, and similarities in treatment.

Like coronary artery disease, migraine is a familial disorder, with a positive family history in two-thirds of cases. Three-quarters of patients will have a family history of migraine on the maternal side only, 20% on the paternal side only, and 6% on both the maternal and paternal sides. There is approximately a 70% risk of migraine in offspring when both parents suffer from migraine, 45% risk when only one parent is affected, and less than 30% risk when both parents are unaffected. The genetic basis for migraine is probably multifactorial; the genetic component is polygenic with the added effect of a number of genes which render the individual more or less susceptible to developing the disorder in response to a number of environmental trigger factors.

The increased risk of stroke in migraine patients is not associated with the age of onset of migraine—the risk of stroke is elevated regardless of the age of the migraine patient. Ten years after regularly using headache medications, patients had a risk ratio for stroke of 1:7. When comparing adjusted risk ratios for stroke, migraine was the third most common contributing factor at 1:7, behind hypertension at 2:1, and diabetes mellitus at 1:9, but ahead of heart disease and male sex at 1:4.

Circadian rhythms are those repetitions of biologic phenomena that occur at about the same time each day. Circulating catecholamines, platelet aggregability, pericranial-musculature pain sensitivity, and vasospastic events all follow circadian rhythms that may have an impact on migraine.

Migraine attacks follow a circadian rhythm, with a marked increase in attacks between 6 AM and 8 AM, a peak migraine frequency between 8 AM and 10 AM, and a dramatic decrease in frequency between 8 PM and 4 AM. A recent review of 28 migraine patients revealed that of 329 migraine attacks, 160 (49%) occurred between 6 AM and noon.

It has been demonstrated that nonfatal myocardial infarction, variant angina, exertional angina, and sudden cardiac death are all more likely to occur between 6 AM and noon than at other times of the day. Platelet aggregability also shows an increase between 6 AM and 9 AM.

Cerebral infarction has been reported to have a circadian pattern with an increased frequency in the late-morning hours. This pattern mimics that of migraine. This is in contrast to subarachnoid hemorrhage, which has been reported to peak between 6 PM and midnight.

The circadian pattern observed in migraine may also be related to changes in the firing rate of serotonergic neurons in the dorsal raphe nucleus. Raskin has proposed that the core abnormality of migraine is unstable serotonergic neurotransmission leading to increased raphe neuronal firing rates. Dorsal raphe units maintain a slow, regular firing pattern as long as there is no change in arousal level. They become totally silent during rapid eye movement sleep. The serotonergic neurons increase their firing rate in response to visual, auditory, or somatosensory stimuli. It is possible that early morning arousal and the marked increase in sensory stimuli may trigger increased dorsal raphe nucleus firing rates, causing the increased frequency of morning migraines via serotonergic effects on platelets and vascular tone.

Nonfatal myocardial infarction, angina, and sudden cardiac death are vascular events that share some similarities with migraine. Both the cardiac events and migraine are associated with changes in vasomotor tone and ischemia. Platelet hyperaggregability has been associated with both conditions. The similarities in circadian rhythm of these phenomena raise the question of the relationship of migraine to other vascular events. Both migraine and coronary artery disease are more common in patients with hypertension and are amenable to prophylactic therapy with aspirin, beta-blockers (without intrinsic sympathomimetic activity), or calcium channel blockers.

The association between myocardial infarction and migraine may also relate to the pathogenesis of the two events. Platelet aggregability has a circadian variability that parallels nonfatal myocardial infarction and sudden cardiac death. The migraine data also suggest that the circadian variability of platelet aggregability parallels that of migraine. Platelet hyperaggregability may lead to the release of chemical mediators, such as serotonin, which may induce vasospasm. Increased sympathetic nervous system activity may also play a role in both cardiac events and migraine. Catecholamine levels in plasma rise between 6 AM and noon, and can induce vasospasm. Vasospasm may be the initiating step in migraine, either through the induction of ischemia, platelet changes, or the release of neurochemical mediators, all of which can activate the trigemino-vascular system.

Migraine and cardiovascular disease share clinical associations, circadian rhythms, pathophysiologic mechanisms, and therapies. It is hoped that advances in the pathophysiology and treatment of cardiovascular disorders will bring benefits to migraine sufferers.

Selected Readings

Askmark H, Lundberg PO, Olsson S. Drug-related headache. Headache 1989;29:441–4.

Dalessio DJ. Beta-blockers and migraine. JAMA 1984;252:2614.

Featherstone HJ. Medical diagnoses and problems in individuals with recurrent idiopathic headaches. Headache 1985;25:136–40.

Hanington E. The platelet theory. In: Blau JN, editor. Migraine: clinical and research aspects. Baltimore: Johns Hopkins University Press; 1987. p. 331–53.

Iversen H, Nielsen T, Olesen J, Tfelt-Hansen P. Arterial responses during migraine headache. Lancet 1990;336:837–9.

Merikangas KR. Comorbidity of migraine and other conditions in the general population of adults in the United States. Cephalalgia 1991;11 Suppl 11:108–9 .

Merikangas KR. Migraine and stroke: association in large-scale epidemiologic study. London: Migraine Trust; 1992.

Muller JE, Stone PH, Turi ZG, et al. Circadian variation in the frequency of onset of acute myocardial infarction. N Engl J Med 1985;313:1315–22.

Raskin NH. Headache. 2nd ed. New York: Churchill Livingstone; 1988. p. 109.

Solomon GD. Comparative review of calcium channel blocking drugs in migraine. Headache 1985;25:368–71.

Solomon GD. Concomitant medical disease and headache. Med Clin North Am 1991;75:631–9.

Solomon GD. Circadian variation in the frequency of migraine. Cleve Clin J Med 1992;59:326–9.

Tofler GH, Brezinski D, Schafer AI, et al. Concurrent morning increase in platelet aggregability and the risk of myocardial infarction and sudden cardiac death. N Engl J Med 1987;316:1514–8.

Editorial Comments

Headache and comorbid medical disorders are common. Management of the patient's headache cannot be done in isolation, and requires considerable knowledge and expertise of numerous medical disorders to effect good overall care. Dr. Solomon presents us with such a case and lends us his considerable knowledge and experience in dealing with such patients. The exact neurobiologic association between migraine and the disorders mentioned, as well as the relationship to biologically induced circadian rhythms, particularly in migraine and cardiovascular disorders, requires further thought and study, as suggested by Dr. Solomon in this chapter.

CHAPTER 10

THE PATIENT WITH MIGRAINE AND TRANSIENT WEAKNESS

NAGANAND SRIPATHI, MD

MARK GORMAN, MD

NABIH M. RAMADAN, MD

Case History

A 23-year-old man presented to one of us with a recent increase in the frequency of his migraines. He described attacks of severe, throbbing, holocephalic pain that would last all day and that would be aggravated by movement. Typically, the headache would build up over 30 to 45 minutes, and it was associated with nausea, vomiting, photophobia, and phonophobia. He did not have any visual changes or diplopia but with some of the headaches he would develop either right or left hemiparesis which would evolve into complete hemiplegia over 45 minutes. Additionally, he experienced vertigo and slurred speech with these attacks.

He had a strong family history of similar events, with three of his siblings (ages 15, 12, and 6 years) all having migraine associated with hemiplegia. A paternal great-aunt had migraine. He neither smoked nor drank alcohol. He had no other neurologic complaints and his only medical problem was a gastric ulcer.

His physical and neurologic examinations between attacks were normal.

Questions about This Case

- What are the diagnostic possibilities in this case?
- What are the minimum investigations that are needed to arrive at the diagnosis?
- What special tests can be ordered to evaluate the familial nature of the disease?
- Is the management of this disorder different from migraine with aura?

Case Discussion

The four important key points in this patient's clinical presentation are (1) headache; (2) transient right or left hemiparesis; (3) vertigo and slurred speech; and (4) similar complaints in several members of the family. The diagnostic considerations in this case are:

- Migraine with aura
- Familial hemiplegic migraine (FHM)
- Cerebral autosomal dominant arteriopathy with subcortical infarcts and leukoencephalopathy (CADASIL)
- Headache associated with vascular disorders
- Mitochondrial myopathy, encephalopathy, lactic acidosis, and stroke-like symptoms (MELAS)
- Epilepsy

The most characteristic feature of migraine with aura is an episode of transient focal neurologic symptoms. The patient's recurrent headaches and the slow build-up of the symptoms over a period of an hour associated with nausea, vomiting, photophobia, and phonophobia are in keeping with the typical migraine headache. Transient focal neurologic symptoms occur in approximately 20% of adult migraine patients. The symptoms of aura may vary from patient to patient and from attack to attack in the same patient. The duration of aura ranges anywhere from 5 to 60 minutes. The most common symptoms are visual but in about 20% of patients, motor symptoms are predominant. The weakness may be focal and may spread to involve an entire limb or side, and sometimes it is bilateral. There may be impaired coordination in addition to the weakness.

The presence of vertigo and slurred speech may suggest basilar migraine. The patient does not have all the classic features of basilar migraine. The symptom of slurred speech may be aphasia or dysarthria. The incidence of speech abnormalities in hemiplegic migraine is close to 50% and both aphasia and dysarthria are described. Attacks of Bickerstaff's (basilar) migraine are more common in childhood and adolescence, and become less frequent in early adulthood. Motor symptoms of basilar migraine are also usually bilateral and visual complaints are very prominent.

A strong family history of headaches and transient neurologic dysfunction could point to FHM, CADASIL, or MELAS.

Hemiplegic migraine, sporadic or familial, can be easily confused with migraine with aura. The resemblance is only superficial as the hemiparesis or hemisensory deficit often precedes the headache and persists throughout the headache phase. A very strong family history with autosomal dominant transmission strongly supports the diagnosis of FHM. Familial hemiplegic migraine is a rare autosomal dominant disorder which manifests in the teens or early twenties. Speech problems are noted in more than 50% of patients. Aphasia is usually mixed and dysarthria is also reported. Brainstem signs and coma have also been reported. The symptoms of vertigo and slurred speech in this patient may also be consistent with hemiplegic migraine and do not necessarily imply basilar migraine. Familial hemiplegic migraine shares many of the features of

migraine, such as headache characteristics, triggers, and the aura.

CADASIL is also a familial disorder of the small vessels manifesting as recurrent strokes, cerebral white-matter ischemic changes, and migraine-like headaches. Our patient had a normal neurologic examination and cranial magnetic resonance imaging (MRI), which disprove the diagnosis of CADASIL.

Associated with point mutations, MELAS is transmitted maternally. The attacks consist of migraine-like headaches and strokes with seizures. The deficits are generally prolonged and permanent. Our patient's symptoms were unlike the clinical presentation of MELAS.

Complex partial seizures may cause vertigo, slurred speech, and sometimes complex motor activities. Generally, there is cognitive impairment during the ictus of a complex partial seizure. Our patient did not develop any ictal cognitive abnormality and never developed complex motor behavior.

Headaches associated with vascular disorders such as arteritis, transient ischemic attacks (TIAs) caused by conditions such as thromboembolism or a connective tissue disorder, unruptured arteriovenous malformations (AVMs), or saccular aneurysm enter into the differential diagnosis of transient focal neurologic deficits and headache. Stereotyped events, repetitive attacks with no permanent sequelae, a strong family history of similar events, absence of systemic manifestations of connective tissue disease, and a younger age at onset are uncommon features of headaches associated with vascular disorders.

A normal cranial MRI excludes symptomatic headaches (e.g., headache with AVM), CADASIL, or MELAS. This is especially important during the evaluation of a first attack. The erythrocyte sedimentation rate (ESR), antinuclear antibody titer (ANA), and anticardiolipin antibody are helpful tests to screen for arteritic diseases that could present with headache and ischemic stroke or TIA. A resting lactate level is useful to evaluate patients with suspected MELAS. A skin and/or brain biopsy may also offer clues to the arteriopathy with osmophilic inclusions in the case of CADASIL. Cerebral blood flow, electroencephalography, and nuclear magnetic resonance spectroscopy are some additional investigations that could be helpful in understanding the mechanisms of the attacks.

Familial hemiplegic migraine was recently linked to chromosome 19p13 and the disease results from mutations in a neuronal P/Q calcium-channel α-1 subunit gene. In approximately 55% of the families known to have FHM, it is linked to chromosome 19. Recently, a new locus for FHM was mapped to chromosome 1q3. This region of chromosome 1 contains another type of neuronal calcium-channel subunit, α-1E supposedly associated with an R- and possibly a T-type of calcium channel.

The importance of making the diagnosis of FHM and distinguishing it from migraine cannot be overemphasized. Important issues to consider are genetic counseling and treatment options. Serotonin (5-HT) agonists that are routinely used in the management of migraine may have adverse effects on patients with FHM. There are no controlled studies to suggest a rational therapy. Calcium channel blockers, antiepileptics, and acetazolamide may cut short the duration of the attack. Prophylactic therapy is rarely needed for the hemiplegic attacks since they are infrequent.

Approximately 15 to 20% of patients with migraine have transient focal neurologic symptoms (aura) along with the other classic symptoms of headache, vomiting, photophobia, and phonophobia. The aura typically consists of visual symptoms, such as fortification spectra. Familial hemiplegic migraine is a subtype of migraine with aura, in which hemiparesis or hemiplegia usually precedes the headache and may persist throughout and beyond the headache phase of the attack. Liveing was probably the first to describe hemiparesis with a migraine attack. Whitty coined the term FHM when he described patients from the same family who would develop stereotyped attacks of migraine with hemiparesis. Since then over 40 families with this autosomal dominant disorder have been described.

Clinical Presentation

The age of onset of FHM is about 13 years (range 2 to 37) but the correct diagnosis is often delayed for many years (the mean age of diagnosis is 31 years). Clinical features of FHM include typical symptoms of migraine with aura in addition to hemiparesis which lasts seconds to hours and in some cases even weeks. Appendicular involvement (arm and leg) is more common than facial weakness.

The weakness often progresses slowly. Other symptoms may include hemisensory loss (which is frequently cheiro-oral with a marching pattern), dysarthria, hemianopsia, dysphasia, and dysmetria. In severe episodes, confusion, fever, drowsiness, or even coma may accompany the other symptoms. The majority of the neurologic symptoms of FHM are reversible, but rare cases of permanent neurologic deficits have also been described. Familial hemiplegic migraine has been associated with retinitis pigmentosa, sensorineural hearing loss, essential tremor, ocular saccadic movement, dysarthria, horizontal nystagmus, and limb ataxia. Certain families manifest a progressive cerebellar syndrome with the clinical hallmarks of horizontal nystagmus and limb ataxia. People in these families have a high chance of a genetic abnormality on chromosome 19. Magnetic resonance imaging findings of affected persons in these families reveal vermian atrophy, but are otherwise unremarkable. The association between infantile convulsions and FHM was recently suggested.

Both the frequency and severity of the attacks may vary within and between families. Patients with FHM generally suffer from episodes of migraine with aura as well as migraine without aura; the episodes of migraine usually occur more frequently than the attacks of hemiparesis.

Trigger factors may include mild head injury, cerebral angiography, emotional or physical stress, or the symptoms may be timed with the menstrual cycle. The presentation may change in some patients over time. They may have FHM in adolescence, migraine with aura in early adulthood, and migraine without aura at a later stage in their lives.

Differential Diagnosis and Investigations

The diagnosis of FHM is a diagnosis of exclusion, and it is necessary to be certain that the transient neurologic symptoms, in association with headache, do not represent other, more ominous processes.

Headache with migrainous infarction can present in a similar manner but the neurologic deficit is usually permanent and/or there is a lesion visible on a brain scan, particularly an MRI scan. A familial mitochondrial disorder, MELAS can present with a stroke-like episode. Elevated levels of lactic acid in the blood can aid in the diagnosis.

Cerebral emboli such as from a carotid artery or cardiac source often cause transient neurologic deficits. There is no familial tendency in these cases. Echocardiography, carotid Doppler ultrasonography, Holter monitoring, and long-term transcranial Doppler (TCD) monitoring can help rule out an embolic source. Infectious etiologies may mimic hemiplegic migraine, especially since attacks of FHM and concomitant fever have been reported. Appropriate serologic tests will help in this regard. Cerebrospinal fluid (CSF) analysis is necessary when an infectious etiology is suspected, but may be confusing as some cases of FHM have been reported with mononuclear pleocytosis and elevated protein levels. A rare condition of **h**eadache mimicking migraine, **n**eurologic **d**eficits, and cerebrospinal **l**ymphocytosis (HANDL) can be appropriately diagnosed by the elevated count of lymphocytes in the CSF and the monophasic course of the illness. Heterozygotes to ornithine transcarbamylase deficiency may have transient neurologic deficits and headache that could be confused with migraine. Ictal elevation of arterial ammonia levels is a clue to the diagnosis.

Genetics

Familial clustering of migraine has been known for centuries but the first writings on the familial nature of this condition date back to Sir Thomas Willis. It has been extremely difficult to define the pattern of transmission of migraine because of its high prevalence in the general population. Familial hemiplegic migraine is the only subtype of migraine with a well-established autosomal dominant transmission. It was observed that some patients with CADASIL also suffered from recurrent headaches and transient focal neurologic symptoms, suggesting that FHM and CADASIL may be allelic. CADASIL was already localized to chromosome 19 and a linkage analysis of two families with FHM was indeed mapped close to the CADASIL locus. Families may have pure FHM or some may have an associated cerebellar syndrome. Also, Ophoff et al. studied five families with FHM and noted that migraine with and without aura occurred among members of those families.

Different families with strong linkage to the short arm of chromosome 19 (19p13) have different clinical presentations. This raises the possibility that FHM and FHM with cerebellar syndrome are either allelic mutations with variable expression of the gene defect or represent a defect in which two genes are involved. Linkage analysis of additional families provided strong evidence for the genetic heterogeneity of FHM. Overall, 55% of the families with FHM are linked to chromosome 19p13, 16% are linked to chromosome 1q, and 29% are not linked; cerebellar ataxia and nystagmus occurred in the linked families. Penetrance was also incomplete in the unlinked families.

Another autosomal dominant disorder, episodic ataxia type 2 (EA-2), was also mapped to chromosome 19p13 in the same interval as that of the FHM locus. Patients with EA-2 have attacks of cerebellar ataxia and migraine-like symptoms. They also have interictal nystagmus and cerebellar atrophy. These attacks respond to acetazolamide, suggesting a common etiopathogenesis, perhaps a channelopathy similar to periodic paralysis. A specific search for ion channel genes within the FHM and EA-2 candidate region revealed mutations in the gene for a voltage-sensitive calcium channel CACNL1A4. The gene is a brain-specific P/Q-type calcium α-1 channelsubunit gene.

Calcium channels are of two classes: low-voltage T-type and high-voltage channels, which are further divided into L, N, P, Q, and R subtypes. The N, P/Q, and R subtypes are neuronal channels. The P/Q channels are most abundant in the cerebellum but recent data indicate their presence in brainstem nuclei (median raphe, reticular formation, deep pontine nuclei), a discovery of major relevance to migraine since the "migraine generator" is believed to encompass some of these areas. Four subunits (α-1, α-2, β, and δ) form the voltage-dependent calcium channels. Studies to this date indicate that missense mutations in the α-1 gene cause FHM and that truncating mutations in the same protein result in EA-2. The CAG expansion in the 3′ untranslated portion of the α-1 gene causes spinocerebellar ataxia type 6. May et al. used subpair analysis to show significant involvement of the 19p13 locus in migraine with and without aura.

Pathophysiology

Genetic factors may be part of a multifactorial mechanism initiating migraine attacks. The recent genetic mapping of a significant proportion of families with FHM to the locus of a voltage-sensitive calcium channel places many of the cases into the category of a channelopathy. Familial hemiplegic migraine, EA-2, and migraine with and without aura may all be ion channel disorders. This concept has profound implications for the understanding of the etiopathogenesis of migraine and for the development of therapeutic interventions. The P/Q neuronal calcium channels mediate the release of neurotransmitters including serotonin; a defective channel would result in abnormal neurotransmitter release, probably lowering the threshold for a migraine attack. Also, Ophoff suggests that defective cortical channels may be involved in triggering cortical spreading depression.

It has been postulated that magnesium may play a part in the pathophysiology of migraine, and indeed magnesium plays an important role in the regulation of calcium channels. Calcium and other ion channels are also involved in the mechanism of spreading depression. Intracellular and plasma magnesium levels were found to be unchanged in 38 patients with FHM. On the other hand, a spectroscopic imaging study revealed that patients with FHM have reduced interictal magnesium in the posterior brain regions. This apparent discrepancy may be explained by the inaccuracy of plasma magnesium levels in predicting intraneuronal levels.

Single photon emission computed tomography (SPECT) scanning has revealed diminished ipsilateral cerebellar blood flow during an attack of hemiplegia in a patient with hemiplegic migraine and ataxia. At the same time, an ipsilateral frontal cortical decrease and a contralateral frontoparietal cortical increase in blood flow were observed. The authors postulated activation of the nitric oxide pathway, via serotonin dysregulation, as a possible mechanism for the symptoms, blood flow changes, and cerebellar degeneration in patients with FHM and ataxia.

Magnetic resonance spectroscopy has identified deficient brain and muscle energy metabolism in affected, as well as some unaffected, family members of patients with FHM. The defect was felt to be in the mitochondrial respiratory chain leaving the individual somewhat impaired in his or her metabolic condition and less able to respond to the high energy demands encountered in metabolic stress. Further research will, it is hoped, clarify the roles these diverse findings play in the picture of FHM.

Treatment

Most of the treatment options for patients with FHM are based on small studies and case reports. Prophylactic treatment for hemiplegic attacks is rarely required as the attacks are infrequent but it may be necessary for the nonhemiplegic spells. It is prudent to avoid beta-blockers, although opinion is divided regarding the safety of this medication. Calcium-channel-blocking agents seem to be a reasonable choice but there are no large controlled studies to confirm their efficacy. Verapamil, nimodipine, and flunarizine have been tried with variable success. It can be argued that these medications have limited efficacy because they act on the L- and not the P/Q- or R-subtype channels. The antiepileptic medications phenytoin and phenobarbital have also been used.

Symptomatic treatment should focus on improving the pain relief of the FHM attack and shortening the duration of the episode. It is recommended that serotonin agonists be avoided. The role of ergotamine is controversial. Intravenous verapamil and naloxone have been shown to improve the outcome. Acetazolamide may reduce the frequency and intensity of the attacks of FHM.

Selected Readings

Ahmed MAS, Reid E, Cooke A, et al. Familial hemiplegic migraine in the west of Scotland: a clinical and genetic study of seven families. J Neurol Neurosurg Psychiatry 1996;61:616–20.

Athwal BS, Lennox GG. Acetazolamide responsiveness in familial hemiplegic migraine [letter]. Ann Neurol 1996;40:820–1.

Campbell KP, Leung AT, Sharp AH. The biochemistry and molecular biology of the dihydropyridine-sensitive calcium channel. Trends Neurosci 1988;11:425–30.

Jensen TS, De Fine Olivarius B, Kraft M, Hansen HJ. Familial hemiplegic migraine—a reappraisal and long-term follow-up study. Cephalalgia 1981;1:33–9.

Joutel A, Bousser M-G, Biousse V, et al. A gene for familial hemiplegic migraine maps to chromosome 19. Nat Genet 1993;5:40–5.

Joutel A, Ducros A, Vahedi K, et al. Genetic heterogenicity of familial hemiplegic migraine. Am J Hum Genet 1994; 55: 1166–72.

Kramer PL, Yue Q, Gancher ST, et al. A locus for the nystagmus-associated form of episodic ataxia maps to an 11-cM region on chromosome 19p. Am J Hum Genet 1995;57:182–7.

Lee TG, Solomon GD, Kunkel RS, Raja S. Reversible cerebellar perfusion in familial hemiplegic migraine. Lancet 1996; 348:1383.

May A, Ophoff RA, Terwindt GM, et al. Familial hemiplegic migraine locus on 19p13 is involved in the common forms of migraine with and without aura. Hum Genet 1995;96:604–8.

Motta E, Rosciszewska D, Miller K. Hemiplegic migraine with CSF abnormalities. Headache 1995;35:368–70.

Ophoff RA, Van Eijk R, Sandkuijl LA, et al. Genetic heterogeneity of familial hemiplegic migraine. Genomics 1994;22:21–6.

Ophoff RA, Terwindt GM, Vergouwe MN, et al. Familial hemiplegic migraine and episodic ataxia type-2 are caused by mutations in the Ca^{2+} channel gene CACNL1A4. Cell 1996;87:543–52.

Ramadan NM, Halvorson H, Vande-Linde A, et al. Low brain magnesium in migraine. Headache 1989;29:416–9.

Smeets MC, Vernooy CB, Souverijn JHM, Ferrari MD. Intra-cellular and plasma magnesium in familial hemiplegic migraine and migraine with and without aura. Cephalalgia 1994;14:29–32.

Uncini A, Lodi R, Di Muzio A, et al. Abnormal brain and muscle energy metabolism shown by ^{31}P-MRS in familial hemiplegic migraine. J Neurol Sci 1995;129:214–22.

Editorial Comments

In certain rare types of migraine, such as familial hemiplegic migraine, it is essential to get the diagnosis correct, particularly since the differential diagnoses involve other rare and sometimes serious neurologic disorders. More importantly, the diagnosis of FHM carries with it restrictions on the use of certain abortive migraine medications, such as the triptan class, and a need for genetic counseling. These authors lead us through a review of the clinical evaluation, treatment, and genetics of similar cases, and carefully describe the significance of calcium channelopathy in neurologic disease states.

CHAPTER 11

THE PATIENT WITH HEADACHE AND DEPRESSION

SEYMOUR DIAMOND, MD

Case History

A 39-year-old male patient came to the clinic having had a daily headache for 3 years. He denied any precipitating factors. The headaches were located in the bitemporal and biparietal regions, and were described as a constant pressure alternating with throbbing pain. He also complained of an almost constant dull ache in his shoulders and neck muscles radiating to the occipital region. The headaches were exacerbated by bright lights, loud noise, and physical exertion. He denied any aura or premonitory symptoms. The headache continued throughout the day, and he experienced recurrent dizziness also during the day. The patient noted difficulty in falling asleep and frequent awakening, after which he experienced difficulty returning to sleep.

On examination, the patient demonstrated a flat affect. He complained of loss of interest in daily activities and admitted to suicidal thoughts—he stated that he wanted to "chop off his head." The patient is married with two sons. He smokes one pack of cigarettes daily, and drinks a 12-pack of beer per week. He previously worked as a factory assembler, and is currently unemployed, stating that he "could not work."

Previously, the patient had been unresponsive to many medications, including acetaminophen, hydrocodone, ibuprofen, ketorolac, hydroxyzine pamoate, sertraline, isometheptene, fluoxetine, amitriptyline, verapamil, and paroxetine. Currently, the patient uses diazepam, 10 mg twice daily as needed, and meperidine, 100 to 200 mg every 12 hours.

The physical examination was normal. The patient's blood pressure was 120/80 and his pulse was 84 beats per minute. His neurologic examination revealed subjective dizziness but no nystagmus. The Dix-Hallpike maneuver for benign positional vertigo was negative on both sides.

A negative laboratory evaluation included electroencephalography (EEG), brainstem auditory evoked potentials, and electronystagmography. A computerized dynamic posturography indicated a nonphysiologic, i.e., a functional, pattern of abnormality. These findings suggest a nonorganic component to the patient's complaints.

Questions about This Case

- Is the presence of a sleep disturbance (difficulty falling asleep and frequent awakening) significant in diagnosing depression?
- This patient complained of somatic symptoms (subjective dizziness), and diagnostic testing was normal. What diagnosis could be considered?
- What symptoms described by the patient are typical of chronic tension-type headache?
- The patient noted an exacerbation of the pain with physical exertion and stated he "was unable to work." Is this characteristic typical of the "migraine personality?"

Case Discussion

This patient represents a classic example of many similar cases that I have encountered in my practice. The patient provides a history of coexisting migraine without aura and tension-type (muscle-contraction) headaches. The daily headaches are described as a constant pressure with an almost dull ache in the shoulders and neck muscles, radiating to the occipital region. He also experiences recurrent throbbing headaches, associated with photophobia and phonophobia—characteristic of migraine.

The term, "muscle-contraction headaches" was used for many years to describe chronic, daily headaches of a nonspecific type that are neither vascular in origin nor associated with traction and inflammation. The Classification Committee of the International Headache Society describes these headaches as "tension-type headaches" and divides them into two categories—episodic and chronic. Episodic tension-type headaches occur fewer than 15 times per month, usually result from the localized contraction of the head and neck muscles, and are associated with fatigue and temporary stressful situations in life. The pain is eased or abolished usually with over-the-counter analgesics and is rarely treated by a physician. The chronic form refers to those headaches occurring more than 15 times per month. Physicians frequently treat patients with these headaches—a headache symptom complex due in part to psychologic problems and associated with concomitant anxiety or depression.

A chronic tension-type headache is a steady non-pulsatile ache, often distributed in a band-like pattern around the head. It may be described as vice-like, a steady pressure, a weight, soreness, or a distinct cramp-like sensation. The location is variable but most often involves the forehead and temple or the back of the head and neck. The type of sleep disturbance present will determine the origin of the headaches. Difficulty falling asleep indicates headaches due to anxiety. Early or frequent awakening is linked to depression. Other factors present in the headache history may indicate an underlying depression. These headaches often have a diurnal variation, increasing in severity in the morning or early evening—times associated with increased stress in families. Headaches may occur or increase on weekends, holidays, and vacation—times when family issues often become prominent. The headaches do not usually respond to standard analgesics. Patients will relate headache onset to a specific event (some insignificant)—a surgical procedure, an infection, an accident, or the death of a loved one.

When interviewing the patient, the physician will observe manifestations of depression, such as dysphoria, flat affect, sleep disturbances, and suicidal tendencies. The depressed patient often presents with a wide variety of complaints, many vague, which can be characterized as physical, emotional, and psychologic. The physical complaints include chronic pain and headaches, sleep disturbances, appetite changes, anorexia, weight loss, and a decrease in sexual activity—impotence in the male and amenorrhea or frigidity in the female. Emotional complaints range from "feeling blue" to feelings of anxiety and rumination over the past, present, and future. Finally, psychologic complaints include statements such as "morning being the worst time of the day," suicidal thoughts, and death wishes.

In a 1966 study by Martin, emotional factors were considered of primary importance in the causation of muscle-contraction headaches. In that study, psychiatric evaluations were provided for a selected series of 25 patients with this complaint. No single psychologic determinant was identified for tension-type headaches. Multiple conflicts are usually evident in patients suffering from such headaches, and poorly repressed hostility was often present. Unresolved dependency needs and psychosexual conflicts were also frequently cited.

Our patient did exhibit symptoms of depression such as sleeplessness, loss of interest in daily activities, and suicidal tendencies. His inability to work due to the headaches may also have aggravated his symptoms. The patient had previously consulted a neurologist and general practitioner for the treatment of his headaches. He denied prior hospitalization for his headaches but reported over 100 emergency department visits because of intense headache pain.

The patient's previous work-up had included a computed tomography scan, a magnetic resonance imaging of the brain with gadolinium, EEG, brainstem auditory evoked potentials, and electronystag-

TABLE 11–1. Criteria for Admission to Inpatient Headache Unit

- Prolonged, unrelenting headache with associated symptoms such as nausea and vomiting that, if allowed to continue, would pose a further threat to the patient's welfare
- Status migrainosus
- Dependence on analgesics, caffeine, opioids, barbiturates, and tranquilizers
- Habituation to ergots; ergots if taken on daily basis, when stopped, cause a rebound headache
- Pain that is accompanied by a serious adverse reaction or complications from therapy; continued use of such therapy may aggravate or induce further illness
- Pain that occurs in the presence of significant medical disease; appropriate treatment of headache symptoms aggravates or induces further illness
- Chronic cluster headache that is unresponsive to treatment
- Treatment requiring copharmacy with drugs that may cause a drug interaction and necessitate careful observation (MAOIs and beta-blockers)
- Patients with a probable organic cause to their headaches requiring appropriate consultations and perhaps neurosurgical interventions
- Severe, intractable pain in the presence of dehydration, electrolyte loss, or prostration
- Severe pain in association with severe psychiatric disease and necessitating frequent parenteral medications

mography. These investigations were all within normal limits, thus excluding an organic cause for the headaches.

On admission to the inpatient headache unit, a long-acting corticosteroid (dexamethasone) was administered intramuscularly to reduce the sterile inflammation usually present in prolonged headache attacks. Intravenous dihydroergotamine mesylate was used as adjunctive therapy, and promethazine was prescribed as an antinauseant. Phenelzine, a monoamine oxidase inhibitor (MAOI), was started concurrently with nimodipine, a calcium channel blocker. A phenothiazine and a nonsteroidal anti-inflammatory drug were given parenterally, as needed, during the first 72 hours of hospitalization to assist with the management of the acute pain.

A neurology consultation obtained for the evaluation of the patient's dizziness was inconclusive and a diagnosis of vestibular dysfunction, probably related to migraine, was suggested. The psychiatric consultation described the patient as having a dependent personality, an anxiety disorder with major depression,

and a chronic pain disorder. A psychologist evaluated the patient for disorders regarding personality, mood, lifestyle, coping styles, and the possible presence of comorbid disorders that may have been contributing to the headache. Psychologic intervention for depression and marital counseling were recommended. The patient steadily improved and was asked to follow up on an outpatient basis after discharge.

Management Strategies

- Obtain a thorough and detailed history and inquire about stressful situations at home or work, relationships (marital, family, work, or school), and coping strategies.
- Observe the patient to determine if depression is manifesting itself as somatic signs and symptoms.
- Inquire about prior or family history of anxiety disorder and/or depression.
- Order neuroradiologic scanning and other laboratory tests to exclude an organic cause for the headaches.
- Discontinue excessive analgesic use (caffeine-containing analgesics, barbiturates, or opioids).
- Consider admission to specialized inpatient headache unit. Criteria for admission are listed in Table 11–1.
- During hospitalization, consider the following therapies:
  1. Intravenous DHE therapy
  2. Analgesics within appropriate limits
- Initiate antidepressant therapy for prophylaxis of both forms of headaches:
  1. Start with a tricyclic, and increase to the maximum allowable dose; look for side effects.
  2. If one tricyclic is not effective, try another tricyclic.
  3. If the patient remains unresponsive, consider a trial on selective serotonin reuptake inhibitors (SSRIs).
  4. If the patient remains refractory, consider the MAOIs. The patient must be instructed on the dietary and pharmacologic restrictions associated with MAOI use. For the patient with coexisting migraine and tension-type headaches, concomitant therapy with a tricyclic antidepressant, other than imipramine, and an MAOI should be considered.

- If indicated, use other prophylactic agents, such as beta-blockers or calcium channel blockers, in combination with the antidepressants.
- If warranted, neurologic, psychiatric, and psychologic consultations must be ordered.
- Use nonpharmacologic modalities, such as biofeedback therapy and physical therapy.

Overview of Migraine and Depression

Depression may be classified into three main categories. The first category is normal grief related to illness or death, which we have all probably experienced. The second is reactive depression, which may be associated with a physical illness or the use of medications, and may occur in association with a psychiatric illness; it is often self-limited, and usually responds well to therapy with tricyclic antidepressants. The third is endogenous or primary depression, which may be unipolar, bipolar, or cyclic mania alone, and is the most difficult to treat.

A significant similarity exists between the epidemiology of migraine and that of the so-called "neurotic" psychiatric disorders, including depression and anxiety. Lifetime prevalence estimates of migraine range from 4 to 19% for adult males, and from 8 to 29% for adult females. Major depression is also a common disorder with lifetime prevalence estimates ranging from 5 to 25% for women, and from 2 to 12% for men. Rates of depression are higher in women and young adults, ages 18 to 25 years, and they tend to increase with age. Several studies have systematically examined the association between migraine and psychiatric symptom patterns, disorders among patients undergoing treatment for migraine, patients in treatment for depression, and subjects from the general population. Despite variation in the methods and design, most studies indicate an association between migraine and depression. During the 1930s, Wolff noted extreme physical fatigue and apathy as characteristic traits of patients with migraine. Since then, clinical descriptions of people suffering from migraine have consistently depicted depression as a characteristic feature that occurs during the migraine prodrome as well as during the interim periods. Wolff attributed a vast

majority of discomforts and pains in the head to dissatisfaction and resentment. Migraineurs are said to resemble the anxious-depressive subtype in which depressive symptoms are accompanied by prominent anxiety.

Over a period of years, migraine patients often develop a coexisting syndrome of migraine and tension-type headaches. Prolonged and excessive contraction of the muscles of the face, scalp, neck, and shoulders, and the reduced blood supply to these muscles play a role in the pain syndrome of depressive headaches. Headaches may become a masochistic manifestation of suffering endured for pity, sympathy, and attention. Past experiences set the model for psychic activity which substitutes pain to replace unfulfilled dependence and need for love and affection. Provocative situations may be created which set the stage for the psychophysiologic changes which produce the headache.

The physician must obtain a thorough history from the patient, including a detailed psychiatric history and information about the patient's marital relationship, occupation, social and family relationships, life stressors, personality traits, habits, methods of handling stressful situations, and any sexual problems. Clues to a possible depression may be provided through inquiries made about a family or personal history of prior depression and inquiries about the onset of symptoms or any precipitating events.

Typically, migraine patients report more life stressors than their "normal" counterparts. In general, migraine patients are intelligent and sensitive people who are methodical and often perfectionists, and will use intellectual techniques to deal with stress. It is hypothesized that during their childhood, these headache sufferers did not express their emotions of anger and rage because of rigid parental attitudes towards uncontrolled behavior. Also, the patient with migraine has often been extended beyond the individual's capacity to produce, which increases feelings of inadequacy and frustration, and causes a response with anxiety. Migraine also increases the risk for substance abuse disorders and suicide attempts. Suicide attempts, affective and anxiety disorders, and alcohol or drug abuse/dependence have stronger associations in patients with migraine with aura than with those experiencing migraine without aura.

Some biochemical features may be common to both migraine and depression. During the past few years, the biochemical determinants of depression have been greatly researched. In the 1950s, tubercular patients treated with isoniazid were observed developing euphoric states. Isoniazid is an MAOI which increases the level of norepinephrine and serotonin in the brain and body tissue. At about the same time, a small percentage of patients being treated for hypertension with the *Rauwolfia* alkaloid, reserpine, were observed to develop severe depression indistinguishable from endogenous depression. These alkaloids were noted to deplete the brain of biogenic amines.

These putative neurochemical features might be at a general level of pathophysiologic predisposition which gives rise to different disorders when repressed or triggered in different sexes, ages, or according to some authors, in different environments. Low platelet monoamine oxidase activity, previously suggested to indicate a generalized vulnerability to psychiatric disorders, has been observed in patients with migraine. Alternatively, the neurotransmitter, serotonin, might provide a neurochemical basis for these associations, as serotonin abnormalities have been separately implicated in the pathogenesis of migraine, depression and mania, obsessive-compulsive disorder, anxiety, panic disorder, and suicide.

Researchers are investigating biochemical methods to measure depression. The measurement of 3-methoxy-4-hydroxyphenylethyleneglycol (MHPG) in the urine is of major concern, as it is the main metabolite in the central nervous system, and urinary loads are monitored to reflect norepinephrine metabolism. However, some controversy remains over the precise amount of MHPG that is derived from the central nervous system. It has been observed that certain subgroups of depressed patients have decreased MHPG in their urine, while other groups of depressed patients have normal or greater than normal levels of MHPG. The possibility has been suggested that two groups of depression exist: in the first group, norepinephrine metabolism is disrupted and serotonin and dopamine systems are normal; whereas in the second, patients have a disorder of serotonin but norepinephrine or dopamine is not affected. The MHPG level may be valuable in the selection of drug therapy.

Another test which may be employed in the differential diagnosis is the dexamethasone suppression test (DST), which is used to establish a diagnosis of Cushing's syndrome. Basically, the test involves the administration of a small amount of dexamethasone to the patient at night and the measurement of the serum cortisol level the next day. In a patient with Cushing's syndrome, the cortisol level is not suppressed. It has been found that in a subgroup of patients with endogenous depression, there is nonsuppression of the morning cortisol level. Approximately 45% of endogenously depressed individuals have an abnormal DST; however, the test is 96% specific for endogenous depression. The most useful value of the DST is to monitor the patient's response to therapy.

Another useful test is the thyroid-stimulating hormone (TSH) response to thyrotropin-releasing hormone (TRH). It has been noted that a large percentage of endogenously depressed patients have a blunted TSH response to the administration of TRH. The mechanism for this blunted response is unknown, and the clinical value of this test has yet to be demonstrated.

In many patients, electromyographic (EMG) studies have demonstrated increased levels of activity correlating with pain in the scalp and neck muscles. However, several other studies have failed to demonstrate any specific correlation between the amount of muscle contraction measured with the EMG recordings and pain. In reviewing the extensive literature concerning the EMG findings and tension-type headache, it was felt that the vast majority of studies failed to show an association between pain and increased muscle tension as measured by surface EMG recordings.

The cornerstone of treatment is twofold. First, continuity of care is essential. Most patients have seen numerous practitioners, and have either referred themselves or have been referred by another provider. The patient must be confident that he or she will remain under the care of one physician and should understand that seeking additional help will only sabotage the treatment. The second essential element of treatment is education. The patient will experience great relief when advised that the condition is a recognized entity and that treatment is available. Patients should be instructed that some agents tried previously will be tried again, only this time in combination with other medications. Patients must also be advised that withdrawal from opioids is mandatory, and that these agents will not be used in their future care.

The research mentioned above serves as the foundation for current drug therapy, primarily involving the tricyclic antidepressants (TCAs), the SSRIs, and the MAOIs. All of these drugs function by increasing the amount of biogenic amines available to the receptor sites. The MAOIs accomplish this action by decreasing their destruction, whereas the TCAs and SSRIs function by decreasing cellular reuptake of the biogenic amines.

The use of antidepressants in the treatment of migraine was first suggested during the late 1960s. In 1969, with Bernard Baltes, I studied 167 patients presenting with a chief complaint of headache and treated them with TCAs. The patients were diagnosed as suffering from migraine (91), depression (52), and coexisting migraine and depression (24). Excellent results were demonstrated in 80% of these patients. Subsequently, the role of antidepressant compounds in both the prophylaxis and relief of pain has become increasingly recognized. It has been suggested that if the antidepressant drugs had been studied for pain relief before they were experimentally administered to depressed patients, these agents would have been classified as analgesics. The manner in which antidepressant drugs control pain has been attributed to their effects on the synthesis and metabolism of serotonin (5-hydroxytryptamine) and norepinephrine. Neurons containing serotonin and norepinephrine have been identified as part of the brain'sanalgesia system. Virtually all antidepressants alter the synthesis or reuptake of the neurotransmitters serotonin and norepinephrine.

Initially, TCAs are usually the drugs of choice, and include amitriptyline, imipramine, desipramine, nortriptyline, doxepin, and protriptyline. The tricyclics are considered more effective for endogenous depression and less beneficial if the depressed patient has many accompanying neurotic traits. Each of these drugs has unique characteristics. Generally, amitriptyline possesses the greatest sedating effect, whereas doxepin is equally sedating but has fewer anticholinergic side effects. The other TCAs are listed according to the strength of their sedative effects: desipramine, nortriptyline, and imipramine. Protriptyline and desipramine generally have little sedative effect.

Amitriptyline is probably the most widely used antidepressant in office practice. Its common side effects include weight gain, weakness, fatigue, drowsiness, dizziness, dryness of the mouth, blurred vision, constipation, and muscle tremors. However, amitriptyline is rarely discontinued due to side effects, since most symptoms subside during continued therapy. Patients must be instructed that the occurrence of these listed side effects provides evidence that an adequate dose is being given. The patients should also be advised that the onset of a beneficial response often requires several weeks. Treatment failure is primarily caused if the dose is too low or the trial is too brief. A single daily dose at bedtime is compatible with known pharmacokinetics, may help insomnia, lessens anticholinergic effects during the day, and may improve patient compliance. Full doses should be maintained for 3 to 4 weeks before deciding that the patient is unresponsive.

A 1979 study compared amitriptyline with a placebo in the prophylaxis of migraine. A statistically significant improvement was demonstrated with amitriptyline therapy. The patients exhibiting the best response to amitriptyline were nondepressed subjects with severe headaches and depressed subjects with less severe attacks of migraine. It has been proposed that the antimigraine effect of amitriptyline is independent of its antidepressant effect. However, it has not been determined whether this effect is due to blocking of the reuptake of serotonin and to a lesser degree norepinephrine at the nerve endings, or due to its anticholinergic, antihistaminic, and antiserotonergic effect.

The SSRIs—fluoxetine, paroxetine, sertraline, and fluvoxamine—are a family of structurally diverse agents that exhibit pharmacodynamic and pharmacokinetic heterogeneity. The longer half-life of an SSRI provides for single daily dosing. When considering the half-life, it is important to recognize the production and activity of drug metabolites. The advantages of an SSRI with a longer half-life include greater protection against patient noncompliance, postdiscontinuation relapse, and abrupt withdrawal syndromes. Conversely, these drugs require greater physician vigilance for drug interactions, postdiscontinuation reactions, and drug accumulation with chronic treatment. The SSRIs have similar side-effect profiles, including nausea. However, as food does not decrease absorption of the SSRIs, taking these medications with meals can reduce nausea. In addition, sexual dysfunction, especially delayed ejaculation or anorgasmy, is not uncommon. Other side effects include somnolence, dry mouth, dizziness, insomnia, nervousness, sweating, anorexia, and diarrhea.

The newer generation of antidepressants includes venlafaxine, nefazodone, and bupropion. Their use is indicated in patients refractory to the other antidepressants or in individuals experiencing unacceptable side effects. However, each of these drugs is replete with side effects and should be used with caution.

The MAOIs are generally considered to be the "third tier" of treatment. In 1969, Anthony and Lance reported on the usefulness of MAOIs in the control of migraine. The MAOIs appear to be useful in the prophylaxis of vascular headaches in some patients but have not been widely accepted and may well be underutilized. The MAOIs are used less frequently because of the need for the patient to avoid tyramine-containing foods and certain drugs that may interact with the MAOIs. Phenelzine sulfate is the most commonly used MAOI. Despite the problems associated with MAOIs, these drugs are often found to be effective when the TCAs fail. In studies comparing the TCAs and the MAOIs, the latter seem to exert a stronger antianxiety action, whereas the former were more effective in reducing weight loss and improving sleep.

Most physicians avoid combination therapy with the MAOIs and TCAs. Isolated instances of hypertensive or hyperpyretic cases leading to death have been associated with combination therapy. A 1971 review by Schuckit et al. described 25 reported cases of morbidity secondary to combination therapy. The results of the study indicated that the risks of combination therapy had been greatly exaggerated. Many of the reported complications were attributed to drug overdose or could be associated with the concomitant use of other drugs which act on the central nervous system. In seven cases, the involved TCA was imipramine. The current feeling is that combination therapy may be of value when all else fails but it should be used with caution, and imipramine should never be used in combination with an MAOI.

The most common reason for treatment failure is underdosage of the antidepressant. Drugs should be given on a fixed time schedule, and multiple drug usage should be reduced to a minimum. Before initiating treatment, habituating agents should be slowly tapered off. Patients should be encouraged to continue normal daily activities and not focus on their headache. Finally, and most importantly, the patient should receive a detailed explanation of the treatment plan. Without the patient's understanding and cooperation, the treatment is destined to fail.

Nonpharmacologic treatment modalities are beneficial in addition to pharmacologic agents. Biofeedback training in the well-motivated patient is effective in reducing tension and promotes relaxation. This technique combines modern instrumentation with ancient Eastern practices and modern psychology. Instruments are used to monitor various bodily functions, such as heart rate, blood pressure, temperature, muscle tension, and brain-wave activity. By relating the status of these various functions back to the individual, biofeedback enables that person to learn to control a previously unused or involuntarily controlled bodily function. In our work with headache patients, temperature feedback and EMG feedback training are used. We find that using both techniques helps achieve a higher success rate with patients prone to various forms of headache. Our results in both psychogenic and coexisting migraine and tension-type headaches show that we can help close to 50% of patients with biofeedback therapy.

Because of the chronic depression in these patients, referral to a psychologist or psychiatrist may be necessary. Prolonged psychotherapy may be required to uncover suppressed anger or unresolved grief. Therapy is most effective when multiple techniques are used, including pharmacologic, psychologic, and physiologic modalities.

Selected Readings

Anthony M, Lance JW. Monoamine oxidase inhibition in the treatment of migraine. Arch Neurol 1969;21:1263.

Asberg M, Schalling D, Traskman-Bendz L, Wagner A. Psychobiology of suicide, and related phenomena. In: Meltzer HY, editor. Psychopharmacology: the third generation of progress. New York: Raven Press; 1987. p. 513–26.

Breslau N, Davis GC, Andreski P. Migraine psychiatric disorders, and suicide attempts: an epidemiologic study of young adults. Psychiatry Res 1991;37:11–23.

Buchsbaum MS, Coursey RD, Murphy DL. The biochemical high risk paradigm: behavioral and family correlates of low platelet monoamine oxidase activity. Science 1979;194:339–41.

Couch JR, Hassanein RS. Amitriptyline in migraine prophylaxis. Arch Neurol 1979;36:695–9.

D'Andrea G, Welch KMA, Riddle JM, et al. Platelet serotonin metabolism and ultrastructure in migraine. Arch Neurol 1989;46:1187–9.

Diamond S. Depressive headaches. Headache 1964;4:255–9.

Diamond S. The masks of depression. Clin Med 1965;72:1629.

Diamond S. Depression and headache. Headache 1983;23:122–6.

Diamond S, Baltes B. The office treatment of mixed anxiety and depression with combination therapy. Psychosomatics 1969; 10:360–5.

Freitag FG, Diamond S, Solomon GD. Antidepressants in the treatment of mixed headache: MAO inhibitors and combined use of MAO inhibitors and tricyclic antidepressants in the recidivist headache patient. In: Rose FC, editor. Advances in headache research. London: John Libbey; 1987. p. 271–5.

Gray JA. Issues in the neuropsychology of anxiety. In: Tuma AH, Maser D, editors. Anxiety and the anxiety disorders. Hillside (NJ): Lawrence Earlbaum Associates; 1985. p. 5–25.

Innis RB, Charney DS, Heninger GR. Differential ^{3}H-imipramine platelet binding in patients with impulsivity, panic disorder and depression. Psychiatry Res 1987;21:33–41.

Insel TR, Murphy DL. The psychopharmacological treatment of obsession-compulsive disorder; a review. J Clin Pharmacol 1981;1:304–11.

International Headache Society. Classification and diagnostic criteria for headache disorders, cranial neuralgias and facial pain. Cephalalgia 1988;8(Suppl 7):1–96.

Lance JW, Curran DA. Treatment of chronic tension headache. Lancet 1964;1:1236–9.

Littlewood J, Prasad A, Gibb C, et al. Psychiatric morbidity, platelet monoamine oxidase and tribulin output in headache. Psychiatry Res 1989;30:95–102.

Mahloudji M. Prevention of migraine. BMJ 1969;1:182–3.

Martin MJ. Tension headache, a psychiatric study. Headache 1966;6:45–54.

Meltzer HY, Lowy MT. The serotonin hypothesis of depression. In: Meltzer HY, editor. Psychopharmacology: the third generation of progress. New York: Raven Press; 1987. p. 513–26.

Norman TR, Judd FK, Gregory M, et al. Platelet serotonin uptake in panic disorder. J Affect Disord 1986;11:69–72.

Pfaffenrath V, Kellhammer U, Pollman W. Combination headache: practical experience with a combination of a beta-blocker and an antidepressive. Cephalalgia 1986;6:25–31.

Schuckit M, Robins E, Feighner J, et al. Tricyclic antidepressants and monoamine oxidase inhibitors. Arch Gen Psychiatry 1971;24:509–14.

Stewart WF, Linet MS, Celentano DD, et al. Migraine headaches and panic attacks. Psychosom Med 1989;51:559–69.

Weissman MM, Leckman JF, Merikangas KR, et al. Depression and anxiety disorders in parents and children. Arch Gen Psychiatry 1984;41:845–52.

Wolff HG. Personality features and reaction of subjects with migraine. Arch Neurol Psychiatry 1937;37:895.

Editorial Comments

Dr. Diamond presents a case of migraine and depression. He overviews the historic, clinical, and putative biochemical and pharmacologic relationships between these disorders, and he makes many useful and insightful suggestions. He utilizes a complex polypharmacy which, although beneficial in his experience, is not recommended for the novice. Most doctors can begin with simpler approaches but for the difficult or intractable patient with these disorders, referral to a comprehensive headache or pain management clinic is advisable.

CHAPTER 12

THE PATIENT IN THE EMERGENCY ROOM: CASE 1

DAVID W. DODICK, MD, FRCPC, FACP

Case History

This 37-year-old married accountant and mother of two presented to the emergency room (ER) with a 2-day history of headache, nausea, and intractable vomiting. She had awoken 36 hours previously with a moderately severe, throbbing, bifrontal headache which escalated in intensity as she began to move around. The headache was associated with nausea, recurrent emesis, unusual light and sound sensitivity, and severe throbbing headache exacerbations with even minimal head movement. Only vomiting and remaining absolutely still provided her with mild amelioration of the pain. She denied having neck stiffness or focal neurologic symptoms during the course of this headache.

She had immediately taken an ergotamine/caffeine suppositories and an extra-strength acetaminophen tablet but her nausea and headache continued to worsen. She then tried various analgesics which she had at her disposal, including acetaminophen with codeine, naproxen sodium, and metoclopramide but was afforded little pain relief. She remained as still as possible for the next 36 hours except for quick dashes to the lavatory to vomit. She had been unable to keep food or fluids down and was in fact anorexic and repelled by the odor or even the thought of food.

This patient began having headaches at the age of 13, around the time of menarche. Her headaches were episodic for several years, occurring perhaps only three to five times per year. During her twen-

ties, she had very infrequent headaches but after the birth of her second child at the age of 31, her headaches began to assume a periodicity of two to four headaches per month with a prolonged headache invariably occurring at the time of her menses. She had a thorough evaluation at that time and had a normal computed tomography scan of the brain. She was diagnosed with migraine and treated with various abortive agents, as listed above. One or more of these in combination would often relieve her headache within 3 to 4 hours, except for those headaches that were present upon awakening. These often proved refractory to her usual remedies and perhaps once every 3 months, a visit to the ER would be required for an injection of a parenteral opioid (narcotic) and antiemetic.

She attributed this headache to sleep deprivation and the stress of tax deadlines. She is in good health otherwise, takes only multivitamins, and has no allergies. She is a nonsmoker and cannot drink alcohol because it is a potent trigger for her headaches. A general and neurologic review of systems was remarkable for orthostatic lightheadedness. Family history is noteworthy for migraine in both her sister and mother.

The general examination was significant for prostration; blood pressure 100/60 supine, 80/40 standing; pulse, 94 beats per minute and regular supine, 110 standing; and temperature 37°C. She was in obvious discomfort and preferred to be in darkness. A neurologic examination was normal. Her fundi were well visualized with normal spontaneous venous pulsations, her neck was supple but there was mild tenderness over the posterior skull base and cervical paraspinal muscles, and she had diffuse but symmetric hyperreflexia.

Questions about This Case

- What is the diagnosis?
- Are there differential diagnostic considerations in this particular case?
- What are the historical and/or physical findings which should raise red flags and necessitate further investigation in a patient presenting to the ER with headache?
- Are any ominous features present in this patient from the information provided?
- How would you manage this patient?
- Do you have any final recommendations before the patient leaves the ER?

Case Discussion

The diagnosis of this particular headache is migraine. Indeed, the question seems rhetorical, self-evident, and almost redundant. However, the importance of an accurate diagnosis, particularly in a patient with a prior history of migraine, cannot be overemphasized. It is precisely this type of case which engenders diagnostic complacency and has led to many unfortunate outcomes. It is not the purpose of this discussion to consider the differential diagnosis of headache in a migraineur presenting to the ER. It is, however, critical to review the process of how the diagnosis is confidently made. An accurate diagnosis will ensure that sinister mimics are not overlooked and that treatment is not delayed by ordering unnecessary diagnostic tests. Not only can serious causes for headache present with features strikingly similar to those of migraine, but conditions such as meningitis and subarachnoid hemorrhage may respond to specific antimigraine therapy with medications such as dihydroergotamine or a triptan.

The diagnosis is made by ascertaining a careful history of the characteristics of past headaches in order to make a relative comparison to the features of the current headache and by methodically eliminating historic features and physical findings which might reflect an organic cause.

The history of prior headaches must take into account the age of onset, the approximate frequency and evolution over time, the associated features which are typical of an individual attack, and perhaps most importantly, the time from onset to peak headache intensity. The various treatments used in the past as well as an approximation of their effectiveness must also be outlined. Only after this background information is obtained can the clinical profile of the patient's current headache provide meaningful diagnostic information. Migraine is well known to vary from one headache to the next in terms of severity, duration, and response to medication. However, the similar mode of onset and associated features between individual headaches are relatively consistent.

Therefore, there is always a differential diagnosis for any patient with a headache presenting to the ER, irrespective of their prior history of headache. The patient arriving in the ER with the chief complaint of headache does so because the headache is
- the worst ever,
- the first ever,
- different from the rest, and
- typical of previous headaches, but refractory to typical remedies.

If it is the worst (unusually severe) or first-ever headache, even if it resembles a migrainous headache, further investigations are obligatory to exclude sinister intracranial causes such as subarachnoid hemorrhage, meningitis, encephalitis, raised intracranial pressure, stroke, arterial dissection, and venous sinus thrombosis.

The following "red flag" features should be part of every headache inquiry since the cost of mistaking these deleterious headaches for another migraine or "sinus" headache can be devastating:
- Abrupt (split-second or "thunderclap") onset
- Subacute or progressive headache over days to months
- Headache associated with nausea, vomiting, and fever which is not explained by a systemic illness
- New onset headache in adult life (>40 years), or a significant change in a longstanding headache problem

- Headache which is precipitated by a Valsalva maneuver (cough, sneeze, bending, straining, position change, head turning), exercise, and sexual intercourse
- Nocturnal or early morning headache
- Headache associated with symptoms/signs suggestive of temporal arteritis (scalp sensitivity, jaw claudication, fever, myalgias, chills, sweats, weight loss, tender/pulseless temporal artery, transient visual loss, middle age)
- Headache associated with neurologic signs or symptoms such as confusion, decreased level of consciousness, alertness, or cognition, meningismus, or papilledema. These features may be observed or mentioned by others (family members) or may be so subtle as to be overlooked.

Once these sinister features have been eliminated, the patient will invariably turn out to have migraine. Tension-type headaches, although more prevalent in the general population, are rarely of sufficient intensity to require emergency attention. Cluster headaches, although perhaps the most severe of all primary headache disorders, seldom present to the ER because of their brevity (<180 minutes). Their features are also distinctive enough to rarely cause diagnostic confusion.

This patient clearly has a long history of migraine attacks which began at menarche but have become increasingly frequent since her early thirties. The attacks are triggered by menses, sleep deprivation, stress, and alcohol and are usually relieved with specific abortive agents and antiemetics. This particular headache is atypical of the majority in that it is refractory to her usual remedies and was present upon awakening. However, similar morning headaches have proved refractory in the past for this patient and have necessitated visits to the ER for parenteral opioid injections. A migraine attack is more likely to be refractory to the individual's usual remedies if the attack is already present upon awakening, as in our patient. This early morning headache should be differentiated from the acute nocturnal headache which awakens a patient from sleep. This type of headache, particularly if it is not typical of an individual's previous migraine attacks, is a cause for concern and warrants further investigation.

This headache gradually intensified with movement, was associated with nausea, vomiting, photophobia, phonophobia, osmophobia, and anorexia, and possibly was generated by stress and sleep deprivation. These features are typical of migraine in general but, more importantly, are typical of this patient's migraine attacks. The location of the headache is also important. Migraine is often thought by definition to be unilateral, and indeed, being unilateral is one of the International Headache Society's (IHS) diagnostic criteria. However, up to one-third of migraineurs will complain of bilateral (often bifrontal or bitemporal) headaches. Migraine location is usually consistent within each individual so that a sudden side to side change or a unilateral headache in a migraineur whose headaches are typically bilateral may warrant further investigation. This patient's neurologic and systemic review of systems and examination were benign except for postural hypotension which almost certainly is due to volume depletion secondary to the decreased oral intake and recurrent emesis.

The treatment of an acute attack of migraine is a decision upon which several variables will influence the choice of drug therapy. Treatment will depend on both the severity and the duration of the attack, as well as the time during the attack when treatment is initiated. Treatment should also consider the patient's prior response to various therapies' specific contraindications, the most disabling symptoms of the attack, efficacy versus side effects, convenience, cost, and appropriate route of administration.

In general, patients who arrive in the emergency department with migraine have almost always made failed attempts to alleviate the pain and nausea with their usual medications and will usually require parenteral medication. Although most patients with an acute uncomplicated attack of migraine can be given adequate relief in the course of a relatively brief stay in the ER, a minority will be acutely ill and require admission to hospital. The guiding principals of treatment, however, will remain the same and should include the following:

- General measures: vital signs, electrocardiography, electrolytes, discontinue potentially offending medications

- Reassurance and rest in a quiet darkened room, if possible
- Replace fluids and electrolytes, if necessary
- Treat nausea, vomiting, and diarrhea
- Treat agitation and anxiety, if necessary
- Implement acute parenteral pain management
- Start with nonhabituating medications, whenever possible
- Use an adequate dose of analgesic

This patient should be sequestered in a private area with as little ambient light and noise as possible, reassured that the headache is migraine, and that effective therapy is available and relief is inevitable. She should be rehydrated with 500 cc normal saline, and the nausea and vomiting treated with an antiemetic. In this particular case, several attempts with metoclopramide at home had failed. I would use an antiemetic which, in addition to causing the desired sedation, might also alleviate the headache or at least potentiate the effect of more specific antimigraine drugs. Prochlorperazine, 5 to 10 mg IV (maximum concentration of 1 mg per mL and rate of 1 mg per minute), can provide prompt relief of headache and nausea. If no response or a suboptimal response is seen within 30 minutes, dihydroergotamine is given at a dose of 0.5 to 1.0 mg, depending on the patient's tolerance, by slow IV push, and repeated every 30 to 60 minutes until headache relief or 3 mg IV is given. The patient is observed in the ER for several hours before being dismissed with a family member or friend to ensure a safe return home.

The migraine sufferer who arrives in the ER often has a long history of migraine with increasingly frequent attacks, deteriorating control of symptoms, and failed attempts at self-treatment with prescription and nonprescription measures. Therefore, once the acute attack is terminated, outpatient referral to a physician with expertise in the long-term management of headaches is essential. Implementation of preventive measures including migraine prophylaxis, appropriate use of outpatient symptomatic therapies, and instruction and education of the patient and family members in the use of treatments and self-help measures will improve their overall control and prognosis, and will help them avoid future visits to the ER and subsequent hospitalizations.

The decision to make a referral to a specialist will depend upon the practitioner's familiarity and comfort with migraine management. The following guidelines are useful in deciding to refer:
- When the diagnosis is suspect
- Warning or "red flag" signals are present
- Migraine attacks are occurring with a frequency or duration sufficient to impair the patient's quality of life
- Headaches fail to respond to previously effective remedies
- The patient is in status migrainosus

Overview

Headache is a serious health burden with an estimated 95% of women and 91% of men experiencing headache within the last 12 months. About 2% of all emergency department visits are for a primary complaint of headache. Despite the assorted primary headache syndromes and various underlying organic disorders which may present with headache as a primary complaint, migraine accounts for over two-thirds of all headache complaints to the ER.

The approach to management will depend upon the nature of the patient's presentation which can be categorized into one of the following:
A. An acute, protracted migraine attack which is refractory to simple outpatient therapeutic maneuvers
B. Status migrainosus
C. A migraine attack which has punctuated a chronic daily headache which is part of a medication-induced/analgesic-rebound phenomenon or a transformed migraine pattern
D. Emotional decompensation or emotional/physical dependence upon analgesics and/or sedatives with "drug-seeking behavior"

The emergency department is not the appropriate venue in which to attempt to provide a solution to the often longstanding and complex problem presented by the latter two clinical scenarios. However, the ER physician can provide some relief of pain, vomiting, anxiety, and a brief sanctuary for the patient from the situation which may have precipitated the attack of headache and the ER visit. The most important strategy in patient management, however, is referral to an appropriate physician with expertise in the care of patients with chronic daily headache or analgesic dependence.

Emergency Room Treatment of an Acute Migraine Attack

These patients arrive in the emergency department because self-treatment with prescription or nonprescription measures has failed. The most appropriate treatment regimen will depend on individual patient circumstances such as medical comorbidities which contraindicate certain medications (e.g., triptans and ergots and ischemic heart disease), potentially dangerous medication interactions (e.g., dihydroergotamine [DHE] and triptans; meperidine and monoamine oxidase [MAO] inhibitors; ergots and macrolide antibiotics), efficacy versus side effects, and previous adverse reactions to certain medications.

When initial therapy is ineffective, or the migraine attack is associated with significant disability, serotonin agonists should be considered. Sumatriptan, a serotonin (5-HT 1B/1D) receptor agonist, is effective in about 60% (oral formulation) to 80% (subcutaneous administration) of migraine attacks. Although several triptans are now available for the acute treatment of migraine (zolmitriptan, naratriptan, rizatriptan), these are available as oral preparations. Subcutaneous administration is the preferred route of administration in the ER because of its rapid absorption and effectiveness, often providing relief within 20 minutes. Sumatriptan has also been reported to be effective in early morning migraine, a feature which would be of relevance to the patient discussed in this case as well as other migraineurs who habitually awaken with a severe early morning headache. The medication is generally well tolerated, with chest pressure and sensations of heaviness being the most common adverse effects. Nausea is often ameliorated after sumatriptan administration without the concomitant use of an antiemetic. Limitations to its use include expense and headache recurrence which occurs in approximately 40% of patients. Ischemic heart disease, uncontrolled hypertension, and pregnancy are contraindications to its use. Triptans should not be administered within 24 hours of receiving either ergotamine, DHE, or another triptan.

Dihydroergotamine can be an extremely useful agent in terminating a prolonged migraine attack. DHE can be given subcutaneously, intramuscularly, or intranasally but is more likely to be effective in an emergency setting if given intravenously. Since gastric emptying is often impaired in an acute migraine attack and the nausea and vomiting may at times be more disabling than the headache pain, it is wise to pretreat the patient with an antiemetic prior to DHE administration because of the risk of producing or exacerbating nausea. Intravenous access is established with a butterfly needle and kept open with 500 mL of 5% dextrose in normal saline. Metoclopramide (10 mg) is given intravenously 10 minutes prior to the DHE injection. Promethazine, available in tablet, liquid, suppository, and injectable forms (25 to 50 mg), is also useful for the control of nausea and vomiting but, unlike metoclopramide, does not promote gastric emptying. DHE is then administered intravenously at a dose of 0.5 to 1.0 mg slowly over 3 to 5 minutes. DHE can also be mixed in the same syringe with 3.5 to 5.0 mg of prochlorperazine, diluted to 3 cc with normal saline, and injected over 3 to 5 minutes. Either of these regimens can be repeated in 1 hour if suboptimal relief is obtained after the first injection, and a maximum of three injections within a 24 hour period may be used.

Common side effects of DHE are nausea, vomiting, diarrhea, abdominal cramps, and leg pain. Diarrhea can be ameliorated with diphenoxylate. Nausea and vomiting can often be prevented with antiemetics, and leg and abdominal cramps can be eliminated with reductions in the dosage. The drug should not be used in patients with a history of Prinzmetal's angina, ischemic heart disease, or during pregnancy. It should never be combined with sumatriptan.

Controlled studies have shown that intravenous chlorpromazine and prochlorperazine are effective in terminating an intractable migraine attack (Appendix 12–1). Prior to neuroleptic therapy, the patient must be cautioned about the possible side effects of hypotension, akathisia and/or acute extrapyramidal reactions, and sedation. Necessary precautions must therefore be taken to avoid these by administering 250 to 500 cc of 5% dextrose in normal saline, mixing the neuroleptic with 25 mg of diphenhydramine or have 1 mg of benztropine available for intramuscular (IM) injection, and observing the patient for several hours or overnight in the ER. It is especially important that the patient be prohibited from operating a motor vehicle for the next 24 hours.

Droperidol, a butyrophenone with strong neuroleptic and antiemetic properties, has also been shown to be highly effective for treating refractory migraine and status migrainosus. After adequate hydration, droperidol can be administered as a 2.5 mg dose intravenous push for 1 minute every 30 minutes until either a total of three doses has been given or the patient becomes almost or completely headache free.

Unfortunately, despite these effective and widely available treatment regimens, opioid therapy is the most frequent treatment in headache patients presenting to the emergency department and is an especially common treatment in migraineurs. Unfortunately, opioids do not address the underlying pathophysiology, often provide suboptimal relief of pain and nausea, and may set in motion a cascade of increasingly frequent ER visits and the ultimate application of a stigmatizing label—"drug-seeker." The administration of meperidine in some patients with infrequent severe migraine attacks may, however, be the most effective regimen, but the treating physician must know the patient well and be acutely aware of potentially dangerous drug interactions (MAO inhibitors). If meperidine is used, it must be given at an adequate dose intramuscularly or intravenously (75 to 100 mg), administered with an antiemetic (metoclopramide 10 mg, promethazine 50 mg, or prochlorperazine 10 mg), and the patient observed for several hours and prohibited from driving home.

Ketorolac, an injectable nonsteroidal anti-inflammatory drug (NSAID), can also be useful in some migraineurs during an acute severe migraine attack. The drug is administered as a 30 to 60 mg IM injection, premedicated with an antiemetic as listed above. The existence of renal insufficiency and the potential for gastrointestinal side effects including hemorrhage should be considered in each patient prior to administration.

Status Migrainosus

Status migrainosus is defined by the IHS as an attack of migraine, the headache phase of which lasts in excess of 72 hours, whether or not treatment is initiated. The headache is either continuous or interrupted by headache-free intervals lasting no longer than 4 hours. The provocative factors for this syndrome are usually nonspecific but may include stress, depression, diet, hormonal factors, and medication abuse. Patients suffering from migraine status have invariably made failed attempts at treatment with multiple medications and are often suffering from severe prostration and dehydration as a result of vomiting and reduced oral intake of fluids. If initial ER treatment as outlined results in significant relief from pain and vomiting, the patient may be managed as an outpatient. Usually, however, a brief hospital admission is required for pain control, rehydration, and relief of nausea and vomiting.

Repetitive intravenous DHE has enjoyed the most success as a means to terminate a truly intractable migraine attack or migraine status. Raskin found that repetitive DHE was effective in eliminating chronic intractable headache within 48 hours in 89% of patients. This method of administration has also been found to be effective in terminating an acute cluster headache and chronic daily headache with or without analgesic rebound.

Figure 12–1 outlines a DHE/metoclopramide protocol, which consists of 0.3 to 1.0 mg of DHE plus 10 mg of metoclopramide in 50 mL of normal saline, infused over 20 to 30 minutes every 8 hours for a total of 2 days. Some patients may be treated for up to 3 to 5 days, if needed. To ensure stability, DHE or DHE/metoclopramide should be diluted in normal saline just prior to administration. Recently, continuous DHE therapy has been shown to have comparable efficacy to repetitive DHE treatment. A 3 mg dose of DHE is mixed in 1 liter of normal saline and infused intravenously at a rate of 42 mL per hour, with adjustments made in the rate of delivery (21 to 30 mL per hour) depending on side effects (nausea, diarrhea), and metoclopramide, 10 mg, infused IV in 50 mL of normal saline over 30 minutes, every 8 hours or on an as-needed basis for nausea for up to six doses.

In those for whom DHE is contraindicated, ineffective, or not tolerated, repetitive intravenous use of chlorpromazine (12.5 mg) or prochlorperazine (5 to 10 mg) infused slowly over 20 to 30 minutes, given every 6 hours for up to 2 days, may be effective in intractable cases.

Corticosteroids can be a useful rescue or adjunctive treatment but should be employed as a "last resort" because of the potential for serious adverse events such as avascular necrosis of the femoral head. Parenteral administration of corticosteroids such as dexamethasone (4 to 20 mg), as a one-time dose, or methylprednisolone (250 mg) every 6 hours for 24 to 48 hours can be effective in aborting migraine status. Corticosteroids can also poten-

tiate the effect of other medications used for the treatment of migraine status as discussed above.

Summary

Prior to initiating treatment for migraine in the emergency department, it is critical that each individual headache be evaluated in the context of the patient's prior migraine attacks. In other words, the most important question is whether the headache which brings the patient to the ER is familiar to the patient from previous attacks. If the headache is unlike any headache experienced in the past, then further investigation is warranted. The practitioner must also remain alert to the possibility of sec-

Intravenous DHE Protocol

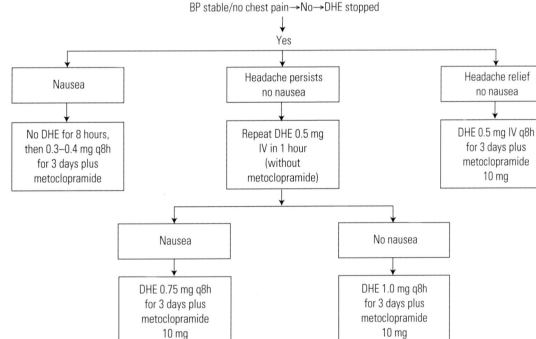

FIGURE 12–1. Inpatient DHE protocol for status migrainosus and refractory migraine. Caution: DHE must not be given to patients with the following conditions: pregnancy, history of ischemic disease, history of Prinzmetal's angina, severe peripheral vascular disease, or onset of chest pain following administration of test dose, or within 24 hours of receiving sumatriptan. (From Raskin NH. Treatment of status migrainosus: the American experience. Headache 1990;30[Suppl 2]:550–3.)

ondary causes which may mimic a "vascular" headache, particularly when there is an established history of migraine. If the history is scrutinized, especially with reference to the abruptness of headache onset, associated symptoms, and "red flag" features, and the neurologic examination is normal, ominous headaches can be identified and the potential for catastrophe avoided.

In the emergency department, rest, reassurance, and rehydration are essential prerequisites to successful treatment. Specific therapy is directed toward the relief of nausea, vomiting, and pain. Antiemetics (metoclopramide/ neuroleptics), often combined with serotonin agonists (triptans/DHE), are delivered parenterally and represent the treatments of choice. Injectable NSAIDs (ketorolac), parenteral opioids, or parenteral corticosteroids can provide useful adjunctive therapy in treatment-resistant cases but the routine use of these medications should be avoided. Patients can often be managed and observed for a brief period in the ER, but for those who are refractory to initial attempts at therapy or are already in status migrainosus, inpatient treatment for up to 3 to 5 days may be required. The final step in the management of these patients is referral to a physician with expertise in the long-term management of headaches.

Selected Readings

Edmeads J. Emergency management of headache. Headache 1988;28:675–9.

Ferrari MD, and the Subcutaneous Sumatriptan International Study Group. Treatment of migraine attacks with sumatriptan. N Engl J Med 1991;325:316–21.

Ford RG, Ford KT. Continuous intravenous dihydroergotamine in the treatment of intractable headache. Headache 1997; 37:129–36.

Gallagher MR. Emergency treatment of intractable migraine. Headache 1986;26:74–5.

Jones J, Sklar D, Dougherty J, White W. Randomized double-blind trial of intravenous prochlorperazine for the treatment of acute headache. JAMA 1989;261:1174–85.

Lane PL, Ross R. Intravenous chlorpromazine—preliminary results in acute migraine. Headache 1985;25:302–4.

Raskin NH. Treatment of status migrainosus: the American experience. Headache 1990;30(Suppl 2):550–3.

Saddah HA. Abortive headache therapy in the office with intravenous dihydroergotamine plus prochlorperazine. Headache 1992;32:143–6.

Silberstein SD. Evaluation and emergency treatment of headache. Headache 1992;32:396–407.

Wang SJ, Silberstein SD, Young WD. Droperidol treatment of status migrainosus and refractory migraine. Headache 1997;37:377–82.

Editorial Comments

This case and discussion by Dr. Dodick presents a comprehensive and excellent review of the clinical features and management options for migraine patients in the emergency room and beyond. As emphasized, correct diagnosis is essential, but when established, management options are several and must be individualized. Caution in the use of neuroleptics is always advised, as is the overuse of opioids, but it is hoped that newer efficacious medications will prove safe and beneficial in this setting.

Appendix 12–1

Initial emergency room treatment:

1. Sumatriptan 6 mg subcutaneously. If this has failed in the past, or is not effective after 30 minutes from administration, or is contraindicated, or not available, then

2. Metoclopramide 10 mg IV/IM (direct IV over at least 1–2 minutes or in 50 mL of compatible diluent over 15 minutes), or

3. Prochlorperazine 5 to 10 mg IV/IM (maximum IV concentration of 1 mg per mL and rate of 1 mg per minute), or

4. Chlorpromazine 1 mg per kg or 0.1 mg per kg IV (or 10 mg IV) diluted in 50 mL of normal saline (maximum concentration 1 mg per mL) and given slowly at a rate of 1 mg per minute (may be repeated every 15 to 30 minutes for up to 3 doses or 30 mg total), then

5. DHE 0.5 to 1.0 mg IV (slow IV push over 3 to 5 minutes) with repeat doses every 30 to 60 minutes, as required, up to a maximum of 3 mg IV per 24-hour period.

6. Droperidol 2.5 mg IV over 1 minute every 30 minutes until headache free or three doses given.

Other options include:
- IM/IV opioid (meperidine) plus an antiemetic
- IM NSAID (ketorolac)
- IM/IV dexamethasone

Inpatient Management

1. Dihydroergotamine (repetitive or continuous IV administration) plus antiemetic (see Figure 12–1)
2. Parenteral neuroleptic protocol
3. Parenteral corticosteroids

THE MAN WITH DAILY HEADACHES

DAVID KUDROW, MD

Case History

The patient is a 42-year-old attorney who came into the office with the chief complaint of excruciating headaches that have been occurring with remarkable regularity for the past 3 weeks. The frequency of headaches has been one to three times per day with at least one of the attacks occurring in the middle of the night, awakening him from a "dead sleep."

Three weeks ago, when the headaches began, they were more sporadic and less severe but within a few days each attack had become unbearable. He indicates that the pain is located always on the same side of the head, in this case on the left. It is centered behind the eye, above the eye, slightly frontal, and temporal and at times even seems to involve the preauricular area and the zygomatic region. There is also an ipsilateral occipital component. The pain builds rapidly and is described as a constant, non-throbbing, boring type of pain that feels as though a stake is being driven directly through the center of his eye. He must stop what he is doing and "escape" from the pain. His need is to be left alone in a closed room. Unable to lie still, he paces or rocks to and fro. He has even put his fist through the door in desperation.

Accompanying the severe pain is a profuse tearing from the left eye and an uncontrollable rush of watery mucus from the left nostril. He has observed a slight redness of the eye and a slight drooping of the left eyelid and a smaller pupil on the left side

while looking at himself in the mirror in the midst of his headache. Rarely does he experience nausea during an attack, though there may be some photophobia. His wife who accompanies him to the clinic notes that there is nothing she can do to help. She recalls that his reaction to her entering the room to offer moral support was similar to her reaction to him when she was in labor. Finally, the pain relents after about 60 minutes and it rapidly diminishes. He is left with a slight soreness over the area affected by the headache.

His past medical history is unremarkable except for prior episodes of these headaches that first began at the age of 28 while in his last year of law school. They would occur seemingly twice per year, lasting 6 to 8 weeks at a time and oddly enough around the fall and spring. He had been to several doctors, none of whom seemed concerned and all of whom prescribed various pain killers with little or no success. On one visit to the emergency room he had been given oxygen with no improvement in his headache. He had stopped going to doctors 5 years before and he just dealt with the headaches with large amounts of over-the-counter medications with no measurable success.

He had been a 2-pack-per-day smoker until the age of 30 and since then has had no cigarettes. He was a heavy drinker of alcohol in college and a weekend drinker in law school. He rarely has any alcohol now. "Even the smell of alcohol" is enough to bring on a headache. There is a family history of migraine in his mother and one of his sisters.

His blood pressure is 130/82 and his general physical examination is normal. His neurologic examination is entirely normal except for a slight miosis on the left side and what may be a mild ptosis also on the left. He has not undergone any neuroimaging procedures.

Questions about This Case

- What is the diagnosis?
- Is the incidence related to age and sex?
- Identify the clinical characteristics.
- What is the differential diagnosis of this headache?
- What further diagnostic tests are needed for this patient?
- What is the treatment of this headache?
- What is the prognosis?

Case Discussion

Cluster headache is certainly one of the most recognizable syndromes in medicine due to its constancy in presentation and its features which include characteristic pain location and character, duration of attack, accompanying symptoms and most identifiably, its periodicity.

Definition

Cluster headache is a primary headache disorder of two major types, episodic and chronic. In the former, patients are beset by self-limiting periods of headache attacks. On average, such periods, called cluster periods, may last 1 to 3 months. This is followed by attack-free periods, called remissions, that have a usual duration of 6 months to 2 years.

Incidence Related to Age and Sex

This condition occurs in both sexes, but five times more frequently in males. The incidence of cluster headache in the general population is estimated at approximately 0.4%. Mean age of onset is approximately 30 years for episodic and 35 years for the chronic type.

Clinical Characteristics

The aforementioned case history is quite typical for episodic cluster headache. The patient's condition had its onset during his twenties while in law school. Cluster periods recurred twice yearly, each period lasting 6 to 8 weeks. At the age of 42, he presents with the worst cluster period yet. The earliest cluster periods are shorter in duration and the attacks are the least painful. As the condition matures, subsequent periods lengthen and the attacks become more severe.

As noted, attacks may often occur in the middle of the night. Many patients will be awakened about 1 to 2 hours after sleep onset in association with oxyhemoglobin desaturation, often during rapid eye movement (REM) sleep. The most frequent time of onset of an attack is while at rest, upon returning home from the day's work. Attacks may also occur at the same times of the day, and with uncanny precision among some patients.

The location of pain is consistent from patient to patient and from attack to attack. With an occasionally reported exception, headache attacks are always unilateral, affecting the eye, the supraorbital, and temporal regions. Many patients report that there is an occipital component as well. In the majority of patients and as exemplified by our 42-year-old attorney, the pain may last from 30 to 90 minutes. It is of exquisite intensity, of boring quality, nonpulsatile, and associated with ipsilateral lacrimation, rhinorrhea and/or nasal stuffiness, and conjunctival injection. In some patients, there may be a noticeable miosis and ptosis, and rarely, this may persist as a complication of this disorder. Importantly, what sets this syndrome apart from other headache disorders is that the headaches are discreet occurrences of relatively short duration followed by intervals of no headache until the next attack. Cluster headache tends to improve spontaneously in the sixth or seventh decade. Cluster attacks may become shorter, less frequent, and less severe, while cluster periods may become farther apart and shorter in duration.

During cluster periods, patients are particularly susceptible to substances such as alcohol, nitroglycerin, and histamine. Sometimes as little as 5 mL of alcohol can precipitate an attack. Sublingual nitroglycerin, as little as 0.4 mg, will with few exceptions provoke an attack during cluster periods. While cigarette smoking does not seem to affect attacks or the disorder in general, the prevalence of this habit, either current or in the past, among cluster patients far exceeds that of the general population, as does the use and abuse of alcohol.

Differential Diagnosis

PAROXYSMAL HEMICRANIAS

Few conditions mimic cluster headache as closely as paroxysmal hemicrania. This disorder differs from cluster headache in that the frequency of the attacks is greater (10 to 30 or more per day), while their duration is shorter (5 to 30 mins). The chronic type is more common than the episodic and it affects females more than the males. All other features, including associated autonomic signs and symptoms, are common to both disorders. The paroxysmal hemicranias are also distinguished by their absolute response to indomethacin.

RAEDER'S PARATRIGEMINAL SYNDROME

Features in common with cluster headache include severe ipsilateral supraorbital pain associated with a partial Horner's syndrome, often awakening the patient in the middle of the night; this condition may last from weeks to months. Unlike cluster headache, attacks may recur daily for only the first couple of weeks. Thereafter, pain is continuous becoming only dull in intensity.

TRIGEMINAL NEURALGIA

In this condition, the pain, while severe, has a different quality than that of cluster headache. It is lancinating or lightning-like. Also, it lasts only seconds and is often triggered by touching certain regions of the face. Further, attacks are not likely to occur in the middle of the night to awaken the patient. This disorder occurs among older people, with equal frequency in men and women.

TEMPORAL ARTERITIS

Its similarity to cluster headache is limited to the site of pain, which is most often unilateral and temporal. The pain, however, is constant. The involved artery on palpation may be nonpulsatile, tender, markedly firm and tortuous, particularly later in the course of the disease. One of the most consistent features of this disorder is jaw claudication upon chewing. The erythrocyte sedimentation rate is usually markedly elevated, and the finding of giant cells on temporal artery biopsy is diagnostic. Untreated, this condition may cause blindness.

Mechanisms of Cluster Headache

There appear to be three clinicopathologic phases to this disorder: failure of the central circadian and circannual pacemakers associated with autonomic nervous system impairment; impairment of chemoreceptor response to sustained hypoxemia; and trigeminal-vascular inflammatory responses involving several cranial nerve pathways and neuropeptides. These three phases are respectively associated with the cluster period, attack induction, and attack signs and symptoms.

Further Diagnostic Tests

In this particular case (our 42-year-old attorney), further studies are not necessary in view of his 14-year history of cluster headache, typical clinical presentation, and negative neurologic examination. It should be cautioned, however, that any unusual features or abnormal neurologic findings in an otherwise typical case may be an indication for imaging studies such as magnetic resonance imaging (MRI) and/or magnetic resonance angiography (MRA). Cluster headache, it should be noted, has been reported to result from intracranial disease, such as arteriovenous anomalies, aneurysms, and meningiomas. In these symptomatic cases, the site of structural abnormality is most often in the area of the ipsilateral cavernous sinus. Psychometric testing, while optional, may help define certain parameters that enable more precise treatment choices and serve as a baseline in the event of subsequent changes. In our clinic, the Minnesota Multiphasic Personality Inventory (MMPI) has served these purposes well.

Treatment

The treatment of cluster headache consists of avoidance and prophylactic and symptomatic management. Thus, patients are strongly advised that if they have not already noted, alcohol is to be avoided during cluster periods. They are further advised to avoid daytime naps, bursts of anger, and excessive physical activity as these may precipitate cluster attacks during the cluster period.

PROPHYLACTIC TREATMENT

The medications of choice for the prophylactic control of episodic cluster headache are verapamil, 80 mg four times a day, spread evenly over twenty-four hours, and ergotamine tartrate, 1 mg an hour before bedtime. Where daytime attacks are not sufficiently controlled, it may be necessary to increase verapamil use to five times a day. Attacks that continue to awaken the patient in the middle of the night may be prevented by an increase in the dose of ergotamine to 2 mg, an hour before bedtime.

Unlike the episodic type, significant resistance to treatment may occur in chronic cluster headache. In the event that the above regimen proves inadequate, even shortly after initiation of treatment, a triple therapy prophylactic regimen is recommended. This includes verapamil, ergotamine, and lithium carbonate, 300 mg. The last-named is to be taken twice daily at 8 AM and 5 PM, and may be increased to three times a day if necessary. If renal function is normal, blood lithium levels at the twice-daily dosage are unlikely to fall in the toxic range. Toxic levels are also unusual when the dosage is three times daily, but slight hand tremor is not uncommon. There appears to be little correlation of "therapeutic" blood levels with responsiveness to treatment. Further resistance to treatment may indicate replacement of either verapamil or lithium with divalproex sodium, up to 1500 mg per day in divided doses.

When patients are no longer having any cluster attacks and they feel that they are in a remission period or they have not had even a slight cluster attack for a period of a week, they may taper off the medications slowly, over several weeks.

When all attempts at medical control of cluster headache have failed, the surgical procedure of choice is radiofrequency trigeminal gangliolysis. Complications from this procedure may include sensory and secretomotor changes or anesthesia dolorosa. [*Editors' note: Other surgical procedures have shown some success in selected cases.*]

SYMPTOMATIC TREATMENT

Cluster headache attacks may be rapidly aborted with oxygen inhalation, 5-HT agonists, or dihydroergotamine. Intranasal 4% lidocaine has a variable success rate, but when successful, may abort an attack within 1 to 2 minutes.

A rapid-acting modality with no side effects is oxygen inhalation. When used properly it has been shown to abort 70% of cluster attacks in under 10 minutes, 80 to 90% within 15 minutes, and over 95% in 20 minutes. Its proper use is outlined below:

1. Equipment includes a standing or portable tank of 100% oxygen, facial mask, and flow regulator, all of which can be rented from medical suppliers.
2. Set flow rate at 7 L/min.
3. With mask loosely held to the face, the patient assumes a sitting position, facing the floor, with elbows on knees.
4. The patient breathes normally for 20 minutes or less, when the attack ends.

Sumatriptan, a 5-HT 1B/1D receptor agonist, is effective in the symptomatic treatment of cluster attacks. In a long-term study, over 95% of attacks were aborted within 15 minutes following the subcutaneous injection of 6 mg of sumatriptan. While side effects are common, they are reported to be transient and of mild to moderate intensity. Most importantly, this medication should be withheld in patients with coronary artery disease or those with significant cardiac risk factors.

Ergotamine tartrate, 0.5 mg by mouth, or dihydroergotamine, 1 mg intramuscularly or subcutaneously,are similarly effective in the acute treatment of cluster attacks. Nausea is the foremost side effect of these preparations, particularly with the former. Ergotamines are also contraindicated in the presence of coronary artery disease.

Intranasal lidocaine hydrochloride 4%, when effective, is the most rapid acting of all symptomatic treatment medications. Many attacks (or patients), however, are not responsive to this preparation. The successful delivery of lidocaine to the sphenopalatine ganglion requires a proper intranasal anatomy, correct positioning of the patient, and slow intranasal administration (in the supine position, the neck should be hyperextended and rotated toward the side of the headache). Unfortunately, these variables prevent a greater treatment success.

Selected Readings

Dimitriadou V, Henry P, Brochet B, et al. Cluster headache; ultrastructural evidence for mast cell degranulation and interaction with nerve fibers in the human temporal artery. Cephalalgia 1990;10:221–8.

Ekbom K. Lithium for cluster headache: review of the literature and preliminary results of long-term treatment. Headache 1981;21:132–9.

Ekbom K, Olivarius B. Chronic migrainous neuralgia-diagnostic and therapeutic aspects. Headache 1971;11: 97–101.

Ekbom K, Monstad I, Prusinski A, et al. The sumatriptan cluster headache study group. Long term acute treatment of cluster headache attacks with sumatriptan—an interim review. Cephalalgia 1993;13 Suppl 13:36.

Gabai IJ, Spierings ELH. Prophylactic treatment of cluster headache with verapamil. Headache 1989;29:167–8.

Gardner WJ, Sowell A, Dutlinger R. Resection of the greater superficial petrosal nerve in the treatment of unilateral headache. J Neurosurg 1947;4:105–14.

Hering R, Kuritzky A. Sodium valproate in the treatment of cluster headache: an open clinical trial. Cephalalgia 1989; 9:195–8.

Kudrow L. Cluster headache. Mechanisms and management. Oxford: Oxford University Press; 1980.

Kudrow L. Response of cluster headache attacks to oxygen inhalation. Headache 1981;21:1–4.

Kudrow L. A possible role of the carotid body in the pathogenesis of cluster headache. Cephalalgia 1983;3:241–7.

Kudrow L. Cluster headache. In: Goadsby PJ, Silberstein SD, editors. Blue book of practical neurology. Headache. Boston: Butterworth-Heinemann; 1997. p. 227–42.

Kudrow L, Kudrow DB. Association of sustained oxyhemoglobin desaturation and onset of cluster headache attacks. Headache 1990;30:474–80.

Kudrow L, McGinty DS, Phillips ER, Stevenson M. Sleep apnea in cluster headache. Cephalalgia 1984;4:33–8.

Moskowitz MA. The neurobiology of vascular headche pain. 1984;16:157–68.

Nappi G, Ferrari E, Polleri A, et al. Chronobiological study of cluster headache. Chronobiologica 1981;2:140.

Sachs JE. The role of the nervous intermedius in facial neuralgia. Report of four cases with observations on the pathways for taste, lacrimation and pain in the face. J Neurosurg 1968; 23:54–60.

Stowell A. Physiologic mechanisms and the treatment of histaminic or petrosal neuralgia. Headache 1970; 9:187–94.

Editorial Comments

Cluster headache represents one of the most easily identifiable primary headache disorders. It truly is a "suicide headache," as it has been called, but there are fairly effective therapies for it including the new triptans. Chronic cases are more difficult to manage. Dr. Kudrow's case makes all the major clinical issues regarding cluster headache clear and, importantly, he outlines differential diagnostic considerations, the need to avoid missing serious disorders, and many useful clinical pearls regarding management. The exact pathophysiology of this disorder eludes us at present but one suspects that a major breakthrough will come in the next few years.

CHAPTER 14

THE MAN WHOSE SEVERE HEADACHES WOULD NOT QUIT

J. KEITH CAMPBELL, MD, FRCP

Case History

When he was aged 26, just after he began to work as a newspaper reporter, the patient was awakened each night with a severe pain on the left side of his forehead and temple. The pain was so intense that he feared he would die if it persisted. He was forced to get out of bed and pace about. Putting several cubes of ice wrapped in a cloth against his left eye gave a little relief, but the pain quickly got worse and reached a peak of intensity after 10 minutes. Tears rolled from the left eye, and he could not breathe through the left side of his nose.

His wife was distraught at her husband's plight and her inability to help him. In fact, he pushed her away and retreated to the basement when she tried to comfort him.

After about half an hour of severe pain, which he described as a burning or tearing pain that made him fearful that his eye would "explode," he noticed a slight reduction in the pain. This was followed by several brief peaks of increased pain which, in turn, were followed by a sudden lessening of the pain, then complete relief. He felt exhausted and for a few minutes his nose ran copiously with a clear watery discharge. After a little while, he was able to return to bed and fall asleep. This drama was repeated almost every night for 5 weeks in the spring. During this time, he was fine during his waking hours except for one evening when he developed a similar attack shortly after drinking a beer with some of his

fellow reporters to celebrate his promotion to the "city desk." He was, at that time, not in the habit of drinking but his two-pack-a-day smoking habit worried his wife.

During the evening attack, she noted that her husband's left eye was very red and that he seemed to be unable to open the eye fully. On closer inspection, she noticed his pupils were different sizes. The right pupil looked dilated. He consulted his doctor about a week after the nightly headaches began. Noting nothing abnormal on examination and not getting a family history of headaches, nor any prior history of headaches, his doctor suggested that the painful attacks might be due to sinus problems, possibly due to allergies to pollen. He advised using a decongestant nasal spray before going to bed. The patient tried this, but the attacks continued. Several courses of antihistamines also failed.

After several visits, the physician advised a long-acting corticosteroid injection to treat the supposed allergies. He was given a shot of triamcinolone. That night he slept through until morning, and after several nights with mild pain, the attacks ceased. He remained well for the next few years but continued to smoke heavily and began to drink several cans of beer daily.

In the spring, 2 years later, the nightly attacks returned, only on this occasion, he noted he would get similar attacks during the evening. He also quickly realized that he would develop an attack shortly after drinking a beer. He stopped drinking, but the nightly attacks persisted. This time he studied the attacks in more detail and observed that he would be awakened about an hour and a half after going to bed, that the attacks lasted about 90 minutes, and that trying to remain in bed during the pain made it worse. Sitting, standing, or pacing seemed to be helpful. Acetaminophen, acetylsalicyclic acid, and other over-the-counter pain relievers seemed to help, but only after an hour. He had several attacks by day and by night. A triamcinolone injection gave relief for only about 5 nights. A course of antibiotics was ineffective. He requested a referral to a headache specialist but before the appointment, the attacks ceased. They had been present for 7 weeks. He did not keep the appointment. Similar attacks occurred in the fall of that year, in the spring of the next year, and then in the winter. On this occasion, he anxiously awaited relief after the, by now, characteristic 5 or 6 weeks. He was disappointed and alarmed when the attacks continued for almost 7 months. This was despite seeing a specialist and being tried on several medications including beta-blockers, antidepressants, lidocaine nose drops, various potent analgesics, and tablets containing ergotamine.

After a brief remission in the fall of that year, the attacks returned, with up to 6 in 24 hours. By the time he was referred to another specialist, he had been suffering daily attacks for almost 18 months. He was desperate and had several times begged his wife to shoot him when the pain was at its peak. He had lost his job, was depressed, and he and his wife were under great stress.

Questions about This Case

- What is the exact International Headache Society (IHS) classification of this headache pattern?
- Why are the attacks no longer coming in groups?
- What investigations should be made?
- Which of the medications mentioned in the vignette were unlikely to have been helpful?
- Does the beneficial response to triamcinolone confirm the suspicion of an underlying allergy?
- How would you manage this patient's headaches for the short and long terms?
- What is the likely natural history?

Case Discussion

Having the benefit of considering this patient's situation after several years have passed, it is easy to conclude that he began with typical episodic cluster headache which, over the course of a few years, changed to chronic cluster headache. This occurs in 10 to 15% of patients with the episodic form of the disease. In a very small percentage (1% or 2%), the chronic form develops from onset—so-called *primary* chronic cluster. Our patient switched from episodic cluster to *secondary* chronic cluster.

The description of his individual attacks includes most of the characteristic features of cluster headache—strictly unilateral attacks without side switch in any particular series of attacks, severe pain around the eye, with intensity peaking in 10 minutes and relief in 60 to 90 minutes. Other features typical of cluster headache include the restlessness, inability to remain in bed during the attack, a desire to be left alone, temporary relief from the application of intense cold, the seasonal attacks initially, and the nocturnal preponderance.

The associated autonomic symptoms are also typical: the injection of the conjunctiva, nasal obstruction due to vasodilatation of the mucosa with overflow of tears secondary to blockage of the nasolacrimal duct, and the ptosis and pupillary inequality typical of a partial Horner's syndrome.

Attacks triggered by alcohol, the history of heavy tobacco use, the fact that the patient is male, and attacks occurring about 90 minutes after going to bed are all typical of cluster headache.

Thus, the diagnosis of episodic cluster headache slowly switching to secondary chronic cluster is clear. The remote possibility of symptomatic cluster headache due to an intracranial lesion such as an arteriovenous malformation or other lesion around the cavernous sinus cannot be excluded without a neuroimaging study— preferably a magnetic resonance imaging (MRI) scan. Certainly, such a study is indicated for the chronic form of cluster headache even if the study is only obtained for reassurance that there is no potentially lethal intracranial cause. Blood tests, electroencephalography, cerebrospinal fluid analysis, and allergy tests are all unnecessary with a history as clear-cut as that presented here.

Sinus disease does not present in this fashion regardless of the underlying condition, be it allergic, infective, or structural. Similarly, temporomandibular joint dysfunction, dental disease, migraine, and other primary headaches are excluded by the periodicity, the presence of the autonomic manifestations, and the temporal profile. Angle-closure glaucoma can present with nocturnal eye pain, but the other features of cluster headache are generally absent— nevertheless, glaucoma should be excluded, especially in somewhat older patients.

With the clear-cut diagnosis of cluster headache, one would not expect any benefit from antidepressants, beta-blockers, oral analgesics, antibiotics, antihistamines, or decongestant nasal sprays. [*Editors' note: Vasoconstrictors occasionally terminate an attack acutely.*]

The apparent response to triamcinolone is not unexpected as corticosteroids almost always provide some protection against cluster headache, at least for the short term. The mechanism is not understood but is presumed to be due to their anti-inflammatory effect. The beneficial response does not suggest an allergic causation.

Ergotamine preparations, if appropriately used, can be beneficial in cluster headache (more on this later) but, in the chronic phase, dosage restrictions limit their usefulness.

The management of chronic cluster headache can be especially difficult as the agents used for prophylaxis are either not easily tolerated for prolonged use or are ineffective in many cases. The high frequency of the attacks often limits the usefulness of those few agents such as dihydroergotamine and sumatriptan, which are effective in shortening individual attacks, to occasional use for exceptionally severe attacks.

Despite the difficulty of treating chronic cluster headache, several prophylactic programs should be tried. These include the use of verapamil, lithium, methysergide, valproate, and even ergots (for limited periods).

Management Strategies

- After an imaging study to exclude the possibility of an intracranial lesion, the patient and his spouse were reassured that cluster headache, although extremely painful and debilitating, is a benign disorder.
- While there is no cure at present, symptomatic relief, and some degree of prophylaxis are available. This should be explained to the patient and spouse or other relatives.
- Avoidance of alcohol and smoking cessation should be encouraged.
- Prophylactic therapy with verapamil should be started after a general physical evaluation and electrocardiography.
- Symptomatic measures, such as the inhalation of oxygen at the onset of an attack, the use of nasal lidocaine drops, and the use of injectable serotonin agonists [dihydroergotamine mesylate (DHE) or sumatriptan], or other triptans by mouth or nasal spray, should be considered. A brief tapering course of corticosteroids may be tried as this occasionally provides temporary respite from the attacks while prophylactic agents are introduced.
- A period of inpatient management may be needed to "break" the pain cycle. Hospitalization can be combined with such options as intravenous DHE or short-term high-dose corticosteroids.
- Referral to a headache specialist should be undertaken if the attacks persist despite the appropriate use of both prophylactic and symptomatic measures.

Detailed Treatment Options

Essentially the same treatment strategies are used for both episodic and chronic cluster headache; however, the details and the expectations of success differ in these two manifestations of the same disorder. Chronic cluster headache tends to be much more resistant to modification by prophylactic programs.

Symptomatic Measures

These have been described in the previous chapter on episodic cluster headache and will not be repeated in detail.

To be of benefit, an abortive or symptomatic preparation has to be administered by a route which enables the drug to reach therapeutic levels very quickly as cluster headache peaks in intensity in 5 to 10 minutes and generally subsides in 45 to 90 minutes. Injectable preparations, nasal sprays, topically applied agents such as local anesthetics, and breathable oxygen are essentially the only useful options.

DIHYDROERGOTAMINE

Many patients are ready to try self-injected DHE, others have a spouse or another person give the injection. A subcutaneous or, preferably, intramuscular injection of DHE 0.5 to 1 mg will shorten most episodes of cluster headache and indeed provide some protection against a recurrent attack for 8 to 12 hours.

Unfortunately, the high frequency of attacks in many patients rapidly precludes using DHE for each and every attack as dosage limits are rapidly exceeded. However, it is a common clinical observation that cluster headache sufferers can tolerate much larger amounts of DHE and other ergots than migraineurs and almost never develop rebound headaches (of any type), nor do they readily develop the signs of early ergotism such as cold extremities, elevated blood pressure, or muscular cramps which often limit the use of these agents in migraine. For several weeks, two or three doses of DHE a day may be easily tolerated and very effective and can provide a period of control while a prophylactic program is introduced.

The nasal spray form of DHE recently approved for migraine may be a useful agent in cluster headache, but the same dosage concerns will apply.

SUMATRIPTAN

The injectable form of sumatriptan given as a 6-mg subcutaneous injection aborts cluster headache in an average of about 12 minutes, and, often, in less than 5 minutes. The short half-life of 2 hours does not provide significant protection against a further attack, but the rapid relief it provides is invaluable. The high cost and the recommended daily dosage limit of 2 injections restricts its widespread use in chronic cluster headache, but it is a useful agent for providing relief when an attack occurs in inconvenient circumstances. It should not be given in the same 24 hours as DHE. The nasal spray of sumatriptan should also be useful.

NASAL LIDOCAINE

Some have found this helpful. It can be prescribed as the 4% topical preparation and either sprayed into the nose on the painful side or, preferably, it can be dripped into the nose with the head tipped backwards and turned slightly to the affected side so as to try to trickle the local anesthetic to the posterior nasopharynx in the region of the sphenopalatine ganglion.

OXYGEN INHALATION

As described in the previous chapter, inhalation of oxygen at a flow rate of 6 to 8 liters per minute from a loose-fitting face mask will abort many attacks. There are no side effects of this inconvenient method of treatment. Many chronic suffers complain, however, that after some time, the oxygen only postpones the attack and they often prefer to get it over with so as to enter a short period during which they can sleep or get on with some other activity.

OPIOIDS

There is very little place for opioids in the treatment of cluster headache in view of the need for frequent doses and the requirement for an injectable form with a tremendous risk of addiction. The nasal spray of butorphanol has been used effectively, especially given the ease with which it may be administered, but this potent analgesic also has the risk of dependence and also has the disadvantage of causing drowsiness. Despite these reservations, there is a place for the occasional use of this preparation in selected patients.

Prophylactic Strategies

CORTICOSTERIODS

While not suitable for long-term prophylaxis, corticosteroids in moderately high doses will often give several weeks of relief from attacks of cluster headache. Such a break is very welcome to an individual who has been having one or more attacks day and night for months. The period of relief may allow re-establishment of a normal wake-sleep cycle which is often greatly disturbed in cluster headache. Overcoming sleep deprivation will occasionally seem to "break" the cluster so that the attacks do not return immediately once the corticosteroids are withdrawn.

ORAL PREDNISONE

A tapering course of prednisone by mouth can be used. For example, 80 mg as a single morning dose for 3 days followed by a 10 mg reduction in dose every fourth day is one such empiric regimen. If there is no medical contraindication, a repeat course can be tried. The side effects of corticosteroids are well known and the patient should be made aware of them including those that are unpredictable, such as aseptic necrosis of the femoral head.

TRIAMCINOLONE BY INJECTION

Sixty to 80 mg by intramuscular injection provides a decreasing blood level for 7 to 10 days and frequently provides a temporary respite from attacks of cluster headache. The precautions and side effects are those of any corticosteroid.

VERAPAMIL HYDROCHLORIDE

This calcium channel blocker, which is not approved for the treatment of cluster headache, has proved to be, arguably, the best prophylactic agent to date. Many patients who have failed other prophylactic programs respond to verapamil. Available as regular and sustained-release tablets, verapamil should be started at 240 mg per day, given as three doses of 80 mg of the regular tablets. The dose can be titrated upwards over several weeks to 360 mg daily. Some patients have only responded to larger doses, but the side effects of constipation, orthostatic hypotension, fatigue, and peripheral edema usually limit the dose to 360 mg per day. Heart block and bradycardia with hypotension are more potentially serious side effects.

In the prophylaxis of cluster headache, verapamil may not become effective for 2 to 3 weeks and, therefore, it is important to persist with this method of treatment for at least a month at full dosage before concluding that it is not effective. This latent period can be covered with the use of corticosteroids described above or, alternatively, with the use of regular doses of ergots as described below. If the attacks cease on verapamil, it is appropriate to continue it for 6 to 8 weeks before initiating a slow tapering of the dose to see if a remission has developed. Recurrence of the headaches as the dose is lowered or discontinued indicates that the patient is not in remission, and full-dose verapamil should be reinstituted. For some patients, long-term prophylaxis is appropriate even when they appear to be in a short remission. The past history of the individual is the best way to judge whether or not to discontinue verapamil.

The agents described under "Symptomatic Measures" are compatible with verapamil.

ERGOTS

While waiting for verapamil to become effective and for other periods of short-term prophylaxis, DHE and ergotamine tartrate can be used judiciously for prophylaxis. For example, 1 mg DHE by injection every 12 hours or 1 mg of ergotamine tartrate by mouth every 8 to 12 hours for several weeks can be effective. Signs of ergotism are rare but should be sought, and this treatment is obviously contraindicated by coronary or peripheral vascular insufficiency and uncontrolled hypertension.

A very useful ploy for patients having nightly attacks of cluster headache is the use of a rectal suppository of ergotamine tartrate 2 mg prior to going to bed. The use of prophylactic ergots precludes the use of sumatriptan for 24 hours but does not prohibit the abortive use of DHE.

METHYSERGIDE

If verapamil fails to provide relief or is contraindicated, or not tolerated, methysergide is an appropriate alternative. Available as 2-mg tablets, this agent can be an effective prophylactic in divided doses of 6 to 8 mg per day. It should be started slowly. One technique is to crush a single tablet and have the patient swallowall the fragments over the course of the first day. If tolerated, a single whole tablet can be tried the next day followed by a gradual increase to one tablet three or four times a day. It may take several days for the patient to feel the benefit. Occasionally, higher doses are required. High doses and the excessively rapid introduction of methysergide can lead to many transient side effects including altered mentation, hallucinations, and confusion as well as leg pains, cramps, and gastrointestinal upsets.

Because of the possibility of the development of fibrotic complications of methysergide, an electrocardiogram, chest radiograph, and serum creatinine should be obtained prior to treatment. It has been recommended to stop methysergide every 6 months for a "drug holiday" as a way of lessening the likelihood of fibrotic complications. There is little evidence to support this plan. The alternative is to continue the drug for as long as it is effective and as long as it is needed but to check for the complications by electrocardiography, chest radiography, heart auscultation, and computed tomography or MRI scan of the retroperitoneal spaces every 6 to 12 months. Tapering the dose every few months to see if a remission has developed is also appropriate. While methysergide is employed, great care must be taken if DHE or ergotamine tartrate are also employed. The physician should be aware that these agents are synergistic. Care should also be exercised if sumatriptan is used for similar, but less well-documented reasons.

Methysergide and verapamil can be combined if either is not fully effective when used singly.

LITHIUM CARBONATE

The next prophylactic medication to try is lithium. It is difficult to take, has a narrow therapeutic range, and needs careful monitoring.

Like most of the prophylactic agents, it should be started slowly and only after the renal function of the patient has been shown to be normal—by a serum creatinine estimation and urinalysis. The dose can be built up to 900 to 1200 mg per day, given as two or three divided doses depending on the actual preparation being employed; controlled-release preparations can be given twice a day. After 2 weeks, the trough serum lithium should be measured and the dose adjusted to achieve a serum concentration of approximately 0.6 to 1 mEq per L. Levels above 1.5 mEq per L are associated with increasing side effects including tremor, polyuria, thirst, and gastrointestinal disturbances. Thyroid and renal function should be monitored periodically and the serum lithium level measured monthly until the level is stable, and then less frequently. Although lithium can be an effective prophylactic treatment of chronic cluster headache, it is often poorly tolerated or only partially effective. It can be combined with the other prophylactic treatments and is compatible with DHE, sumatriptan, and ergotamine. As with other preventive treatments, it is appropriate to periodically taper the dose of a patient whose cluster headaches are completely controlled to see if they have gone into remission.

OTHER AGENTS

Indomethacin is very occasionally effective in cluster headache, but not as specifically as in chronic paroxysmal hemicrania. If indomethacin in doses of 50 mg three times a day is not effective in a week, it is unlikely to help and should be withdrawn.

Valproate (valproic acid or divalproex sodium) has been known to exert a prophylactic effect on episodic cluster headache but rarely helps in the chronic phase. If other treatments are ineffective, a trial of valproate in full anticonvulsant doses is reasonable.

There have been anecdotal reports of other drugs helping in chronic cluster headache, for example, clonidine, chlorpromazine, acetazolamide, and carbamazepine. The reports concern small numbers of patients and are generally uncontrolled.

The DHE protocol described by Raskin, as used for migraine, has been effective in breaking clusters of headache and should be tried if the prophylactic regimens already described are not helpful.

Surgical Options

For the absolutely medically resistant patient who is desperate for relief, the final consideration should be a surgical procedure on the trigeminal pathway on the affected side. The procedure that is most likely to be helpful is a radiofrequency thermocoagulation of the gasserian ganglion. The thermal lesion must be suitably placed to cause complete loss of sensation to all modalities in the ophthalmic division of the nerve. In two large series of patients so treated, relief was provided to 66% of cases. Anesthesia dolorosa, trigeminal motor weakness, damage to adjacent cranial nerves and other structures are all potential risks. Loss of the corneal reflex puts the eye at definite risk. Finally, despite sensory loss in the appropriate division, there is no guarantee that the pain of the cluster attack will not be felt. Despite these serious shortcomings, a trigeminal procedure can be very successful for several years or longer.

Selected Readings

Campbell JK. Diagnosis and treatment of cluster headache. J Pain Symptom Manage 1993;8:155–64.

Ekbom K, Sakai F. Cluster headache: management. In: Olesen J, Tfelt-Hansen P, Welch KMA, editors. The headaches. New York: Raven Press; 1993. p. 591–9.

Kudrow L. Cluster headache. In: Goadsby PJ, Silberstein SD, editors. Blue books of practical neurology: headache. Boston: Butterworth-Heinemann; 1997. p. 227–42.

Mather PJ, Silberstein SD, Schulman EA, Hopkins MM. The treatment of cluster headache with repetitive intravenous dihydroergotamine. Headache. 1991;31:525–32.

Mathew NT, Hurt W. Percutaneous radiofrequency trigeminal gangliorhizolysis in intractable cluster headache. Headache 1988;28:328–31.

Raskin NH. Repetitive intravenous dihydroergotamine as therapy for intractable migraine. Neurology 1986;36:995–7.

Editorial Comments

As a unique headache disorder, cluster headache requires special attention. Diagnosis is relatively easy if the clinical profile is typical, yet differential diagnoses are always necessary, as are occasional investigations. Dr. Campbell outlines excellent diagnostic and treatment strategies in his discussion of this case. He discusses various management options for all types of cluster headache, identifying the problem areas and reasonable therapeutic options.

Further, it is noteworthy that intranasal capsaicin has been helpful in some patients in decreasing headaches when used daily as a preventive medicine. As well, a recent report describes a small number of people who have benefited from gamma knife surgery of the root entry zone of the ipsilateral trigeminal nerve.

CHAPTER 15

THE MAN WITH NEVER-ENDING HEADACHES

LAWRENCE C. NEWMAN, MD

Case History

The patient is a 36-year-old man who reports an 8-year history of daily, constant headaches. The pain is described as a steady ache or squeezing sensation involving the forehead bilaterally, with radiation into the vertex and the occiput. When severe, the pain has a throbbing quality. The severity of the pain ranges from moderate to severe and tends to worsen as the day progresses. There is no worsening with activity. The patient reports pain upon awakening each morning but denies that he suffers from sleep disruption secondary to the headaches.

The headaches are associated with difficulty concentrating and irritability, but photophobia, phonophobia, nausea, and vomiting are not experienced. No identifiable triggers are noted. There is no family history of headache.

Over the years the patient has consulted with his internist, two neurologists, a dentist, and an allergist. He has been treated with a variety of medications including propranolol, amitriptyline, antihistamines, and decongestants, all without benefit. Trials of over-the-counter analgesics and prescription pain-relievers were unhelpful. The patient takes no medications at this time as, "They don't help, so why should I take anything?" Magnetic resonance imaging (MRI) of the brain, performed 1 year ago, was normal.

The patient's general medical and neurologic examinations are normal.

Questions about This Case

- What are your diagnostic considerations?
- What is your differential diagnosis?
- How would you manage this patient's headaches, and what specific therapies would you recommend?
- What long-term management strategies would you suggest for this patient?

Case Discussion

Approximately 35 to 40% of patients seeking treatment at a headache subspecialty center suffer from daily or near daily headaches. The classification of frequent severe headaches is controversial and has not yet been adequately addressed by the International Headache Society (IHS). Using the current IHS guidelines, our patient would receive the diagnosis of chronic tension-type headache (CTTH). These headaches, as reported by our patient, are typically described as a bilateral throbbing or pressure sensation of mild to moderate severity. The complete IHS criteria for CTTH may be found in Appendix 15–1.

Comparing our patient's symptoms with the IHS criteria, however, it becomes obvious that the diagnosis of CTTH is not adequate. The patient reported in this case describes daily bilateral headaches but complains at times of severe pain that has a throbbing quality. The presence of a throbbing component excludes CTTH using current IHS guidelines. Yet, throbbing pain, while characteristic of migraine, may occasionally be seen in tension-type headaches (TTHs). In clinical practice, the distinction between migraine and tension-type headaches may be difficult. Some investigators have suggested that TTHs may in fact represent two distinct headache syndromes; one would be a form of mild migraine and the other a headache disorder in which all features of migraine headache are absent. Employing that scenario, this patient would be diagnosed with the first form of TTH.

Although not recognized by the IHS, many clinicians prefer the term chronic daily headache (CDH) when referring to headache disorders that occur on a daily or near daily basis. Chronic daily headache represents a heterogeneous group of disorders. Epidemiologic studies suggest that these disorders are rare, affecting only 0.5% of the population, yet they account for the majority of patients consulting headache centers. [*Editors' note: Recent studies indicate the prevalence of these disorders is about 4% of the population.*] Silberstein et al. recently proposed revisions to the IHS criteria for these frequent headache disorders. In their system, CDH is divided into primary and secondary disorders. The primary subtypes are further classified by duration: those occurring for fewer than or more than 4 hours per day. Those headaches occurring on a daily basis with an average duration of more than 4 hours include transformed migraine (TM), CTTH, new daily persistent headache (NDPH), and hemicrania continua (HC). Each disorder may be subclassified depending on the presence or absence of medication overuse. Appendix 15–2 lists the IHS criteria revisions proposed by Silberstein et al.

As our patient has denied overusing symptomatic medications, the management of his headaches should be less complicated than it otherwise might have been. The majority of patients with CDH overuse symptomatic medications. This pattern of overuse by headache patients often induces "rebound headaches," whereby medication overuse leads to the development of CDH in patients prone

to episodic migraine or tension-type headaches. Interestingly, our patient has never experienced prior episodic headaches; instead he reports an 8-year history of daily, unrelenting headaches from the onset. Therefore, the diagnoses of transformed migraine and new daily persistent headaches have been excluded.

The management of CTTH without analgesic overuse is multifactorial. Factors that are imperative in the treatment of this disorder include a long-term commitment on the part of the patient and physician, an understanding that control of headache not a "cure" is the goal of treatment, and possibly a team approach.

Successful treatment depends in large part on establishing the correct diagnosis; secondary causes of CDH must always be excluded. Comorbid medical and psychiatric conditions, if present, must be identified and addressed. After a thorough history and examination, a simple explanation of the diagnosis and underlying pathogenesis of the patients' headache disorder should be presented. Terms attributing the disorder solely to stress or tension should be avoided. Most patients can be appropriately treated on an outpatient basis, although sometimes hospitalization is required.

The most efficacious treatment plans incorporate both pharmacologic and nonpharmacologic therapeutic modalities. Mood disturbances are common in patients suffering from daily headaches and need to be appropriately managed. When appropriate, stress management, relaxation techniques, biofeedback, and individual and family psychotherapy all have a role in treating CTTH. Occasionally, physical therapy (including hot and cold compresses, massage therapy, stretching, and nerve blocks) is employed.

Treatment strategies employing simple analgesics, either alone or combined with caffeine, i.e., butalbital, isometheptene, or codeine, and nonsteroidal anti-inflammatory agents (NSAIDs), are the mainstay of acute therapies. Limits must be set, and patients educated, regarding the potential for medication overuse leading to the development of "rebound" headaches. The choice of acute treatment depends upon the frequency and severity of the patient's headaches and the associated symptoms.

For patients complaining of mild to moderate pain, the use of simple analgesics including oral acetaminophen, or acetylsalicylic acid, nonsteroidal anti-inflammatory agents, or caffeine-containing medications often suffice. For more severe headaches or when the above agents are ineffective, it may be appropriate to use prescription medications such as the more potent NSAIDs (ketoprofen, naproxen, indomethacin, ketorolac), butalbital-containing medications, or the combination of acetaminophen, isometheptene, and dichloralphenazone. Once again, strict limits must be set as these agents are capable of producing "rebound headaches," and butalbital has a high addiction potential. If nausea is present, the concurrent use of an antiemetic (metoclopramide, chlorpromazine, or prochlorperazine) or suppository analgesic formulations (indomethacin) is useful.

Prophylactic therapy is warranted in patients in whom headache frequency is greater than twice weekly or when the duration of the headache exceeds 4 hours daily. Preventive therapy is also indicated to prevent overuse of symptomatic medications with subsequent "rebound" in patients with frequent headaches. The choice of preventive agent should take into account other comorbid conditions. Medications frequently prescribed for this condition include the tricyclic antidepressants, selective serotonin reuptake inhibitors (SSRIs), beta-blockers and calcium channel blockers, and anticonvulsants.

The tricyclic antidepressants amitriptyline, nortriptyline, desipramine, and doxepin are the most often prescribed. Dosages required are usually much lower than for depression. We generally begin with 10 to 25 mg at bedtime, gradually increasing the dose by 10 to 25 mg every week. Side effects include sedation, dry mouth, and weight gain.

The SSRIs are more easily tolerated than the tricyclic antidepressants and they too can be prescribed in lower doses than are required for depression. Commonly prescribed SSRIs include fluoxetine, paroxetine, and sertraline.

The typical "antimigraine" medications may also be used as preventive therapy for CTTH. The use of the beta-blockers propranolol and nadolol and the calcium channel blockers verapamil and diltiazem has been successful according to anecdotal evidence. The dosages employed are similar to those used for migraine. The antiseizure medication divalproex sodium also appears to be useful in the treatment of this disorder. The dosages used are similar to those for migraine. We generally begin with 125 mg, twice daily, and gradually increase to a maximum of 1250 mg per day in divided doses. Table 15–1 lists the commonly prescribed preventive medications.

The patient presented in the case report would not appear to have a secondary cause of CDH as his headaches are longstanding and without progression, his medical and neurologic examinations are normal, and a prior MRI of his brain was normal. He has not been overusing symptomatic medications that could induce headaches; in fact, he takes no medications as they do not help. Therefore, the issue of "rebound" does not come into play.

TABLE 15-1. Selected Prophylactic Medications for CDH

Class	Tricyclic	SSRI	Beta-Blocker	Calcium Channel Blocker	Antiseizure
Medication	Nortriptyline	Paroxetine	Nadolol	Verapamil	Divalproex sodium
Starting dosage (mg)	10–25	10	40	40–80	125–250
Effective dosage (mg)	25–125	10–30	40–120	240–360	500–1250
Contraindications	Urinary retention, glaucoma, cardiac conduction disturbances	Mania	Asthma, CHF, depression, Raynaud's disorder	Heart block, hypotension	Liver disease, bleeding disorders
Potential side effects	Sedation, weight gain, dry mouth	Sedation, weight gain	Sedation, depression, bradycardia	Constipation, bradycardia	GI upset, sedation, alopecia, tremor, liver enzyme abnormalities, platelet dysfunction

Although the patient reports having been treated with propranolol and amitriptyline, we are not told of the doses used or the length of time they were prescribed. All too commonly patients have been prescribed the correct medications but in inadequate doses. Additionally, many patients (or their physicians) prematurely discontinue treatment because of a perceived lack of efficacy. The full therapeutic effect of the preventive medications may take 2 to 6 months to be felt. Therefore, we need to inquire as to past doses and length of treatment. If the prior agents were discontinued prematurely or if subtherapeutic doses were employed, a second trial at an appropriate dosage may be useful.

The patient does not describe features of a mood disorder. If he did, using an SSRI or tricyclic would be helpful. I would probably begin therapy with nortriptyline or an SSRI such as paroxetine first. If there was no benefit after an appropriate trial, I would next consider divalproex sodium. Acute pain could be managed with a long-acting NSAID for milder attacks and isometheptene for more severe pain. Daily and weekly limits should be explained at the time of issuing the prescription. If psychologic issues are uncovered, psychotherapy, behavioral modification, and stress management should be employed.

If outpatient measures fail or are suboptimal, hospitalization for intravenous dihydroergotamine mesylate (DHE) may prove helpful. The DHE protocol has already been discussed in another chapter.

Management Strategies

- Exclude secondary causes of headache.
- Establish the correct diagnosis.
- Ensure analgesic overuse with subsequent "rebound" headache is not present.
- Identify comorbid medical and psychiatric conditions.
- Educate the patient regarding diagnosis and prognosis.
- Review prior medications; were dosing and duration of treatment adequate?
- Limit acute therapies, and match properties of agent to patient's symptoms.
- Begin trial of preventive agent, gradually increasing the dose to limit side effects.
- Continue therapy until therapeutic effects are obtained, side effects become intolerable, or the maximum dose has been attained.
- Employ nonpharmacologic therapies.
- Consider hospitalization for treatment-resistant patients.

Case Summary

- The patient is suffering from chronic tension-type headaches without analgesic overuse.
- The IHS criteria for daily severe headaches does not adequately address this issue.
- Clinically, tension-type headaches may have features of migraine.
- Alternative classifications of CDH have been proposed.
- There is no *best* treatment for this disorder; therapy should be guided by the individual patient profile.
- Management strategies are outlined and serve only as a guide.

Overview of Chronic Daily Headache

The International Headache Society divides tension-type headaches into episodic and chronic varieties. Tension-type headaches can last minutes to days. The pain is usually described as a squeezing or tightening sensation and is of mild to moderate intensity. Patients typically describe the headache as a tight band encircling the head or as a vise squeezing the skull. The pain is invariably bilateral and is not worsened by routine activity. The TTH begins at some point during the day and then increases in intensity as the day progresses; nocturnal awakening secondary to headache is uncommon and should prompt a search for an underlying pathology. The IHS guidelines allow for photophobia and phonophobia individually. Nausea, but not vomiting, is occasionally reported by patients with the chronic form. When headaches meeting these criteria occur more often than 15 days per month for more than 6 months, the IHS terms them chronic tension-type headaches.

Unfortunately, patients presenting to the physician with frequent headaches without any underlying pathology pose a diagnostic dilemma. Typically, patients with CDH are diagnosed as having CTTH using the current IHS guidelines. Newman et al., using data obtained from the American Migraine Study, reported that although 0.5% of the population suffer from severe daily headaches, only 3% meet IHS criteria for CTTH. Further complicating the issue, these daily headache sufferers account for the majority of patients consulting headache subspecialty clinics.

Recently, Silberstein et al. proposed new revisions to the IHS classification. Using their system, CDH is divided into primary and secondary varieties. The primary forms are further subdivided on the basis of average daily duration. According to this classification scheme, CDH with a duration of 4 hours or more per day include transformed migraine, CTTH, new daily persistent headache, and hemicrania continua.

Transformed migraine (TM) occurs in patients with a prior history of episodic migraine. Although the majority of sufferers of TM overuse analgesics or ergotamine-containing medications, a subset of migraineurs spontaneously "transform" without overusing medications. Over time, headache frequency increases so as to occur on a daily or near-daily basis, but as the frequency increases, the typically associated migrainous features lessen, and the headache more closely resembles CTTH. Nonetheless, headaches meeting the IHS criteria for migraine still sporadically occur.

According to this new classification, CTTH adds to the IHS criteria the requirements of either a past history of episodic TTH or the history of an evolving headache which gradually increased in frequency over a 3-month or longer period.

New daily persistent headache (NDPH), unlike CTTH or TM, occurs in patients without a prior history of headache. These patients usually report the abrupt onset of headache beginning over a period of fewer than 3 days and then continuing unabated. Many patients can recall the exact time and day the headache began; in some it may follow a viral illness. Although the characteristic features of NDPH are similar to CTTH, it is distinguished by the absence of a prior history of migraine or TTH.

Hemicrania continua is an uncommon headache disorder characterized by a continuous low-level baseline hemicranial headache with superimposed exacerbations of more severe pain. Exacerbations can last minutes to days and may be associated with the autonomic features of cluster headache. This disorder is uniquely responsive to treatment with indomethacin.

To date, the pathophysiology of CDH is uncertain. Recent evidence points to several putative mechanisms including defective pain modulation, abnormalities within the central pain pathways within the brain stem, and abnormal excitation of peripheral nociceptive fibers.

As CDH represents a heterogeneous group of disorders, treatment must be aimed at the specific headache disorder. Both pharmacologic and non-pharmacologic therapies should be employed, and analgesic overuse must be identified and discontinued. Outpatient strategies employing symptomatic medications and preventive agents combined with behavioral modification (as outlined above) are very useful, although occasionally hospitalization is required. Treatment outcome is generally quite good but requires commitment on the part of the patient and family. While no "cure" exists, it is possible to attain control of the headaches. Treatment failures or resistant cases should be referred to subspecialty centers for comprehensive treatment modalities.

Selected Readings

Featherstone HJ. Migraine and muscle contraction headaches: a continuum. Headache 1985;25:194–8.

Holroyd KA. Tension-type headache, cluster headache, and miscellaneous headaches: psychological and behavioural techniques. In: Olesen J, Tfelt-Hansen P, Welch KMA, editors. The headaches. New York: Raven Press; 1993. p. 515–20.

Newman LC, Lipton RB, Solomon S, Stewart WF. Daily headache in a population sample: results from the American Migraine Study. Headache 1994;34:295.

Sanin LC, Matthew NT, Bellmyer LR, Ali S. The International Headache Society (IHS) headache classification as applied to a headache clinic population. Cephalalgia 1994;14:443–6.

Saper JR. Chronic headache syndromes. Neurol Clin 1989;7: 387–412.

Silberstein SD, Lipton RB, Goadsby PJ. Headache in clinical practice. Oxford: Isis Medical Media; 1998.

Silberstein SD, Lipton RB, Solomon S, Matthew N. Classification of daily and near daily headaches: proposed revisions to the IHS classification. Headache 1994;34:17.

Vanast WJ. New daily persistent headaches: definition of a benign syndrome. Headache 1986;26:317.

Editorial Comments

What exactly is chronic daily headache (CDH)? Does it exist as a separate entity? It is extremely difficult to answer the preceding questions based on our current knowledge. However, the debate continues to find the answers and the concept of CDH has great clinical utility. Dr. Newman's case and discussion allow us to consider CDH in a clinical context. All headache physicians see numerous cases of this nature, and one can only hope that this entity will be ultimately defined in neurobiologic terms, allowing precise and definitive therapy to be applied.

Appendix 15–1
Classification of Headache, after the International Headache Society Classification, 1988

Chronic Tension-Type Headache

A. Average headache frequency >15 days/month (180 days/year) for >6 months fulfilling criteria (B–D)

B. At least two of the following pain characteristics:
   1. Pressing/tightening quality
   2. Mild or moderate severity (may inhibit but does not prohibit activity)
   3. Bilateral location
   4. No aggravation caused by walking up or down stairs or by similar routine physical activity

C. Both of the following:
   1. No vomiting
   2. No more than one of the following: nausea, photophobia, and phonophobia

D. No evidence of underlying disease

Appendix 15–2
Criteria for CDH, Proposed by Silberstein et al., 1994

Primary Headache (duration >4 hours)*

- Transformed migraine (TM)
- Chronic tension-type headache (CTTH)
- New daily persistent headache (NDPH)
- Hemicrania continua (HC)

Proposed Criteria for Transformed Migraine

A. Daily or almost daily (>15 days/month) head pain for >1 month

B. Average headache duration of >4 hours/day (if untreated)

C. At least one of the following:
   1. History of episodic migraine meeting any IHS criteria 1.1–1.6
   2. History of increasing headache frequency with decreasing severity of migrainous features over at least 3 months
   3. Headache at some time meets IHS criteria for migraine 1.1–1.6 other than for duration

D. Does not meet criteria for daily persistent headache or hemicrania continua

E. No evidence of underlying disease

Proposed Criteria for New Daily Persistent Headache

A. Average headache frequency >15 days/month for >1 month

B. Average headache duration >4 hours/day (if untreated); frequently constant without medication but may fluctuate

C. No history of tension-type headache or migraine which increases in frequency and decreases in severity in association with the onset of NDPH (over 3 months)

D. Acute onset (developing over >3 days) of constant unremitting headache

E. Headache is constant in location? (Needs to be tested)

F. Does not meet criteria for hemicrania continua

G. No evidence of underlying disease.

---

* May occur with or without medication overuse.

CHAPTER 16

THE WOMAN WITH DAILY HEADACHES

NINAN T. MATHEW, MD, FRCPC

Case History

The patient is a 44-year-old woman with frequent headaches that have been occurring for almost 6 days a week for the past 3 years. Some of the headaches are more severe than others. Severe headaches are predominantly one-sided, either on the left or the right. A headache can switch sides during the same attack or headache sites can be different during different attacks. The headaches are pulsating at times. At other times, the patient feels a pressure-like sensation. She also feels sharp, short-lived head pains in various areas of the head from time to time. The severe head pain lasts for a long time. It may subside to a degree only to have a low-grade nagging pain continuing almost constantly.

The headaches are associated with nausea and, when severe, vomiting. Bright light bothers her. Noise bothers her. She may sometimes become dizzy and there have been instances where she has had near syncopal episodes.

The patient started having headaches as a teenager. The headaches were fairly moderate to start with and they were occasional. They occurred when she was tired or when she missed sleep. In her early twenties, the headache became more frequent and more severe, occurring approximately once a month. In her early thirties, she started having three or four moderate to severe headaches a month and she also started having low-grade headache in between her

severe headaches. She was treated during that time with various medications, mostly pain medications. She would take over-the-counter medications which contained caffeine and aspirin for less severe headaches and codeine for the more severe headaches. By her late thirties, the headache frequency increased and she continued to take pain medications. By the age of 41, she was taking approximately six tablets of over-the-counter caffeine-containing medications and prescription medications which contained butalbital, caffeine, and aspirin with codeine three to four times a day. Since then, her headache continued in an intractable fashion. Between the ages of 39 and 43, she was prescribed various preventive medications including beta-blockers, calcium channel blockers, tricyclic antidepressants, and selective serotonin reuptake inhibitors. During the time that she was on prophylactic medications, she was also taking her pain medications daily. Her history also suggests that there was aggravation of the headache during menstrual times starting about a day or two before menstruation and continuing through the menstrual period.

There is a family history of migraine in her mother and grandmother, and one of her daughters.

She finds it very difficult to relax. She gets depressed and becomes very anxious. She has occasional crying spells. She has been under a lot of stress, both at work and at home. There have been some ongoing marital problems.

TABLE 16–1. Clinical Comparison of Transformed Migraine and Chronic Tension-Type Headache

Transformed Migraine	Chronic Tension-Type Headache
• Headache frequency >180 days/year	• Headache frequency >180 days/year
• Previous history of episodic migraine	• No history of distinct migraine
• Family history of migraine	• Family history of chronic tension-type headache
• Retains migraine features to a significant degree intermittently or continuously	• Migraine features are lacking
• Increased GI and neurologic symptoms	• No GI or neurologic symptoms
• Menstrual aggravation	• No particular menstrual aggravation
• Relief during pregnancy	• No change during pregnancy
• Excessive analgesic intake	• Excessive analgesic intake
• Responds to antimigraine therapy	• Response to antimigraine therapy is less striking
• Behavioral and psychologic comorbidity	• Behavioral and psychologic comorbidity present

Her caffeine intake is very high. She drinks about five cups of coffee a day plus about three or four diet sodas a day. She uses aspartame in her coffee.

A review of systems was negative. She is not hypertensive, diabetic, or hypercholesterolemic. There is no known thyroid disease. There is no other relevant illness. She has had a magnetic resonance imaging scan of the brain before, which was reported normal. On examination, no neurologic abnormality was found except for some tenderness of the suboccipital triangle and tightness of the neck muscles. There is no evidence of increased intracranial pressure or focal neurologic abnormality. A systemic examination, including the blood pressure, was normal. Her Beck Anxiety Scale was 25 which is above the normal scale, indicating moderate anxiety. The Beck Depression Scale was 32, indicating severe depression.

Questions about This Case

- What are your diagnostic considerations in this case?
- Why do you think the patient's headaches are getting worse?
- What is analgesic rebound?
- Do you wish to know more about this particular case; if so, what pertinent information would you like to know?
- How would you manage this patient's headache, and what specific therapies would you suggest? What long-term strategies would you suggest for her?

Case Discussion

At the time the patient presented to the physician, she had a history of daily or near daily headache. Some of the headaches were severe, unilateral, pulsating, associated with nausea, photophobia, and phonophobia, and she had had multiple episodes of such headaches prior to presentation. That type of severe headache fits in with the diagnosis of migraine without aura according to the International Headache Society (IHS) criteria. The low-grade headache she had was more diffuse, nondescript, nagging, without associated features such as nausea, photophobia, or phonophobia. There was neck muscle spasm and tenderness. Applying the IHS criteria, those headaches could be diagnosed as tension-type headache. But, the striking feature is that these tension-type headaches were extremely frequent occurring almost on a continuous basis. They could be also precipitated by situations that would precipitate her migraine. In other words, stress, wrong diet, lack of sleep, too much sleep, etc., could also bring on the second type of headache (tension-type headache).

The previous history is important in making a diagnosis in this case. From the case history, you can see a gradual progression in the frequency and severity of the patient's headaches until, in her late thirties, she developed chronic daily headache (CDH) in spite of taking pain medications frequently. The character of the headache in the initial years, particularly in her early twenties, was that of migraine. So, looking at the progression and the natural history of this disorder in this particular person, it appears that

TABLE 16–2. Proposed Criteria for Transformed Migraine*

A. Daily or almost daily (>15 days/month) head pain for 4 months
B. Average headache duration of 4 hours/day (if untreated)
C. At least one of the following:
   1. History of episodic migraine meeting any IHS criteria 1.1 to 1.6
   2. History of increasing headache frequency with decreasing severity of migrainous features over at least 3 months
   3. Current headache meets IHS criteria for migraine 1.1 to 1.6 other than duration
D. At least one of the following:
   1. There is no suggestion of one of the disorders listed in groups 5 to 11
   2. Such a disorder is suggested but it is ruled out by appropriate investigations
   3. Such a disorder is present, but first migraine attacks do not occur in close temporal relation to the disorder

*Silberstein SD, Lipton RB, Sliwinski M. Classification of daily and near daily headaches. Field trials of revised IHS criteria. Neurology 1996;47:871–5.

she has transformed migraine (TM). Migraine which started out as an occasional episodic phenomenon has now turned into a chronic persistent disorder. Transformed migraine is one of the major forms of chronic daily headache, the other form being chronic tension-type headache (CTTH). Table 16–1 shows the differences between CTTH and TM. Suggested criteria for the diagnosis of TM are given in Table 16–2. If one applies the IHS classification to this case, at least three separate diagnoses, namely, migraine without aura, chronic tension-type headache, and headache due to medication overdose, have to be made.

Multiple factors may be involved. In many patients with migraine, there is a natural progression of the disorder into a chronic state. This natural tendency for migraine to become chronic is probably enhanced by other transformational factors which include the excessive and frequent use of analgesics, particularly those which contain butalbital, analgesics, and caffeine, and ergotamine, comorbid conditions like anxiety, depression, and neuroticism, stress and inability to relax, hormonal factors which may play a part, dietary factors, and hypertension. This particular patient had many of these transformational factors. She was taking an ASA, butalbital, caffeine, and codeine preparation and an analgesic in large quantities for a long time on a daily basis. In spite of taking them daily, she continued to have headaches. We were able to document that she was depressed and anxious and was not able to relax, which also contributed to the problem. Her diet was also probably contributing to her headache because of her excessive intake of caffeine, aspartame, and chocolate. Her inability to relax and the stress also made her condition more persistent. So, the reason why the headaches are getting worse is multifactorial. One of the most prominent and most important and correctable causes is the excessive use of analgesics. In other words, she appears to have analgesic-rebound headache, which complicates the whole clinical picture.

"Analgesic-rebound headache" is a term which is often used to characterize the headache-perpetuating tendency when immediate-relief medications are used frequently.

There appears to be some confusion between the terms "recurrence" and "rebound." Recurrence may be defined as the return of the same headache, which was significantly relieved by an abortive antimigraine agent. Recurrence should take place within the expected natural duration of that migraine attack. Rebound headache, on the other hand, can be defined as the perpetuation of head pain in chronic headache sufferers, which is caused by frequent and excessive use of immediate-relief medication. It can also be defined as "a self-sustaining, rhythmic, headache-medication cycle characterized by daily or near-daily headache and irresistible and predictable use of immediate-relief medications as the only means of relieving headache attacks."

The most convincing evidence for analgesic or ergotamine rebound is the fact that mere discontinuation of these medications results in significant improvement. There are ample data in the literature to support the existence of analgesic or ergotamine-rebound headache. Silverman et al. reported that moderate or severe headache occurred in 52% of patients on caffeine withdrawal based on a double-blind cessation of caffeine consumption. In a recent survey of physicians engaged in the treatment of headache, more than 40% of the respondents (174) indicated that analgesic rebound is present in at least 20% of their patients with headache.

A number of clinical characteristics help us in identifying the occurrence of analgesic-rebound headache in patients with primary headache disorders. The following are the clinical features of analgesic rebound:

- The headache is refractory, daily, or near daily.
- It occurs in a patient with a primary headache disorder who uses immediate-relief medications very frequently, often in excessive quantities.
- The headache itself varies in its severity, type, and location from time to time.
- The slightest physical or mental effort will bring on the headaches. In other words, the threshold for head pain appears to be low.
- Headaches are accompanied by asthenia, nausea, restlessness, irritability, memory problems, difficulty in concentration, and depression.
- There is a drug-dependent rhythmicity to the headaches. Predictable early morning (2AM to 5AM) headaches are frequent, particularly in patients who use large quantities of analgesics, sedatives, caffeine, or ergotamine combinations.
- There is evidence of tolerance to analgesics over a period of time, so patients need increasing doses as time goes by.
- Withdrawal symptoms are observed when the patients are taken off pain medications abruptly.
- Spontaneous improvement of headache occurs on discontinuing the medications.
- Concomitant prophylactic medications are relatively ineffective while the patients are consuming large or excess amounts of immediate-relief medications.

Other important information would be to rule out any chronic organic conditions that would cause increasing headache. Idiopathic intracranial hypertension (IIH) (pseudotumor cerebri) is one of the major considerations when a patient's headache is persistent and chronic without responding to migraine medications. Even though papilledema with no other neurologic signs in a healthy-looking young female with persistent headache may point to IIH, it should be noted that IIH can occur without papilledema, making the diagnosis difficult until a lumbar puncture is done to measure the cerebrospinal fluid pressure.

Adult hydrocephalus from longstanding abnormalities like aqueductal stenosis can cause daily persistent headache.

Other organic conditions that can manifest as chronic daily headache without neurologic signs include untreated sphenoid sinusitis. A computed tomography scan of the sinuses with special attention to the sphenoid sinus is warranted in this situation.

Management Strategies

- Establish the correct diagnosis or diagnoses in this case. If you are not a specialist, then a referral to a specialist may be the best way to sort this case out in the first instance, but once you recognize that the patient has migraine transforming into CDH as a result of analgesic overuse then you know he or she has medication-induced headache.
- No investigations are indicated, as the patient already has had them done.
- You may require several visits to sort out the complex medical history with respect to the headaches.
- The following steps are essential for the successful management of transformed migraine with analgesic rebound.

Step 1: Detoxification

Discontinuation of daily analgesics, opioids, sedatives, caffeine, and ergotamine is the first step. Withdrawal can be done as an outpatient or as an inpatient. Those patients with multiple comorbidities, such as severe anxiety, depression, or neuroticism, in addition to the analgesic overuse are better treated as inpatients for a short period of time. Abrupt withdrawal of analgesics and opioids is possible; however, it should be done under close supervision. To minimize the withdrawal effects, particularly from opioids, clonidine may be used. A 0.1-mg clonidine patch is a convenient form to use and is applied to the skin on the first day of withdrawal and changed after 7 days. Those who consume large doses of barbiturate-containing analgesic combinations have to be withdrawn more gradually to avoid barbiturate withdrawal seizures. Apprehension, muscle weakness, tremors, postural faintness, anorexia, and twitches may occur on the first few days of withdrawal from barbiturate-containing medications. Seizures, which are fortunately rare, may occur on the second or the third day.

Psychosis and delirium have been reported occurring between the third and the eighth day of barbiturate withdrawal.

Step 2: Breaking the Cycle of Headache

For the majority of transformed migraine patients, the daily headache cycle can be broken by the repetitive intravenous administration of dihydroergotamine (DHE). A test dose of 0.3 mL of DHE with 5 mg of metoclopramide or 10 mg of prochlorperazine may be used, followed by 0.5 mL of DHE with one of the above antinausea medications every 6 hours for 48 to 72 hours. Some patients may require the therapy for a few additional days. Approximately 70 to 80% of patients do respond to DHE. Diarrhea, leg cramps, and chest pain are seen as side effects in some patients. Dihydroergotamine is contraindicated in coronary and peripheral vascular disease.

In those who are unable to tolerate DHE or when it is contraindicated, alternative intravenous medications are possible. These include intravenous chlorpromazine or intravenous prochlorperazine. A 12.5-mg piggy-back dose of intravenous chlorpromazine every 6 hours for 2 days has been found to be effective in some patients. Orthostatic hypotension is a possible side effect and precautions should be taken to prevent dizziness and syncope as a result of orthostatic hypotension.

Prochlorperazine, 5 to 10 mg administered intravenously, is also effective and can be repeated. Extrapyramidal dystonic reactions are possible side effects which can be counteracted by benztropine. Anecdotal reports also indicate the use of intravenous dexamethasone. Even though there are no controlled studies to prove its clinical efficacy, those who have prolonged migraine seem to respond to such therapy. It can be combined with DHE.

Diener et al. found that repeated subcutaneous injections of sumatriptan may be useful in breaking the cycle of chronic daily headache which is transformed from migraine. Naratriptan tablets may be worth trying in these cases because of their prolonged effect and low rate of recurrence.

Breakthrough headaches can be treated with nonsteroidal anti-inflammatory drugs or triptans.

Step 3: Prophylactic Pharmacotherapy

Depending on the type of chronic daily headache, prophylactic pharmacotherapy can be planned. Those with transformed migraine may respond to antimigraine prophylactic agents effectively, provided that analgesics have already been discontinued. The clinician may choose a prophylactic agent or a combination of prophylactic agents, depending on the clinical diagnosis and comorbid factors. There is a place for rational copharmacy in the prophylactic treatment of chronic daily headache of the transformed-migraine type. For example, one can combine a primary antimigraine prophylactic agent such as a beta-blocker, methysergide, or divalproex sodium with agents which act on the psychiatric comorbid conditions such as depression or anxiety. A combination of antidepressants or antianxiety agents with antimigraine prophylactic agents is a rational way of approaching the treatment of persistent chronic daily headaches.

Bonuccelli et al. treated patients with analgesic-rebound headache with a combination of intramuscular dexamethasone, 4 mg for 2 weeks, followed by amitriptyline, 50 mg a day, for 6 months. Acute exacerbations were treated with sumatriptan. They reported a good response with this combination treatment. In an open study, divalproex sodium used prophylactically reduced the frequency and the severity of chronic daily headaches of a transformed-migraine type.

Step 4: Concomitant Behavioral Therapy

Concomitant behavioral intervention, including biofeedback therapy, individual behavioral counseling, family therapy, physical exercise, and dietary instructions, is imperative for the successful management of patients with chronic daily headache. Details of these modes of treatment are beyond the scope of this chapter. Physical therapy, with the application of heat, massage, and ultrasound to neck muscles, may help partially. The selected application of trigger-point injections may also help.

Step 5: Education

Adequate instruction about the nature of their disorder, the ill effects of certain medications used in excessive and frequent quantities, particularly analgesics and opioids, should be emphasized to patients. They have to understand the fact that this disorder is biologic in nature with neurochemical and physiologic changes producing the headache. They should also appreciate the fact that behavioral factors such as anxiety, depression, inability to relax, and stress influence this biology a great deal, making headaches more frequent, more severe, and more difficult to manage. Every program which deals with chronic daily headache should include education.

Step 6: Continuity of Care

Chronic daily headache is usually a prolonged problem occupying years of a person's life, and none of the preventive medications is 100% effective. Adverse effects prevent prolonged use of many medications. Patients develop tachyphylaxis to many medications. Therefore, continuity of care with frequent follow-up and adequate physician-patient communication is essential on a long-term basis.

Referral

Primary care physicians should be prepared at some point to engage the help of a neurologist or headache specialty unit in such cases as this one, since such patients are very hard to manage alone.

One should not give up on this type of patient; success can be achieved in most instances.

Selected Readings

Hering R, Steiner TJ. Abrupt out-patient withdrawal of medication in analgesic-abusing migraineurs. Lancet 1991;337:1442–3.

Isler H. Migraine treatment as a cause of chronic migraine. Advances in migraine research and therapy. New York: Raven Press; 1982. p. 159–64.

Kudrow L. Paradoxical effect of frequent analgesic use. Adv Neurol 1982;33:335–41.

Mathew NT. Transformed or evolutive migraine. Headache 1987;27:102–6.

Mathew NT. Chronic refractory headache. Neurology 1993;43 Suppl 3:S26–33.

Mathew NT. Transformed migraine: analgesic rebound and other chronic daily headaches. Neurol Clin 1997;15:167–86.

Mathew NT, Kurman R, Perez F. Drug induced refractory headache: clinical features and management. Headache 1990;30:634–8.

Rapoport AM. Analgesic rebound headache. Headache 1988;28:662–5.

Raskin NH. Repetitive intravenous dihydroergotamine as therapy for intractable migraine. Neurology 1986;36:995.

Raskin NH. Modern pharmacotherapy of migraine. Neurol Clin 1990;8:857–65.

Sheftell FD. Chronic daily headache. Neurology 1992;42 Suppl 2:32–6.

Silberstein SD, Lipton RB, Solomon S, et al. Classification of chronic daily or near-daily headaches. Proposed revisions to the IHS criteria. Headache 1994;34:1–7.

Silberstein SD, Schulman EA, Hopkins MM. Repetitive intravenous DHE in the treatment of refractory headache. Headache 1991;31:334–9.

Silverman A. What are our dangerous drugs? J Hosp Dent Pract 1971 Apr;5:87–9.

Editorial Comments

The evolution of the concepts underlying "chronic daily headache" has taken many years. Terms such as recurrence, rebound, medication-induced headache, and transformational migraine are now part of the lexicon of all physicians dealing with chronic daily headache. In Dr. Mathew's case, the questions and answers as well as the discussion help us review this entity in detail, and he offers useful suggestions and insights into dealing with these problems. All of these concepts, of course, have great utility in daily practice and allow us to manage cases within a rational framework of thinking. The debate on the neurobiologic mechanisms underlying these entities continues to date—are they separate disorders or a combination of many common disorders?

CHAPTER 17

THE WOMAN WITH DAILY PERSISTENT HEADACHES

WILLIAM B. YOUNG, MD

Case History

A previously healthy and headache-free 30-year-old woman developed bronchitis. During a coughing spell she suddenly developed a severe holocephalic headache. Because of the severe pain she came to the emergency department, where she had a normal neurologic examination. Routine laboratory tests were normal, as were a computed tomography (CT) scan and lumbar puncture (LP). The patient then developed a severe lumbar puncture headache and was hospitalized. Magnetic resonance imaging (MRI) of her brain was normal, and an otolaryngology consultation failed to identify any abnormality. The positional component of the headache was successfully treated with intravenous caffeine, but there was no other clinical improvement during her hospitalization.

Several weeks later, the patient went to a headache center. By this time, the severity of her baseline daily holocephalic headache was moderate with exacerbations associated with nausea and photosensitivity. Brief as well as prolonged exacerbations of pain were triggered by coughing, sneezing, and Valsalva's maneuver. She was unable to work.

Questions about This Case

- What are the diagnosis and the differential diagnosis?
- What other tests would you do?
- What treatments would you try?

Case Discussion

The patient developed chronic daily headache without any prior history of headache. The sudden onset prompted the appropriate evaluation for subarachnoid hemorrhage, meningitis, intracranial mass lesion, and most systemic illnesses.

The onset of a daily headache without a background of worsening episodic headaches should prompt a thorough investigation for secondary causes of headache, even with normal general and neurologic examinations. An extensive list of secondary causes of new daily persistent headache (NDPH) can be generated.

Most other diagnostic possibilities were excluded in this patient by the tests performed. We ordered a magnetic resonance venogram to exclude venous sinus thrombosis and a Lyme titer—both were negative. A diagnosis of NDPH was made.

Our patient's acute onset of headache with cough is unusual but is consistent with the proposed criteria for NDPH, which require onset over 3 days or less.

Because of our patient's cough headache, indomethacin was tried but it was unsuccessful. The patient was hospitalized and treated with the repetitive intravenous dihydroergotamine protocol and started on methylergonovine as a headache preventive. She became headache free in the hospital and returned in follow-up with a biweekly episodic headache. She has been weaned off her preventives and continues to have moderately severe episodic headache but is now back at work.

Management Strategies

- Establish the correct diagnosis.
- An MRI and a Lyme titer are indicated in this case to rule out secondary headaches.
- Avoid analgesic overuse—rebound may occur in NDPH.
- Hospitalization is indicated if the patient is disabled and has been refractory to aggressive outpatient strategies.
- Always bear in mind that a secondary headache might exist—with this pattern of headache onset, an extra level of vigilance is indicated.
- Treat with abortive and preventive agents that work for transformed migraine or chronic tension-type headache.

Case Summary

- The patient has NDPH.
- In this case, as with many NDPH cases, onset occurs with a systemic illness; however, the nature and treatment of this systemic illness appear to have little bearing on the treatment and final outcome of the daily headache which persists long after the original illness is gone.
- There is little literature to help the clinician provide the most successful abortive and preventive strategies.
- Inpatient treatment with repeated intravenous dihydroergotamine is often successful.

Overview of New Daily Persistent Headache

Daily headache may begin without a history of evolution from episodic headache. Based upon the absence of identifiable structural or metabolic causes for headache in many of these patients, Vanast proposed an entity that he called new daily persistent headache (NDPH). Silberstein et al. found that NDPH accounts for a significant number of clinic and hospitalized headache patients. NDPH has been found in children and adolescents as well as adults. Silberstein et al. have proposed that NDPH be added to the International Headache Society taxonomy as a separate primary headache disorder and put forward the criteria listed in Appendix 17–1.

Note that these criteria, like those of the other primary headache disorders, require the exclusion of secondary causes of headache (Appendix 17–2).

The clinical features, other than daily headache duration, are not specified in Appendix 17–1. In our experience, NDPH often resembles chronic tension-type headache or transformed migraine. It may develop during the acute or recovery phase of a flu-like illness.

Several investigators have searched for the causes of or trigger factors for NDPH and have suggested that particular viruses may be involved in its genesis. I do not routinely look for these abnormalities since they will not alter therapy.

Unfortunately, little has been written about therapy for NDPH. Many clinicians have the impression that NDPH is quite difficult to treat and less responsive to therapy than correspondingly severe transformed migraine. Several investigators have noted that this headache responds to inpatient repetitive intravenous dihydroergotamine. For the most part, clinicians tend to treat this disorder similarly to chronic tension-type headache or transformed migraine.

Selected Readings

Gladstein J, Holden EW. Chronic daily headache in children and adolescents: a 2-year prospective study. Headache 1996; 36:349–51.

Hamada T, Ohshima K, Ide Y, et al. A case of new daily persistent headache with elevated antibodies to Epstein-Barr virus. Jpn J Med 1991;30:161–3.

Mathew NT. Chronic refractory headache. Neurology 1993;43 (6 Suppl 3):S26–33.

Silberstein SD, Lipton RB, Sliwinski M. Classification of daily and near-daily headaches: field trial of revised IHS criteria. Neurology 1996;47:871–5.

Silberstein SD, Lipton RB, Solomon S, Mathew NT. Classification of daily and near-daily headaches: proposed revisions to the IHS criteria. Headache 1994;34:1–7.

Vanast WJ. New daily persistent headaches: definition of a benign syndrome. Headache 1986;26:317.

Editorial Comments

Sometimes patients develop new headaches out of the blue without a previous history of migraine or other primary headache disorders. These headaches can persist on a daily basis and, in the absence of any specific etiology, have been termed new daily persistent headache or NDPH. Dr. Young presents such an intriguing and interesting case and suggests the diagnosis of NDPH. It is still not certain in our minds that this patient does not have a secondary cause for her headache, but we are in full agreement with the approach taken and the overall philosophy regarding diagnosis, put forward by Dr. Young. Time will be the ultimate judge of whether cases such as this are NDPH or some other disorder that we cannot detect at present.

Appendix 17–1
Criteria for New Daily Persistent Headache, Proposed by Silberstein et al., 1994

4.7 New Daily Persistent Headache (NDPH)[*]

A. Average headache frequency 15 days/month for >1 month

B. Average headache duration >4 hours/day (if untreated). Frequently constant without medication but may fluctuate.

C. No history of tension-type headache or migraine that increases in frequency and decreases in severity in association with the onset of NDPH (over 3 months)

D. Acute onset (developing over <3 days) of constant unremitting headache

E. Headache is constant in location? (Needs to be tested)

F. Does not meet criteria for hemicrania continua (4.8)

G. At least one of the following:
1. There is no suggestion of one of the disorders listed in groups 5–11 (this refers to IHS diagnostic groups)
2. Such a disorder is suggested, but it is ruled out by appropriate investigations
3. Such a disorder is present, but the first headache attacks do not occur in close temporal relation to the disorder

---

[*] May occur with or without analgesic overuse (rebound)

Appendix 17–2
Differential Diagnosis of NDPH

1. Intracranial structural
   - Tumor
   - Stroke—particularly hemorrhagic
   - Epidural, subdural hematoma
   - Venous sinus thrombosis
   - Post-traumatic headache
2. Disease of skull, spine, temporomandibular joints
3. Sinusitis, especially sphenoid sinusitis
4. High and low pressure headaches
5. CNS infection
   - Lyme disease
   - Atypical bacterial/viral (shunt) infection
   - Fungal meningitis
6. Chemical meningitis
   - Noninfectious nonsteroidal-drug-induced meningitis
7. Hypercarbia/obstructive sleep apnea
8. Systemic illness
   - Infections: EBV, Lyme, HIV
   - Autoimmune disease
   - Temporal arteritis
   - Carcinoid syndrome
9. Toxic metabolic
   - Medication-induced
   - Intoxication, especially carbon monoxide
10. Psychogenic

CHAPTER 18

THE PATIENT WHO REFUSED PHARMACOTHERAPY

RANDALL WEEKS, PhD

STEVE M. BASKIN, PhD

Case History

The patient was a 27-year-old, single female who was a teacher. She was referred for nonpharmacologic treatment of her headaches as she was adamant that she did not want to take prophylactic medication and was reluctant to take abortive medication. She had been on tricyclic antidepressants in the past, which had caused significant weight gain, and multiple selective serotonin reuptake inhibitors, which had caused sexual side effects. She had been given beta-blockers, which caused a drop in her blood pressure and dizziness secondary to this. She had been placed on calcium channel blockers, which were not effective and caused constipation. Antiseizure medication caused significant nausea and gastrointestinal distress. Hence, the patient was quite resistant to the use of prophylactic medications to treat her headaches.

Her headache history revealed that she was experiencing severe to incapacitating headaches approximately four times per month. These were especially apparent around her menses each month. The onset of these headaches had been when she was 12 (associated with menarche). The headaches had an intermittent pattern initially and had become more frequent over the past 2 to 3 years.

The pain was located in the bioccipital area of her head and would radiate to behind either eye (the right side more frequently than the left). There was no aura prior to the attack. The pain was described as a throbbing sensation which would markedly escalate with bending or exertion. The duration of the headache would be up to 2 days. The pain was associated with nausea, vomiting, dizziness, sonophobia, and photophobia. In addition to menses, other triggers seemed to be certain perfumes, sleep-pattern changes, and let-down periods from stress.

The patient also noted a daily mild to moderate headache which would wax and wane throughout the day. The pain was described as bifrontal and would localize into both temples. This was a dull ache which would also include a mild throbbing sensation in the temples as pain reached a moderate level. There were no associated symptoms of migraine except occasional sonophobia. The patient would medicate with either aspirin, acetaminophen, or ibuprofen, and, at the time of consultation, she was using six to eight of these over-the-counter preparations on a daily basis. The pain had been daily for the past year and seemed to be more severe as time passed. Fortunately, the patient was able to remain functional with these headaches and would not miss school because of them.

The patient's medication intake included aspirin, acetaminophen, or ibuprofen—6 to 8 tablets, as noted above. She had been given a butorphanol nasal spray to use for her more severe headaches but "I stopped taking it because I couldn't function … it knocked me out." She also took multivitamins.

The patient had been on a variety of agents due to previous efforts to control her headaches. At no point, however, was she told to discontinue the daily use of her over-the-counter medications. She noted numerous side effects, as indicated above. In addition to the above agents, she had used sumatriptan (both subcutaneous and oral) without benefit. Ergotamine preparations created a great deal of nausea. Dexamethasone seemed to offer good relief of her headaches but she was concerned about "using something as strong as a steroid for my pain." She denied having any specific medication allergies.

A medical history revealed that the patient had not suffered any episodes of head or neck trauma, loss of consciousness, or seizure disorder. She noted "low normal blood pressure" with occasional periods of "lightheadedness" with postural changes. She had occasional "burning in the stomach" secondary to aspirin or nonsteroidal anti-inflammatory products. She noted ongoing cervical tightness and bruxism but no apparent temporomandibular joint click or pain. She had not had any Lyme disease testing previously. The patient had no history of psychiatric difficulties or treatment. She had not had any biofeedback or relaxation training previously.

The patient had magnetic resonance imaging (MRI) of her brain approximately 1 year prior to our consultation. This study was read as being within normal limits. She had not had electroencephalography, a computed tomography scan, or a lumbar puncture. A recent neurologic examination was within normal limits. The patient noted that her headaches had not changed qualitatively since her MRI except that they were becoming slightly more severe.

From a habit perspective, the patient did not smoke cigarettes, limited her alcohol consumption (red wine could trigger a headache), and denied having any history of substance use or abuse. She limited her caffeine to one cup of coffee each day (and would consume this every day). She noted some initial insomnia with a 30 to 60-minute sleep-onset time. Sleep was somewhat restless as the patient had nocturnal bruxism as well as a tendency to "toss and turn." Although sleeping 8 hours a night, the patient felt lethargic in the morning.

The patient felt frustrated with her headaches and noted a tendency to reduce the number of pleasurable activities she engaged in due to concerns about the pain. This was especially true in anticipation of the more severe headache associated with her menses each month.

From a family perspective, the patient was single and had never been married. She was involved with a significant other who was said to be quite supportive regarding her headaches. He encouraged the patient not to withdraw socially but "was understanding" when she was unable to function.

The patient has an older sister and a younger sister. She described a good relationship with both. Both her parents were said to be living, and they reportedly shared a good relationship. The patient denied any areas of family conflict which might have been negatively affecting her headaches. Her family history was positive for migraine headaches (both her mother and a sister had an intermittent migraine pattern with frequencies of 2 to 3 attacks per year). They would use an agent containing caffeine, aspirin, and butalbital for each attack. There was no family history of alcoholism or substance abuse, psychiatric difficulties, or other neurologic disorders.

The patient taught seventh grade and, although she enjoyed her work, it was said to be quite stressful. She had relocated to a new school during the previous year and noted some friction with some of her colleagues. The patient had concerns that "some of my peers don't do their job…they don't seem interested in educating the kids." This was quite frustrating to the patient as she took her job quite seriously ("I put in much longer hours than most of the other teachers").

Psychophysiologic profiling revealed that the patient had moderate elevations in electromyographic readings of the frontal muscles, marked elevation in electromyographic readings of the masseter muscles bilaterally, and marked elevation of readings in the trapezius muscles bilaterally. There was also marked evidence of disturbance in the peripheral blood flow.

The patient indicated that she had significantly decreased her exercise program due to the head pain. She had been quite active prior to this—taking aerobic dancing 3 to 4 nights per week. She noted having difficulty relaxing and "unwinding at the end of the day." She seemed to ruminate about her preparation for class and appeared to be a perfectionist in her approach to her job.

Questions about This Case

- What are the tentative diagnoses for this patient?
- Why do you think her headaches are getting worse?
- How would you handle the patient's resistance to pharmacotherapy?
- What do you feel about her prognosis for improvement?

Case Discussion

The patient was given a diagnosis of chronic daily headache potentially consisting of (1) migraine without aura, (2) chronic tension-type headache, (3) analgesic-rebound headache, and (4) rule out an adjustment disorder with mixed emotional features. In reviewing this with the patient, she was adamant that she did not want to take prophylactic medications given the side effects she had experienced previously. Her neurologist suggested that she try a belladonna, caffeine, and ergotamine preparation which she had used before, but this time only after premedicating with an antiemetic metoclopramide. (Treatment of this patient predated the availability of the newer "triptans" and other agents that have become available in nasal spray preparations.)

As our previous research has shown, the "analgesic washout period" (the length of time necessary for the patient to reach significant improvement), may be up to 8 weeks. We agreed to revisit the question of prophylactic medication, if the patient had discontinued her analgesics and had followed through with nonpharmacologic treatment but was not starting to improve over the next 6 to 8 weeks. She agreed to try an ergotamine preparation again with an antiemetic, and agreed to start the Behavioral Medicine Program.

The Behavioral Medicine Program has several goals:

- Education—giving the patient information about current thinking regarding the causes and treatments of headache. This includes a complete discussion about "analgesic-rebound headache" and, if appropriate, the side effects of the medication that was prescribed. Patients are allowed to ask any (and all) questions about their headaches. They must keep headache calendars.
- Dietary and lifestyle changes—putting the patient on a "migraine diet" (if appropriate) and altering other lifestyle factors that could be contributing to headaches.
- Self-regulation/biofeedback—providing instruction in ways to control physiologic responses involved in headache.
- Cognitive/behavior modification—adjusting actions, attitudes, and expectations that can lead to physiologic arousal and headache. This includes trying to create a greater internal locus of control.
- Participation—requiring that patients are active participants in their treatment. They must keep headache calendars to assure compliance to pharmacologic and nonpharmacologic treatments.

Education

This part of the program includes an initial discussion of the patient's diagnosis as well as the anticipated course of treatment. For this patient, the complication of analgesic rebound was discussed as well as the need to discontinue analgesics and she was advised as to what might happen during the 4 to 8 weeks of the analgesic washout. In other words, the patient was told that her headaches might actually increase as she stopped using over-the-counter preparations. We also discussed how the effects of such agents could compromise usually effective pharmacologic and nonpharmacologic treatments that she had tried previously. The patient agreed to taper off over-the-counter agents by one pill each day.

The patient was asked to keep a headache calendar indicating the severity of her headaches on a daily basis. In addition, she was to note the response to any medication that she might have taken with respect to headache relief. She was also asked to note any specific environmental factors that may have been triggers. Finally, she was asked to note her menstrual days on the calendar.

Dietary and Lifestyle Changes

The patient was given an elimination diet to exclude certain foods that have been shown to trigger migraines. She was advised to go on this diet for 1 month and to note any specific foods that might be problematic. At the end of 1 month, she was told that we would begin to "plug back in" her favorite foods and note what, if any, role these foods might be playing as triggers for headache.

The patient was advised that we were trying to keep sleep patterns "as stable and consistent as possible." We would address this issue as part of our biofeedback and self-regulation training. In addition, the patient was encouraged to keep her caffeine consumption constant with no marked variations. Finally, the patient was advised to gradually start to increase her exercise regimen. As she was going through the analgesic washout period, it was suggested that she avoid high impact activities but "build up" to get back to her frequent aerobic activities.

Biofeedback/Self-Regulation

The patient took part in our typical biofeedback and self-regulation program. The first session was spent orienting the patient to the use of the feedback instrumentation and working on forehead relaxation. A relaxation tape was made for the patient incorporating proper breathing strategies (the importance of diaphragmatic breathing) as well as progressive relaxation strategies that incorporated "tense/relax" sequences. The importance of body awareness was noted, and the patient was instructed to note idiosyncratic "stress reactions" and/or "bracing responses" against pain. These typically entail shallow breathing, jaw tightness, and shoulder tension. She was asked to monitor these behaviors once or twice per hour and to try to eliminate them. The patient was able to achieve a much better sense of releasing forehead muscle-tension and a better body awareness. As with many patients, she had been unaware of regularly having jaw tightness.

The patient was next introduced to a passive relaxation strategy and was given a relaxation tape for home practice. This entailed combining proper breathing with the sequential relaxation of different muscle groups. This enables a person to develop self-regulation skills without having to alternately tense and then relax the muscles. By this point in the training, we had begun to work with the patient's jaw muscles. We spent three sessions targeting the release of jaw tension and discussing how "referred pain" occurs. It was important to note that the patient had

a tendency to "clench" her teeth. In addition, she frequently would chew gum which seemed to exacerbate her headache. She was asked to discontinue this behavior as part of relaxing her jaw muscles.

We then spent two sessions working to release tension in the shoulder and neck areas. The patient was taught specific relaxation exercises that involved stretching and then releasing the muscles in this area. She was also taught the importance of correct posture with respect to "a jaw tuck" so as not to unduly strain the muscles in this area. The technique of guided imagery was introduced where the patient was asked to imagine soothing warmth massaging these muscles—allowing the muscles to release more completely. It should be noted, however, that other patients work well with imagery suggestions that incorporate "refreshing coolness" radiating into these areas. A relaxation tape was made for her, using this particular strategy.

The next session targeted the relaxation of the frontal, masseter, and trapezius muscles. The patient demonstrated good skills in the release of these muscles and in her ability to keep these muscles relaxed over extended periods of time.

At that point in the training, we decided to begin thermal or vascular training. Basically, this involved learning to raise hand temperature in an effort to stabilize blood vessels. Feedback modalities included temperature from the tips of her fingers as well as pulse wave amplitude. Both of these measures are highly correlated with changes in autonomic nervous system functioning. A self-hypnotic tape that targeted increase in hand temperature was made for the patient.

As with most patients who typically have migraine, the patient's hands were quite cold (75°F). Early in the training, most individuals experienced little change in hand temperature, and a great many patients have a drop in skin temperature. This seems to occur because simply "monitoring" the response seems to make it worse.

Over the next four sessions, the patient was able to successfully learn to raise her peripheral hand temperature up to 95°F. This was a rapid acquisition of this response as the patient showed a great deal of diligence in practicing using the self-hypnotic tape and imagery techniques that she had learned previously. She was instructed to implement this response prior to and throughout her menses. As mentioned in the history, the patient noted more severe headaches with her menses each month. The importance of using generalization strategies to maintain this response throughout the day was also discussed.

In sum, the goal of biofeedback training was to assist the patient in acquiring physiologic responses that helped to manage and prevent headaches during the "analgesic washout period" and thereafter. These involved both a reduction in muscular tension as well as stabilization of smooth-muscle activity. While the specific underlying agent of change that brings about benefit is unknown (as with most causal and treatment factors in headache), this type of training seems to foster some sort of physiologic, probably biologic, behavioral, and perceptual change within the patient (with respect to an internal versus external locus of control regarding health issues).

Cognitive/Behavioral Modification

The patient was then taught a specific "strategy" to implement with the onset of her pain. She was specifically asked not to take any medication for mild headaches. She was cautioned against using any type of abortive medication more than 3 days per week (except during her menstrual times). This was to avoid the recurrence of either analgesic or ergotamine rebound as well as habituation or rebound from "triptan" agents.

The patient was encouraged to develop an "action plan" that involved a more positive and strategic way of approaching her pain rather than her usual "resignation and helplessness" with respect to the impending pain. Cognitive variables were examined looking at issues such as catastrophizing, magnification, and other cognitive styles that would led to a sense of helplessness. She was taught to identify more quickly the types of headaches that would develop into her typical migraine and to use medications appropriately. The use of headache calendars was especially helpful to note menstrual days.

The patient also benefited from further cognitive therapy with respect to nonpain behavior. More specifically, she was taught to examine some of her tendencies toward perfectionism as well as her somewhat overly self-critical style. As mentioned previously, the patient felt quite stressed and frustrated by some of her colleague's apparent "lack of dedication" to their jobs. It was important to teach the patient to "step back" from her concerns regarding this and to "only attempt to control the things that you can control." Similarly, she was taught that while it was important to be as professional as possible—her job was a job and not her life. This patient (and many others) tend to view their self-worth as being "solely and intimately" related to their performance in every task of life. This presents a great deal of stress and apprehension and leads to a notion of a need to be "perfect."

Behaviorally, the patient was encouraged to increase her exercise (as mentioned above) as well as to increase other pleasurable activities. The patient had numerous life changes over the past year and had "forgotten" some of the specific behaviors that she used to enjoy. For patients with headache (or other types of pain), it is important that they reconnect with the ability to laugh, play, and share pleasurable activities with others. This helps to reestablish the patient's identity as a "person" instead of a "headache sufferer."

Finally, the patient was asked to do some behavior modification with respect to communication patterns within her family. More specifically, the first question she would be asked by her mother or her father would be "how bad is your headache today?" This served to perpetuate an ongoing definition that the patient was, in fact, "a headache sufferer" with a loss of recognition of her personhood. She was instructed to ask her parents (and others) to ask her questions such as "What are you going to do today?" and "How is school going?" which are more typical questions that get the patient out of a defined patient role.

Participation

As can be seen from the model above, it is important that patients are active participants in their treatment. This serves to increase compliance to both pharmacologic as well as nonpharmacologic treatment strategies. Similarly, patients seem to respond better to the collaborative effort more than to the "guinea pig" approach, where they are given medications on a "trial and error basis" looking for the "magic pill." Such behavioral medicine programs typically target the comprehensive management of patients. Obviously, patients with less complex histories may not require such a program. There are, however, many patients who desperately need such a comprehensive approach.

This patient began to have headache-free days 8 days after the total elimination of her consumption of analgesics. Her headache frequency continued to decline throughout the treatment period. At the end of treatment, she was reporting approximately four mild tension-type headaches per month and one severe to incapacitating migraine every 6 to 8 weeks. Interestingly, the ergotamine preparation and anti-emetic combination offered almost total relief of these attacks and the patient reported only minimal side effects of nausea.

The patient was instructed to come in for biofeedback booster sessions once or twice per year. Similarly, she was to follow up with her physician every 4 to 6 months. The patient was agreeable to and compliant with these requests.

Selected Readings

Baskin S, Weeks R. Nonpharmacological treatment of migraine. In: Tolison D, Kunkel R, editors. Headache: diagnosis and interdisciplinary treatment. Baltimore: Williams & Wilkins; 1993. p. 107–14.

Rapoport AM, Weeks R. Analgesic rebound headache. In: Rapoport A, Sheftell F, editors. Headache: a clinician's guide. Great Neck (NY): PMA Publishing Corp; 1993. p. 157–66.

Weeks R. A behavioral medicine approach to the headache patient. In: Rapoport A, Sheftell F, editors. Headache: a clinician's guide. Great Neck (NY): PMA Publishing Corp; 1993. p. 215–22.

Weeks R. The difficult headache patient calls for a multifaceted approach. Neurol Rev 1995;3:15–6.

Weeks R. Psychological assessment of the headache patient. In: Samuels M, Feskes S, editors. Office practice of neurology. New York: Churchill Livingston; 1996. p. 1096–101.

Editorial Comments

All physicians caring for headache patients recognize how important it is to treat all the patient's headache subtypes and to recommend nonpharmacologic therapies along with education. We strongly suggest combining behavioral therapies with pharmacologic treatment in appropriate patients. When used in appropriate patients by individuals such as Drs. Weeks and Baskin, these therapies can be most successful. Even if all the therapies overviewed are not available to each practicing specialist, the discussion in this particular case contains many pearls of wisdom which should benefit the management of headache patients.

CHAPTER 19

THE ADOLESCENT WITH CHRONIC DAILY HEADACHE

JACK GLADSTEIN, MD

Case History

John is a 16-year-old who experienced headache practically every day. His history of headache began when he was 8 years old, and was consistent until this past year. As a youngster, he had intermittent headache occurring about seven to eight times per year. These headaches were bifrontal, throbbing, came to maximum intensity within 30 minutes, and were accompanied by photophobia, phonophobia, nausea, and pallor. They occurred in the afternoon, most often during the school week. John's mother suffers from debilitating migraines, and his father suffers from "tension headaches." John has been depressed in the past, requiring fluoxetine on two previous occasions. Over the past year, he has continued to have one debilitating attack per month but has developed a daily headache that is different. The daily headache is bifrontal and throbbing but is not accompanied by nausea, photophobia, or pallor. His pain is worse in the morning and subsides as the day progresses. It never awakens him from sleep, but it does interfere with his ability to get to school before 10:00 AM. An "A" student, John is the star of many high school plays, and aspires to a career in acting, despite his parents' wishes to see him go to medical school.

John denies alcohol, tobacco, or drug use. He stopped growing about 2 years ago. He denies sexual activity but is in his first serious relationship with a girl he met at a summer camp. He hinted at some conflict with sexual preference, stating that he is just different from almost everyone at school.

He is currently on fluoxetine for a history of depression and tries acetaminophen or ibuprofen occasionally. Physical examination, including blood pressure, eye grounds, skin examination, neurologic examination, and Tanner staging, was completely normal.

Questions about This Case

- What are the diagnostic considerations?
- Why are his headaches getting worse?
- What more would you like to know?
- How would you manage this case?
- How is this scenario different from that of an adult with the same problem?

Case Discussion

It is clear that John's headaches are different from the previous ones. As a young child, he suffered from a typical case of migraine without aura. He had all the findings to meet the International Headache Society (IHS) criteria that were designed for adults, in addition to those qualities more commonly found in children and adolescents. Children more often have bilateral pain, a briefer time to full intensity of headache, relief with sleep, and nausea without vomiting. Although these headaches were quite violent and debilitating, John was doing very well until this year.

John has developed a chronic daily headache (CDH) profile. Could he have a tumor? After all, his headache is worse in the morning and improves as the day progresses. He has finished growing; therefore, growth or pubertal arrest cannot be significant. Could he have pseudotumor, be on drugs, have school avoidance, and/or conflict with his parents regarding independence and other areas of adolescence? He does not seem to be habituated to over-the-counter medications, and his migraine pattern has not changed. This does not sound like the typical transformed migraine that we see in adults. In adults, migraines become more frequent with less autonomic symptoms and are almost always accompanied by medication overuse. John does not fit this picture.

The patient's history was inadequate, and more information was required. In our first interview, John and his parents were interviewed together. His mother tried to answer most of the questions whereas John and his father were quiet and acquiescing. At our second meeting, we interviewed the parents individually and the patient separately, ultimately bringing the three together at the end of the session.

The patient informed us that although he is a good student, he does not like math or science but loves acting, preferring to be in a full-time high school for the performing arts. Although still feeling parental love, John believes that despite parental wishes, he would prefer an acting career. John's parents, however, would be more comfortable if he gave himself more options with a strong academic track. Missing so many mornings, the patient is in academic difficulty at school. John also is being ridiculed by some of his peers who see him in the afternoon looking healthy but know that repeatedly he has been missing in the morning. He feels that nobody believes him anymore and even wonders about his parents believing him. He denied having separation problems when entering grade school.

John's parents are very worried and think he may have a brain tumor. They are convinced that he is a well-adjusted teenager, with a medical diagnosis. They feel that John is not depressed and that the fluoxetine is helping. There is a positive family history for depression on both sides of the family. The parents are currently in marriage counseling.

Chronic daily headache describes a situation where headaches occur practically every day. Silberstein presented a classification scheme for CDH based upon symptoms, and divided patients into four diagnostic categories: (1) transformed migraine, (2) chronic tension-type headaches, (3) new daily persistent headache, and (4) hemicrania continua. Each subtype can occur with or without medication overuse. We looked at 37 children to see if their symptoms would fit into the adult categories. We found that 35% did not. We coined a new diagnostic category called "comorbid headache" to represent those children who displayed concurrent daily tension-type headache along with intermittent migraine. In these patients, no transformation of migraine symptoms had occurred. John meets the criteria for CDH-comorbid type. He still has the same frequency of migraine but now has an underlying tension headache practically every day. He is not habituated to over-the-counter medications. With a normal neurologic examination and no evidence of papilledema, it is unlikely that he has a brain tumor or benign intracranial hypertension. However, with the high level of parental anxiety, an MRI might be therapeutic, if not diagnostic.

A basic knowledge of the tasks of adolescents may shed light on why his situation is deteriorating. An adolescent seeks independence, must be comfortable with body image, develops stronger attachment and interactions with peers, and must develop a sense of self. Cognitively, he moves from a concrete to an abstract thinker, starts to define career options, and develops a sense of values. During this continuum, conflict may arise, which can manifest itself in many ways. Adolescents with chronic diseases are at particular risk for infantilization because their families have developed ways of coping with illness, may hinder independence. In this case, John may fit into this model. He struggles with his parents regarding vocation, goals, and school-related issues. Although not formally a chronic disease, the patient's headaches have become a major source of attention in this household. He has real pain, but, as is the case with many such youngsters, life's stresses may play a big role.

Management for this adolescent should include a combination of medical and psychologic interventions. One must validate the adolescent's pain, and the parental concerns, while allowing the patient to take an active part in his care. The parents must see, via the practitioner's interactions, that the adolescent is almost an adult. The patient must make appointments, fill prescriptions, and answer questions directed at him. At the same time, parental worries need to be addressed. A meeting with the school personnel may be in order to recommend his promotion to the next grade, and to explain to them about chronic headaches. I explain to the family that by the time a patient is so debilitated, both medical and psychologic factors must be looked at together, rather than separately. The "layers of an onion" analogy often works.

Medical management might include the judicious use of tricyclics, calcium channel blockers, beta blockers, or valproate. Behavioral techniques might include biofeedback, imagery, or relaxation. Individual and/or family therapy can begin concomitantly. The use of fluoxetine maybe problematic in this case because fluoxetine itself can cause headaches. One may try starting amitriptyline (75 to 150 mg/d) at 10 mg every 5 hours, working up to doses appropriate to treat "depression," and then stopping the fluoxetine.

If all this does not work, inpatient hospitalization could be tried. Again, a dual approach of medication and psychotherapy could be instituted. Dihydro-ergotamine and metoclopramide could be given every 6 hours, whereas family therapy could begin to look at coping patterns and family dynamics that surround his headache. Again, a good relationship with the school system will help prevent added anxiety over school absences.

John continues to have intermittent headaches that are debilitating, but he has managed to negotiate school, and is coping better. He continues fluoxetine, amitriptyline, and valproate. He plans to return to summer camp. Conflict regarding career choice remains unresolved.

The clinical characteristics of CDH in children are somewhat different from CDH in adults. In both children and adults, however, the frequency of occurrence by definition is similar with daily or near-daily headaches. A generally agreed upon frequency of five or more days with headache per week is necessary for inclusion in current research protocols for both adults and children. The adult literature indicates that location of pain varies in CDH with most subjects reporting either bifrontal or whole head pain. Location also can vary considerably in children due to either developmental constraints on the localization of pain or limitations in the reporting of pain complaints. Bifrontal pain appears to be the norm in childhood headaches. Depending upon the type of CDH encountered in child and adolescent populations, duration of pain will be variable with chronic daily tension-type headache presenting with relatively brief but frequent episodes and new persistent daily headache continuous in duration. This is not dissimilar from adult populations. Finally, severity is likely to vary depending upon the coping characteristics of the individual patient, whether adult or child. Severity in childhood, however, is linked to functional disability indicators such as missed school days, disrupted peer and social activities, and stressful family interactions.

When children and adolescents present with chronic headache, it is important for the primary practitioner and the specialist to be certain that serious pathology is not present. Growth and/or pubertal arrest and amenorrhea are cardinal signs that something is very wrong. Signs of increased intracranial pressure (i.e., blurry vision, morning headache, and headache that awakens a youngster from sleep) are very worrisome. On the other hand, "la belle indifference," history of school phobia, separation anxiety, family problems, or misbehavior, point toward a benign illness. It is crucial to interview the parents and youngster both separately and together, to better understand family dynamics, and to evaluate differences in perception of symptoms and disability. Interviewing the adolescent alone is crucial to establish independence and give credence to the feelings of the youngster. The practitioner also must be comfortable taking a sexual and drug history from an adolescent.

Several general disease categories can result in headache in children and adolescents. These include systemic and intracranial infections, sinusitis, trauma, hypertension, cerebrospinal fluid pressure abnormalities, ocular disorders, and substance abuse. Many of these disease states also are underlying factors that need to be considered when evaluating CDH in children and adolescents. In addition, many medications used to treat disease states in children may produce headache as a side effect.

It is clear from the results of the limited research that CDH presents differently in children than in adults. It is less likely that children will display a transformed migraine pattern and more likely that a comorbid presentation of migraine and daily headache will emerge early in the course of the history of the illness. Children and adolescents also appear to display a mixture of vascular and tension-type symptoms during their daily headache episodes. Higher levels of functional disability are associated with the presence of daily headache regardless of whether or not periodic migraines also occur. The role that psychologic and familial factors play in the expression and progression of symptoms for children with CDH has not been specified but is an important priority for future research in this area. Given the behavioral and psychologic plasticity of children, a clear understanding of the role of environmental factors will be necessary to develop effective treatment regimens.

Even more important than antecedents with children are the consequences that may occur after their headache pain episodes. Immediate reactions both by children and significant others in their environment can reinforce the occurrence of headaches. For example, overly protective parents may allow minimally disabled children to avoid daily responsibilities or inadvertently provide too much attention for the sick-role behavior. Children's immediate coping skills also may exacerbate the experience of pain. Avoidant and negative coping tendencies are likely to create high levels of stress around headache episodes, increasing sensitivity to pain or otherwise exacerbating daily headache symptoms. In recurrent pain syndromes with a high frequency of difficult-to-control episodes, such as CDH, immediate reactions will lead to potential long-term negative effects for the individual sufferer, including altered self-efficacy and deterioration in coping skills. Relationships with parents may become chronically strained, resulting in alternating episodes of great concern and negative responses to pain episodes. Associated emotional and behavioral distress can

occur, leading to even further overall functional disability for the child or adolescent. Missed diagnoses, and applications of ineffective treatment strategies by health care providers can contribute to negative long-term effects that only make the CDH pattern more recalcitrant.

How the occurrence of chronic pain in children alters pain perception and pain generalization is an area for further investigation. Clinically, distorted pain perception and enhanced pain sensitivity are a common accompanying symptom in children and adolescents with CDH as well as children with other chronic illnesses that result in recurrent pain episodes (e.g., sickle cell disease).

There are no known treatment intervention studies for CDH exclusively in children and adolescents. However, there is a large body of literature indicating that cognitive-behavioral stress management and biofeedback interventions are effective treatment modalities for tension-type headaches in pediatric populations. Many of the patients investigated in these studies met the criteria for chronic tension-type headaches, but because they are not separated out by this diagnostic category we can only assume that these intervention strategies may be effective. Controlled treatment outcome trials have been conducted in adults with chronic tension-type headache, which is one form of CDH. Other authors have reported the successful use of verapamil and valproate in adult CDH patients. Anecdotally, physicians on the American Association for the Study of Headache (AASH) Pediatric Committee treat patients with CDH with either tricyclics, calcium channel blockers, beta blockers, or valproate, with varied success. Engel reports the successful use of biofeedback and relaxation in adolescents. McGrath summarizes the numerous reports of the psychologic aspects of diagnosis and treatment of pain in children, with an extensive emphasis on headache.

Over the last few years, we have begun to delineate the differences between adults and children with regard to diagnosis of headache, but have yet to answer the questions regarding efficacy of treatment in this fascinating age group. This case points out the challenge ahead for those that choose to treat adolescents with headache.

Selected Readings

Blanchard EB. Psychological treatment of benign headache disorders. J Consult Clin Psychol 1992;60:537–51.

Congdon PJ, Forsyth WI. Migraine in childhood. A study in 300 children. Dev Med Child Neurol 1979;21:209–16.

Engel JM, Rapoff MA, Pressman AR. Long-term follow-up of relaxation training for pediatric headache disorders. Headache 1992;32:152–6.

Fordyce WE. Behavioral conditioning concepts in chronic pain. In: Bonica JJ, Lindblom U, Iggo A, editors. Advances in pain research and therapy. Vol. 5. New York: Raven Press; 1983. p. 781–8.

Gladstein J. Headaches: the pediatrician's perspective. Semin Pediatr Neurol 1995;2:119–26.

Gladstein J, Holden EW. Chronic daily headache in children and adolescents: a 2 year prospective study. Headache 1996;36: 349–51.

Gladstein J, Holden EW, Peralta L, et al. Diagnoses and symptom patterns in children presenting to a pediatric headache clinic. Headache 1993;33:497–500.

Holden EW, Gladstein J, Trulsen M, et al. Chronic daily headaches in children and adolscents. Headache 1994;34: 508–14.

Holroyd KA, Nash JM, Pingel JD, et al. A comparison of pharmacological (amitriptyline HCL) and non-pharmacological (cognitive-behavioral) therapies for chronic tension headaches. J Consult Clin Psychol 1991;59:387–93.

McGrath PA. Pain in children: nature, assessment and treatment. New York, NY: Guilford Press; 1990.

Prensky AL. Migraine and migraine variants in pediatric patients. Pediatr Clin North Am 1976;23:461–71.

Silberstein SD, Lipton RB, Solomon S, et al. Classification of daily and near-daily headaches: proposed revisions to the IHS criteria. Headache 1994;34:1–7.

Editorial Comments

In adults the concept of transformed migraine producing chronic daily headache has clinical utility and allows appropriate treatments to be instituted. There are many forms of chronic daily headache in adults. In children and adolescents, chronic daily headache may present with different headache types and comorbidities. Dr. Gladstein's case and thoughtful, detailed discussion give us some insight into CDH in adolescence, along with useful management suggestions.

CHAPTER 20

THE MAN WITH COUGH AND HEADACHE

GORDON ROBINSON, MD, FRCPC

Case History

This 62-year-old man had been in good health throughout his life with no history of cardiac disease, hypertension, or diabetes. He rarely attended a physician other than for a "routine check-up" every few years. Recently, he had experienced a winter cold and began to have headache for the first time in his life. The headache was present only when he strained or leaned over to tie his shoelaces. The most severe headaches occurred whenever he coughed and he was now quite fearful of doing so.

Upon coughing, he would develop the onset of a generalized headache which would become severe within 3 to 5 seconds and last for 1 to 2 minutes. If he had a succession of coughs, the pain would remain longer and occasionally persist as a dull ache for up to an hour. He was attempting to avoid any activity that would precipitate the headache.

He denied any other complaints and felt that his cold had resolved months ago. There were no arthritic complaints, or problems with chewing. He was a nonsmoker and drank only on social occasions. He was married with grown children, and the family history was unremarkable. He worked as an office supervisor.

General physical and neurologic examinations were normal aside from his blood pressure which was 160/95 mm Hg. Temporal arteries were pulsatile and nontender.

Questions about This Case

- What is the differential diagnosis in this case?
- Would you investigate this case? If so, with what test?
- What treatment would you offer him?
- Would the response to treatment help you decide on further investigation?

Case Discussion

Cough headache has an unmistakable presentation with its direct precipitation at the time of coughing. A single cough, or at times multiple coughs, will result in the rapid onset of a moderately severe generalized headache that is usually short lived. Sneezing, bending, stooping, and straining also may produce the same headache leading to an avoidance of these activities. Commonly, this headache is seen in individuals not prone to headache and is not a feature of other primary headache disorders such as migraine.

Although cough headache also has been referred to within the context of benign exertion headaches it appears to be a separate entity. Benign cough headache is recognized in the International Headache Society (IHS) classification (1988) and is defined as a bilateral headache of sudden onset that (1) lasts less than 1 minute and is precipitated by coughing, (2) may be prevented by avoiding coughing, and (3) may be diagnosed only after structural lesions such as posterior fossa tumor have been excluded by neuroimaging.

Cough headache may be present as a benign condition or occur secondary to structural disease, usually in the posterior fossa or cranial-cervical junction. The age of presentation may be an important clue in differentiating benign from secondary causes. Although the condition of cough headache has been reported in a wide age range of patients, most with secondary causes are under 50 years of age, and those with the benign variety over 50 years. Males predominate in all reported case series.

Although available literature is conflicting, benign cough headache is the more common entity seen in clinical practice. An older male with typical symptoms and no other neurologic disease is a familiar profile for most headache specialists. Findings of the investigation are most often normal due to the low incidence of secondary causes. Although the mechanism is unknown, treatment is often successful using indomethacin. The response is frequently immediate. Gastrointestinal side effects can be a problem and require other management strategies. No other agents are useful although some patients intolerant of indomethacin may respond to other nonsteroidal anti-inflammatory drugs such as naproxen. There are some recent reports of lumbar puncture being effective in terminating a cough headache. Secondary cough headache is most commonly associated with Arnold-Chiari type I malformations. The mechanism is thought to be due to compression or traction on pain-sensitive dura and other structures as the caudally placed cerebellar tonsils undergo a pulsatile downward movement during coughing. This also may cause a brief obstruction to cerebrospinal fluid flow. Some patients may have an associated syringomyelia with other clinical symptoms and signs. Patients with secondary cough headache do not respond to indomethacin. Decompressive surgery will successfully eliminate cough headache in these patients.

Management Strategies

1. Diagnosis—benign cough headache
   - Characteristic symptoms
   - Older male
   - Normal examination

2. Investigation—probably unnecessary
   - The index of suspicion in this patient is low for finding an underlying structural cause. A therapeutic trial with indomethacin would be the best management strategy.
   - If investigation was deemed necessary magnetic resonance imaging (MRI) scan is the imaging of choice as computed tomography scan would have much lower yield in this clinical problem.

3. Treatment
   - Commence treatment with indomethacin 25 mg t.i.d. after meals and increase to 50 mg t.i.d. if inadequate response after 7 days. Further increases are usually of little value and are poorly tolerated. If gastrointestinal upset is a problem, add cimetidine 150 mg t.i.d. or consider changing to indomethacin 75 mg rectal suppository.
   - Taper or withdraw indomethacin every 4 to 6 weeks and reinstitute if cough headache recurs.
   - For long-term use, 75 mg sustained-release indomethacin may be preferred.

4. Treatment failure
   - Consider MRI in all treatment failures
   - May try naproxen 250 to 500 mg t.i.d. (enteric-coated, if necessary)
   - Consider lumbar puncture (only after normal MRI)

Selected Readings

Pascual J, Oterino A, Berciano J. Headache in type 1 Chiari malformation. Neurology 1992;42:1519–21.

Pascual J, Oterino A, Iglesias F et al. Cough headache. Headache Q 1996;7:201–6.

Raskin N. The cough headache syndrome. Neurology 1995;45:1784.

Sands G, Newman L, Lipton R. Cough, exertional, and other headaches. Med Clin North Am 1991;75:733–47.

Editorial Comments

Cough headache is an interesting benign clinical entity which deserves attention, particularly in relationship to its differential diagnosis and responsiveness to indomethacin. Many rare and unusual headache disorders require careful exploration to ensure the absence of serious disease, and a trial of indomethacin to establish the diagnosis definitively. Dr. Robinson provides us with an overview of such a case. Once recognized, the management of this entity can be rewarding for the patient and their physician.

CHAPTER 21

THE MAN WITH RECURRENT SUDDEN HEADACHES

SEYMOUR SOLOMON, MD

Case History

A 35-year-old male physician diagnosed himself as having a subarachnoid hemorrhage and was seen by a neurologist colleague within 20 minutes of the sudden onset of a severe generalized headache; it was the first and worst such headache in his life. The patient denied a precipitating event or triggering factor. The headache was throbbing but there were no other features of a migraine or cluster headache. There were no associated symptoms or systemic features such as fever or stiffness of the neck. The patient had been in excellent health without a past history of important illness. He did not smoke or drink excessively. His parents and two siblings were living and well; however, his mother had had migraine in her earlier years. The patient was married and had 2 children, neither of whom had headaches.

General physical and neurologic examinations were normal. An emergency computed tomography (CT) scan of the head was normal. By the completion of the test, 2 hours had passed and the headache had gradually disappeared. A lumbar puncture was recommended to rule out a small subarachnoid hemorrhage, but the patient refused, reasoning that serious disease would cause a more prolonged headache. The patient was told to call the neurologist immediately if similar headaches were to occur in the future.

The patient duly reported similar headaches but of only 15 minutes' duration occurring once or twice a week during the next 2 months. Repeated examinations were normal. Finally, the patient sheepishly admitted that the headaches occurred immediately after sexual intercourse with his secretary but not with his wife. Coital headache was diagnosed and the patient was treated with indomethacin, 25 mg three times a day; an extra dose was to be taken before sexual intercourse. This course of therapy usually prevented headaches and those headaches which were not completely prevented were much less intense. After several months, the patient began to have symptoms of upper gastrointestinal distress in spite of daily use of misoprostol. When the indomethacin was discontinued, the headaches following sexual intercourse returned but only occasionally.

Within 2 years, the patient had divorced his wife and married his secretary. The coital headaches did not occur again.

Questions about This Case

- What other diagnostic considerations should be entertained?
- What other laboratory studies should be considered?
- Was the initial evaluation adequate?
- What other therapeutic modalities might be considered?

Case Discussion

There are several terms for coital headache such as "benign coital cephalalgia," "benign orgasmic cephalalgia," or more properly "headaches associated with sexual activity." The latter term is preferred because not all such headaches are associated with sexual intercourse; for example, they may be associated with masturbation. Similarly, orgasm need not occur for the development of headache. Benign coital cephalalgia is also not an ideal term because headaches associated with sexual activity are not necessarily benign.

Five to 12% of subarachnoid hemorrhages occur with the exertion of sexual intercourse. Sexual activity may precipitate a cerebral hemorrhage in a hypertensive patient who experiences an additional rise in blood pressure with coitus; a pheochromocytoma is another consideration. Cerebral or brainstem infarction also may occur. Other diseases in the differential diagnosis are Arnold-Chiari malformation, other abnormalities of the cervical-cephalic juncture and a colloid cyst of the third ventricle. Additional diagnostic considerations are the thunder-clap headache associated with cerebral vasospasm and the sentinel headache preceding a full-blown subarachnoid hemorrhage. Of course, forms of exertion other than coitus may lead to a sudden severe headache. About 1 in 5 patients who have headaches associated with sexual activity also have headaches triggered by exertion.

Headaches associated with sexual activity occur more commonly in men than in women; the ratio is approximately 4 to 1. The headache does not occur with every sexual act. Fortunately, it is infrequent; unfortunately, it is unpredictable. There are three types of headache associated with sexual activity related to associated physiologic changes. An explosive headache occurs approximately 75% of the time, a dull ache 20%, and a post-lumbar-puncture-like headache 5% of the time. Coitus is accompanied by elevated pulse, blood pressure, muscle tone, and intracranial pressure; vasodilation also occurs. The most common headache type is sudden and severe, often likened to an explosion, occurring in association with orgasm. The headaches are not necessarily correlated with the degree of sexual excitement and may occur both before and after orgasm. However, coital headache is often associated with sexual activity that is illicit, as in the case described. The headache associated with sexual activity is more often a throbbing than a steady ache; it may be generalized or predominant over the occipital area. The duration of the headache ranges from several minutes to 1 or 2 hours. Occasionally, a specific position during sexual intercourse may provoke the headache. This first type of headache associated with coitus occurs more often in migraineurs than in the population as a whole. Occasionally, nausea and vomiting are associated with the headache and, when the pain is throbbing, migraine may be misdiagnosed. About two-thirds of people who experience headache with sexual activity have a history of migraine. The sudden increase in intracranial pressure associated with orgasm evokes pain presumably by stretching the meninges and the basilar blood vessels.

A second headache associated with sexual activity is a dull ache throughout the head and neck that intensifies as sexual excitement increases. This headache is probably due to increasing tension of the neck and scalp musculature as part of the generalized increase in muscle tone during sexual activity. The headache associated with the gradual increase in muscle tone can be relieved by deliberate relaxation during sexual activity. The third and least common headache associated with coitus is a postural headache, with pain that occurs when the patient is upright and subsides when the patient is horizontal; the same type of headache may occur after a lumbar puncture. This headache is attributed to a tear in the meninges that rarely occurs with the sudden rise in intracranial pressure during orgasm.

Headaches associated with sexual activity may be difficult to diagnose because patients are often too embarrassed to see a doctor or, as in the case described, too embarrassed to relate the circumstances of the triggering event. Sometimes, fear of headache may cause abstinence or impotence with a consequent feeling of rejection by the sexual partner and associated marital strife. The partner may feel that headache is used as the proverbial excuse to avoid sexual intercourse. The examiner should specifically ask about the relationship of sexual activity to the onset of headache rather than simply asking if there were precipitating or associated events.

Headaches associated with sexual activity are not absolutely responsive to indomethacin, as are the paroxysmal hemicranias and hemicrania continua. But, if not completely effective, indomethacin usually decreases the frequency of occurrence and the intensity of the pain. If indomethacin fails, other therapies are often effective, particularly those used for migraine. Propranolol may be useful as a prophylactic agent; however, it may also impair sexual potency. Ergotamine may be used in anticipation of the headache before sexual intercourse or for treatment of the acute pain, if it is prolonged.

Management Strategies

- Establish the correct diagnosis. Determine whether sexual activity was a factor in the onset of the headache.
- Consider the differential diagnoses, especially subarachnoid hemorrhage and Arnold-Chiari malformation.
- To rule out subarachnoid hemorrhage, a CT scan of the head is usually all that is necessary, but if there is any doubt about the diagnosis, a lumbar puncture should be performed. Cerebral arteriography is rarely necessary.
- If recurrent headaches are frequent, prophylactic therapy with propranolol or indomethacin may be warranted.
- Reassure the patient that this is a benign condition but that any changes should be reported immediately.

Case Summary

Coital headache or, more accurately, headache associated with sexual activity can be diagnosed easily if the patient is forthcoming or the physician is inquisitive. Serious diseases such as subarachnoid hemorrhage and Arnold-Chiari malformation should be considered. Treatment with propranolol or indomethacin is usually effective but not absolutely so. The patient and the patient's partner should be reassured that the condition is benign.

Summary of Types of Indomethacin-Responsive Headaches

There are two headaches that are invariably responsive to indomethacin, namely, episodic or chronic paroxysmal hemicrania and hemicrania continua. Other brief headaches are partially responsive to indomethacin. They include exertional or cough headaches, ice-pick headaches or jabs and jolts of head pain (idiopathic stabbing headache), and headache associated with sexual activity.

Selected Readings

Lance JW. Headaches related to sexual activity. J Neurol Neurosurg Psychiatry 1976;39:1226–30.

Levy RL. Stroke and orgasmic cephalalgia. Headache 1981; 21:12–3.

Lundberg PO, Osterman PO. The benign and malignant forms of orgasmic cephalalgia. Headache 1974;14:164–5.

Porter M, Jankovic J. Benign coital cephalalgia. Differential diagnosis and treatment. Arch Neurol 1981;38:710–2.

Selwyn DL. A study of coital related headaches in 32 patients. Cephalalgia 1985;5 Suppl 3:300–1.

Silbert PL, Edis RH, Stewart-Wynn EG, Gubbay SS. Benign vascular sexual headache and exertional headache: interrelationships and long term prognosis. J Neurol Neurosurg Psychiatry 1991;54:417–21.

Silbert PL, Hankey GJ, Prentice DA, Apsimon HT. Angiographically demonstrated arterial spasm in a case of benign sexual headache and benign exertional headache. Aust N Z J Med 1989;19:466–8.

Editorial Comments

Headaches associated with sexual activity can be a diagnostic problem for the clinician, if the patient is not forthcoming, as Dr. Solomon points out. Serious etiologies are rare but must be considered and excluded in all cases. Treatment strategies are outlined and are of some value. One wonders if some of the newer triptans with a longer half-life leading to less recurrence will be helpful in such cases or if the rapid onset of action of the newer triptans will abort post-sexual-activity severe headache.

CHAPTER 22

THE PATIENT WITH "ICE-PICK" PAINS

NAZHIYATH VIJAYAN, MD

Case History

This patient is a 46-year-old woman who began experiencing recurrent headaches at the age of 13 years. They were infrequent during her teenage years. There were no premonitory symptoms. The pain was described as a unilateral or bilateral pain which would gradually build up in intensity. Eventually this developed into a severe throbbing pain over the entire head. This was associated with nausea, photophobia, sonophobia, and vomiting if the pain was very severe. Sometimes the headaches occurred around her menstrual periods but not consistently. Hunger and decreased amounts of sleep often triggered them.

The frequency and severity of the patient's headaches increased during her twenties. However, during her pregnancy the headache almost completely subsided only to return after delivery.

The headache frequency decreased during her thirties. She then noticed the development of a sharp head pain usually over the frontal regions or in the eye prior to the onset of her regular headache. Occasionally she would experience several of these sharp pains during the entire day and would eventually develop one of her usual headaches. This sharp jabbing pain lasted only for 15 to 20 seconds but was very severe. It virtually jolted her each time it occurred. These painful episodes did not have any

specific pattern or cyclical features. There was no conjunctival injection, tearing, or nasal congestion.

In her forties, the lifelong severe headache almost completely subsided; however, she noticed several of the sharp jabbing pains on an almost daily basis. The frequency fluctuated but she generally had 20 to 30 of these on a single day. The pain still lasted only for 15 to 20 seconds. The location of the pain was either in the eyes or in the temporal regions; however, it did occur in other parts of the head. The pain did not awaken her from sleep. She did not observe any specific triggering factors.

She had no other medical problems. There was a history of recurrent headache in her mother, sister, and daughter. None of them experienced the sharp jabbing pains. A magnetic resonance imaging (MRI) scan of the brain was normal.

Ergotamine tartrate had been used effectively in the past to relieve her regular headache. She was treated prophylactically in her twenties with beta-blockers which reduced the frequency of the headaches. They were re-introduced to control the sharp pains but with no benefit. She tried taking pain medications round the clock without benefit. She was subsequently treated with indomethacin, 25 mg three times a day, resulting in a 50% reduction of the sharp pains. When the dosage was increased to 50 mg, three times a day, the headache became very infrequent. Attempts to lower the dose subsequently lead to increased frequency. She has remained on this dose with intermittent unsuccessful attempts at withdrawal.

Questions about This Case

- What is your diagnosis?
- What are the differential diagnostic considerations?
- Are there any other investigations you want to undertake in this patient?
- How would you manage this patient on a long-term basis?

Case Discussion

This patient developed intermittent headache at the age of 13 years that fluctuated in intensity and frequency over the years. Overall, as she grew older, there was a gradual reduction in the frequency and severity, and in her forties, the headaches almost completely subsided. They were typical of migraine without aura as defined by the International Headache Society (IHS). The major features included a family history of headache in her mother, sister, and daughter, intermittent unilateral headache which eventually became bilateral with a pulsating quality, and associated nausea, vomiting, photophobia, and phonophobia. The history of headache triggered by hunger, change in sleep pattern, relationship to menstrual periods, and subsidence during pregnancy are all typical of migraine headache. Generally speaking, the frequency and the severity of the headache decrease as patients grow older. In this particular patient, these headaches subsided substantially by the time she was 40.

In addition to the migraine, she also noticed the sharp jabbing pains in her thirties. Initially these were associated with the migraine headache. They were either isolated or would occur as multiple episodes prior to experiencing a typical migraine. This is a very common phenomenon and often is overshadowed by the migraine itself because these episodes are very brief and infrequent. However, once the migraine headache subsided she began having 20 to 30 of these in a single day. The pain

lasted only for 10 to 20 seconds. It was located most frequently in either eye or the temporal regions even though it could be located in other parts of the head. There were no symptoms of conjunctival injection, lacrimation, ptosis, or rhinorrhea associated with these head pains. There was an excellent therapeutic response to indomethacin. This type of head pain is typical of "idiopathic stabbing headache," formerly known as ice-pick pains. The headache is described in the IHS headache classification (4.1) as transient stabs of pain in the head that occur spontaneously in the absence of organic disease of underlying structures or of the cranial nerves. The IHS diagnostic criteria for this type of headache are as follows:

1. The pain is confined to the head exclusively or is predominantly felt in the distribution of the first division of the trigeminal nerve (orbit, temple, and parietal area).
2. The pain is stabbing in nature and lasts for a fraction of a second. It occurs as a single stab or a series of stabs.
3. It recurs at irregular intervals (hours to days).
4. The diagnosis depends on the exclusion of structural changes at the site of the pain and in the distribution of the affected cranial nerve.

Stabbing pains are more commonly experienced by people subject to migraine headache, in which case they are felt in the site habitually affected by headache in about 40% of patients and tend to be more frequent at the time of headache. They commonly subside with the administration of indomethacin, 25 mg orally three times daily.

This patient's head pain fits all the diagnostic criteria outlined above including the response to indomethacin.

There is no other condition which causes such sharp pains of short duration without any other neurologic signs and symptoms. However, it is appropriate to discuss some of the other clinical entities that may resemble this particular syndrome, especially if the history of headache available is not adequate and the reader is not familiar with these other disorders.

Chronic or episodic paroxysmal hemicrania (CPH, EPH) is a rare disorder resembling cluster headache but predominantly occurring in females as opposed to the male predominance of cluster headache. Each headache episode lasts for a very short time, generally 2 to 5 minutes but according to IHS classification could be as long as 45 minutes. The frequency of the attacks is more than 5 per day but typically up to 30 attacks per day is more the norm. The headache has the same periorbital or retro-orbital distribution as cluster headache. The pain is associated with all the typical autonomic accompaniments including conjunctival injection, lacrimation, nasal congestion, rhinorrhea, and rarely ptosis and eyelid edema. The headache is always unilateral and responds to indomethacin. Some patients will have cycles of these headaches which are then classified as EPH as opposed to CPH, which is the most common type of presentation.

Short-lasting, unilateral, neuralgiform headache with conjunctival injection and tearing (SUNCT) is a rare syndrome. It occurs more commonly in men. The duration of the pain is from 30 to 120 seconds and is associated with conjunctival injection and tearing just like in cluster headache and CPH. Pain can often be precipitated by turning the head from side to side. The frequency of the headache varies. No specific drug appears to control it consistently.

In trigeminal neuralgia, the pain is confined to one of the divisions of the trigeminal nerve, most commonly the mandibular division. The pain is extremely brief or momentary and has a sharp shooting quality. There are often paroxysms of pain, one after the other like a "machine gun peppering." There are no autonomic accompaniments. Trigger points are often present. Touching, cold air blasts, talking, and eating are the most common triggering factors. The examination is normal unless the neuralgia is one of the rare symptomatic ones. Medical treatment using drugs like carbamazepine is usually very helpful in the majority of patients.

All patients with this type of headache syndrome have a normal neurologic and physical examination. There is no reason to investigate these patients beyond the history and examination unless there are atypical features which raise doubts in the examiner's mind regarding the diagnosis.

Management Strategies

Patients who have infrequent jabbing headache in association with migraine or other benign headaches do not require any specific therapy other than treating the accompanying major headache problem. Generally, if one is able to control the migraine headache, the jabbing pains also come under control. However, if the frequency increases and they seem to occur independent of any other headache syndrome, specific therapy may be required.

Indomethacin appears to be the first choice in treating this syndrome. The majority of patients show significant improvement and some patients attain complete resolution. However, the response is not "absolute" as described in other headache syndromes like CPH. Generally, a dosage of 25 mg, taken three times daily, is effective. The dosage could be doubled if there is no response. Gastric problems are the most common side effects and these should be watched for and treated if necessary. It is possible to evaluate the effectiveness within 2 to 4 weeks. The drug should be discontinued if there is no response within this period of time because of the potential for gastrointestinal side effects in a large proportion of patients. Other non-steroidal anti-inflammatory agents and antimigraine agents like calcium channel blockers have also been found to be effective. Tricyclic antidepressants could also be tried. There have not been any controlled trials of any of these drugs so far.

Case Summary

- This patient has migraine without aura.
- She experienced infrequent "jabs and jolts" either preceding or during a migraine headache.
- The "jabs and jolts syndrome" became the most prominent symptom after resolution of her migraine headache.
- There was significant response to treatment with indomethacin as seen in the majority of these patients.

Overview of Benign Idiopathic Stabbing Headache

This syndrome has been described under various terms including "jabs and jolts syndrome," "ice-pick-like pain", "sharp stabbing head pain," and "needle-in-the-eye syndrome." The name suggested by the IHS is "idiopathic stabbing headache."

The exact incidence of this type of headache is unknown. The coexistence of isolated episodes of stabbing pain in patients with other types of headache is fairly common but patients rarely ever discuss or mention this unless they become frequent. This reportedly occurs in 40% of patients with migraine and often is located in the same territory as the patient's migraine. The frequency increases just prior to or during a migraine headache. It has also been reported with cluster, tension, and post-traumatic headaches. In some patients, however, this type of headache occurs as an independent entity with the frequency varying considerably. A patient may experience one or two episodes a day or there could be as many as 50 a day. Pain may sometimes occur in a cyclical fashion, and rarely is there any fixed pattern as seen in cluster headache. There is no gender predilection as seen in cluster headache or CPH.

The duration of the pain is often a few seconds and almost always less than one minute. However, many patients will describe a very low-grade pain and occasionally tenderness in the same location for minutes to hours after an intense episode of pain. The location of the pain tends to change even though several episodes may occur at the same site. More often, pain occurs at random locations. Temporal, orbital, and supraorbital locations appear to be most common. The intensity is moderate to severe and often jolts the patient especially because of the unexpected occurrence and partly due to the intensity. Each individual episode may not be disabling, but when multiple episodes occur on a daily basis the problem becomes intolerable and patients seek help.

Most of the painful episodes occur without any provocation. Some of Raskin's patients reported a sudden change in posture, physical exertion, dark-light transition, and head motion as probable triggers.

In the vast majority of patients, no specific treatment is required. Management of the associated headache syndromes often relieves the symptoms. Indomethacin appears to be effective in the majority of patients who suffer from the independently occurring episodes. The response is not thought to be absolute as seen in CPH patients. Other nonsteroidal or vasoactive agents similar to those used in the prophylaxis of migraine and cluster headache may also be beneficial in cases where indomethacin fails.

Selected Readings

Drummond PD, Lance JW. Neurovascular disturbances in headache patients. Clin Exp Neurol 1984;20:93–9.

Lansche RK. Ophthalmodynia periodica. Headache 1964;4:247–9.

Mathew NT. Indomethacin responsive headache syndromes. Headache 1981;21:147–50.

Raskin NH. Ice cream, ice pick and chemical headaches. In: Rose FC, editor. Headache. Handbook of clinical neurology. Amsterdam: Elsevier; 1986. p. 441–8.

Raskin NH, Schwartz RK. Ice-pick-like pain. Neurology 1980;30:203–5.

Editorial Comments

The spectrum of symptoms in patients with migraine is remarkable despite relatively precise IHS criteria. Migraine can express itself in a myriad simple and complex symptomatologies, and this case reported by Dr. Vijayan is no exception. The differential diagnosis of such brief, frequent, paroxysmal, painful events is likewise fascinating. Pathophysiologically, one wonders what neuronal or vascular perturbations occur to result in "jabs and jolts," and presumably they are part of the "nerve storms" originally described by Liveing in his book On Megrim. *Much is to be learned from this case, in large part due to the author's clear and concise narrative.*

CHAPTER 23

THE WOMAN WITH CONTINUOUS HEADACHE

EGILIUS L.H. SPIERINGS, MD, PhD

Case History

A 48-year-old woman related the onset of her headaches in her late teenage years. Initially the headaches occurred twice a month and were relieved by a nonprescription analgesic. Over time they gradually increased in frequency and, 2 or 3 years before consultation, became daily. The headaches were present on awakening in the morning and did not have a particular diurnal pattern. They did not awaken her at night. The headaches were located on the right, in the eye, the forehead, the side of the head, and the back of the neck. They were steady in nature like a vise and mostly moderate in intensity. The headaches were not associated with nausea, vomiting, photophobia, or phonophobia. Bending over made the headaches worse, whereas lying down made them somewhat better. They were also worse with her menses, which were regular.

The patient had been taking an analgesic, which contains 250 mg acetylsalicylic acid, 250 mg acetaminophen, and 65 mg caffeine per tablet, every day for the headaches. She had been taking four to six tablets per day until 10 days before her consultation, when she discontinued them because of a lack of benefit. However, since that time the headaches had been severe in intensity, especially in the right eye, despite her taking an isometheptene, dichloralphenazone, and acetaminophen compound, ketorolac, and butorphanol. In addition, she was on nadolol, 60 mg per day, for headache prevention, and levothyroxine, 0.112 mg per day, for hypothyroidism.

Apart from the headaches, the patient felt well generally but had problems falling asleep and, to a lesser extent, sleeping through the night. Her neck and shoulder muscles were tight and sore on the right and she also experienced some soreness in her right upper arm. She had not had any illnesses or surgeries. Seven years before consultation, she had slipped on ice and had fallen on her back but without suffering a head or neck injury. She did not smoke, occasionally drank alcohol, and drank one cup of coffee a day. The family history was unremarkable for headaches in the parents, two siblings, and one child.

The physical and neurologic examinations were without abnormalities. Her blood pressure was 135/90 with a pulse rate of 56 beats per minute. Routine hematology and blood chemistry were unremarkable; her thyroid-stimulating hormone level was 1.27 (normal). A cranial magnetic resonance scan was normal whereas a computed tomography scan of the sinuses showed minimal mucosal thickening in the ethmoidal sinuses and a small osteoma in the right frontal sinus.

The patient was advised to discontinue the analgesics she was taking. She was given a 3-day course of prednisone (60 mg the first day, 40 mg the second day, and 20 mg the third day) with diazepam, 5 mg four times per day, to break the 10-day stretch of severe headaches. In addition, she was given carisoprodol, 350 mg as needed every 4 hours, for the abortive treatment of the headaches. The thought was that she suffered from "chronic daily headache," perpetuated by analgesic overuse. She had withdrawn herself from the caffeine by discontinuing the analgesic she was originally on, causing the headaches to get worse. At the same time, she had continued taking other analgesics, in this way not allowing the headaches to get better, as this requires discontinuation of all analgesics and vasoconstrictors.

The headaches were thought to arise, at least in part, from a vascular as well as a muscular mechanism ("muscle-contraction vascular headache"). A vascular mechanism was assumed on the basis of the history of severe pain in the eye as well as the worsening of the headaches with bending over and during her menstrual periods. A muscular mechanism was suggested by the association of the headaches with tight ipsilateral neck and shoulder muscles. The mechanisms were treated with medications which lack analgesic and vasoconstrictor properties, that is, with prednisone to inhibit the (neurogenic) inflammation associated with the vascular mechanism and diazepam to relax the tight muscles associated with the muscular mechanism. In addition, the patient was given carisoprodol as a fast- and short-acting muscle relaxant to be used for the abortive treatment of the headaches.

The headaches improved on the prednisone and diazepam course to a mostly mild and sometimes moderate intensity but continued to occur daily. They were also still present on awakening in the morning and required the patient to take two or three carisoprodol tablets per day. The neck and shoulder muscles on the right were less tight, and she was prescribed imipramine, 25 mg at bedtime, as a preventive medication to further relax the muscles and improve sleep. The headaches improved further in the sense that they were mild most of the time and sometimes came about shortly after getting up rather than being present on awakening in the morning. The dose of the imipramine was gradually increased to 50 mg at bedtime when the patient developed severe constipation and had a very hard time getting up in the morning. The dose of the nadolol was gradually decreased to see whether that would help reduce the fatigue on awakening in the morning. The headaches became intermittent for a short period of time but returned to their daily occurrence when the nadolol was discontinued. This also caused the

headaches to become more intense which forced the patient to go back to taking the isometheptene, dichloralphenazone, and acetaminophen compound after she had been off all analgesics and vasoconstrictors for 5 months.

The imipramine was continued at a dose of 50 mg at bedtime and, instead of nadolol, she was prescribed atenolol in a gradually increasing dose, up to 100 mg per day, which reduced her pulse rate to 64. She got sick with a "head cold" which increased the intensity of the headaches and went back to taking two to four tablets of the original analgesic daily. In the meantime, the imipramine had been changed to amitriptyline, 25 mg at bedtime, because of the patient's increased problems sleeping at night. As a result of this, she began sleeping much better and did not feel as tired during the day. However, the headaches continued to occur daily and she continued to take two tablets of the analgesic per day. The headaches were located in the right eye and sometimes also on the right side of the back of her head. At this time, which is 1 year after the initiation of the treatment, she also sometimes experienced sharp stabbing pains on the right side of the back of her head. The amitriptyline was changed to an ergotamine, phenobarbital, and belladonna compound, one tablet at bedtime, but without any change in the headaches or the insomnia.

The patient became depressed and saw a psychiatrist who prescribed sertraline, 12.5 mg per day, and clonazepam, 0.25 mg at bedtime. The ergotamine, phenobarbital, and belladonna compound had been discontinued, but she continued to take atenolol, 75 mg per day, and was taking the analgesic every day as well, four to six tablets per day. She was again advised to discontinue the analgesic and was given another course of prednisone but now for 6 days, that is, 60 mg the first 2 days, 40 mg the second 2 days, and 20 mg the third 2 days. The headaches were much better during the prednisone course but came back immediately afterwards and the patient went back to taking four to six tablets of the analgesic per day. She was still experiencing occasional sharp stabbing pains on the right side of the back of her head and claimed 40% relief of the headaches from the analgesic. At this point she was advised to discontinue the analgesic again and was prescribed indomethacin, 25 mg four times per day, with meals and at bedtime. Almost as soon as she started taking the medication, the headaches improved dramatically, in her own words, by 75 to 80%. The headaches did not occur daily anymore and were also much less intense; on average, they occurred 1 or 2 days per week. She continued to use the indomethacin in the dosage indicated above. She discontinued the atenolol and sertraline but continued the clonazepam at a dose of 0.5 mg at bedtime. She has been on indomethacin now for more than a year and continues to do very well with regard to the headaches and without side effects, in particular heartburn or epigastric pain.

Questions about This Case

- On the basis of the presentation, what diagnosis best describes the headaches?
- How is that diagnosis changed by the described response to indomethacin?
- How does the response to indomethacin differ from that to analgesics in general?

Case Discussion

The patient presented with daily headaches which had been present for 2 or 3 years. Daily headaches affect 4 to 6% of the population and may be the presenting symptom in as many as half the patients seeking care from a specialist for their headaches. Daily headaches can be divided into paroxysmal and nonparoxysmal, depending on whether or not they have a well-defined attack pattern. The paroxysmal daily headaches, which constitute such headache syndromes as cluster headache and paroxysmal hemicrania, however, account for only a small fraction of the total daily headaches. The majority lack a well-defined attack pattern and are often referred to as "chronic daily headache." Another requirement for chronic daily headache is that the headaches have been present daily or almost daily for a long-enough period of time. Of course, this is arbitrary but the minimum time considered for the fulfillment of this requirement is generally either 6 months, as with chronic tension-type headache, or 1 year, as with chronic cluster headache (Headache Classification Committee of the International Headache Society, 1988).

About 80% of patients with chronic daily headache initially experienced intermittent headaches. Of these patients, about 20% experienced an abrupt transition into daily headaches and 80% a gradual one, which was the case for our patient. The gradual transition of the initial intermittent headaches into daily headaches takes, on average, a decade. In our patient, the transition took at least 2 decades.

Of the patients who gradually developed daily headaches out of initially intermittent headaches, one-third initially experienced mild (episodic tension-type) headaches and two-thirds severe (migraine) headaches. However, the daily headaches which these patients ultimately developed were the same, regardless of whether the initial headaches were mild or severe. In our patient, the daily headaches seem to have developed out of mild headaches as the headaches were relieved by use of the initial analgesic, which is generally not the case with severe (migraine) headaches.

I diagnosed the headache as muscle-contraction vascular headache, using the old terminology of the so-called Ad Hoc Committee (Committee on Classification of Headache of the National Institute of Neurological Diseases and Blindness, 1962). According to the classification of the International Headache Society, the headaches would have been diagnosed as chronic tension-type headache. In actual fact, they would have fallen into the subcategory of chronic tension-type headache associated with a disorder of the pericranial muscles because of the associated muscular symptoms. This diagnosis would not have done justice, however, to the (migrainous) vascular component of the headaches, as manifested by the, at times, severe pain in the eye and the worsening of the headaches with bending over and during the patient's menstrual periods. On the other hand, referring to the headaches as migraine without aura combined with chronic tension-type headache would not have been right because the patient did not have and, as far as the history goes, never had migraine.

The fixed lateralization of the patient's headaches is generally considered a somewhat unusual feature of chronic daily headache. This is a feature that is considered typical of the paroxysmal daily headache syndromes, that is, cluster headache and paroxysmal hemicrania. However, in an analysis of 258 patients with chronic daily headache, we found almost 30% of the daily headaches to have a fixed lateralization. Fixed lateralization is also a feature of hemicrania continua which, like paroxysmal hemicrania, is an indomethacin-responsive headache syndrome (Sjaastad and Spierings, 1984).

Our patient not only had daily headaches but was also taking analgesics and vasoconstrictors daily. This combination should raise suspicion of analgesic-induced and/or vasoconstrictor-rebound headache (Kudrow, 1982). As is required in proper headache management, this was addressed first by discontinuing all analgesics and vasoconstrictors. In order to diminish the withdrawal headache which often follows the abrupt discontinuation of analgesics and/or vasoconstrictors, the patient was given prednisone with diazepam for 3 days. On this regimen, the headaches became less intense but continued to be daily, although not always present anymore on awakening in the morning. The patient was kept off analgesics and vasoconstrictors for 5 months and was treated with preventive medications but the headaches continued to occur daily. The preventive medications used were beta-blockers and tricyclics which, in combination, are generally considered most effective for the kind of headache syndrome the patient was thought to have (Mathew, 1981). The beta-blockers used were nadolol and atenolol and the tricyclics were imipramine and amitriptyline.

As there was no significant improvement in the headaches after 5 months off analgesics and vasoconstrictors, it can be safely stated that the patient did not suffer from analgesic-induced and/or vasoconstrictor-rebound head-aches. The headaches, in addition, seemed to be unresponsive to the standard preventive antiheadache medications, that is, the beta-blockers and tricyclics. Other preventive medications could certainly have been considered at this point but, instead, attention was focused on the relief the patient obtained from the initial analgesic, an acetylsalicylic-acid-containing medication, which she had fallen back on for the abortive treatment of the headaches. Patients with analgesic-induced and/or vasoconstrictor-rebound headaches take excessive amounts of medications but generally

acknowledge very little if any benefit from these medications. They continue to use the medications despite gaining insignificant relief because of a lack of understanding that the medications, in actual fact, may be harmful to their headaches and because they do not know what else to do. The patient claimed 40% relief of the headaches from the analgesic which was ultimately the reason that she was prescribed indomethacin preventively, under the assumption that she possibly suffered from hemicrania continua. The fast and dramatic response of the headaches to the indomethacin at the relatively low dosage of 25 mg four times per day confirmed the diagnosis.

Overview of Hemicrania Continua

Hemicrania continua is an indomethacin-responsive headache syndrome that was described by Ottar Sjaastad and me in 1984. This was 8 years after Sjaastad and Dale had described the first headache syndrome with an absolute response to indomethacin, that is, chronic paroxysmal hemicrania (Sjaastad and Dale, 1976). Sjaastad and I conceptualized the idea and coined the term hemicrania continua in June 1983 while traveling through Poland after having lectured in Lodz on the invitation of Antoni Prusinski. I brought to Sjaastad's attention a 53-year-old man I had been treating who had daily continuous headaches which were limited to the right side of the head (case 2 of the 1984 publication). The only medication that relieved the headaches was acetylsalicylic acid, of which a 500-mg dose rendered him headache free for 3 hours. This had reminded me of the patients with chronic paroxysmal hemicrania Sjaastad and Dale had described in their publication. I subsequently prescribed that patient indomethacin 75 mg by slow release twice daily. He was headache free the day after he started the medication which gave him, in his own words, 99% relief of the headaches. Sjaastad had treated a similar patient, a 63-year-old woman, also with daily continuous unilateral headaches, who responded well to acetylsalicylic acid and experienced complete relief on indomethacin. In both patients the headaches had been present daily and continuously since the onset.

Sjaastad's patient had occasional "jabs and jolts" associated with the headaches, as was the case with the patient described in the present case history, but this was not the case with my patient. Jabs and jolts, or idiopathic stabbing headache as it is called in the classification of the International Headache Society, is a headache syndrome with a partial response to indomethacin (Spierings, 1990).

Hemicrania continua is like cluster headache and paroxysmal hemicrania, both of which occur in an episodic and chronic form (Kudrow et al., 1987; Spierings, 1992), being a unilateral headache syndrome with fixed lateralization, that is, the headaches always occur on the same side of the head. However, whereas cluster headache and paroxysmal hemicrania have a typical clinical presentation in terms of the frequency and duration of the headaches, hemicrania continua does not. Therefore, it is impossible to diagnose hemicrania continua solely on the clinical presentation; it requires the typical response to indomethacin. Hemicrania continua that is resistant to indomethacin, as suggested by Kuritzky (1992), does not exist; however, there are many patients who have continuous unilateral headaches with fixed lateralization who do not respond to indomethacin. The key to look for in the history is a response to acetylsalicylic acid which seems to predict the responsiveness of the headaches to indomethacin. This is the feature that ultimately leads to the identification of both chronic paroxysmal hemicrania and hemicrania continua as indomethacin-responsive headache syndromes.

Selected Readings

Committee on Classification of Headache of the National Institute of Neurological Diseases and Blindness. Classification of headache. J Am Med Assoc 1962;179:717–8.

Headache Classification Committee of the International Headache Society. Classification and diagnostic criteria for headache disorders, cranial neuralgias and facial pain. Cephalalgia 1988;8 Suppl 7:1–96.

Kudrow L. Paradoxical effects of frequent analgesic use. Adv Neurol 1982;33:335–41.

Kudrow L, Esperanca P, Vijayan N. Episodic paroxysmal hemicrania? Cephalalgia 1987;7:197–201.

Kuritzky A. Indomethacin-resistant hemicrania continua. Cephalalgia 1992;12:57–9.

Mathew N. Prophylaxis of migraine and mixed headache. A randomized controlled study. Headache 1981;21:105–9.

Sjaastad O, Dale I. A new (?) clinical headache entity: chronic paroxysmal hemicrania. Acta Neurol Scand 1976;54:140–59.

Sjaastad O, Spierings ELH. "Hemicrania continua": another headache absolutely responsive to indomethacin. Cephalalgia 1984;4:65–70.

Spierings ELH. Episodic and chronic jabs and jolts syndrome. Headache Q 1990;1:299–302.

Spierings ELH. Episodic and chronic paroxysmal hemicrania. Clin J Pain 1992;8:44–8.

Spierings ELH, Schroevers M, Honkoop PC, Sorbi M. Presentation of chronic daily headache: a clinical study. Headache 1998;38:191–6.

Spierings ELH, Schroevers M, Honkoop PC, Sorbi M. Development of chronic daily headache: a clinical study. Headache 1998;38:529–33.

Editorial Comments

Rarely does one get to view a case where the author was actually one of the original clinicians to describe the entity under discussion. Dr. Spierings along with Dr. Sjaastad coined the phrase hemicrania continua in 1984 and specified its absolute responsiveness to indomethacin. This case goes beyond the usual presentation and discussion to allow the reader to truly understand the evolution of this form of chronic daily headache and its unique therapy.

CHAPTER 24

THE WOMAN WITH SHORT-LASTING, UNILATERAL HEADACHE AND AUTONOMIC SYMPTOMS

TODD D. ROZEN, MD

Case History

A 24-year-old woman began having a stereotypic headache syndrome at the age of 18. Her headache was always right sided, beginning with a twinge of pain over the right eye that could radiate into the right upper cheek and behind the right ear. A tightening, painful sensation at the base of the right side of the neck sometimes preceded the headache by several minutes. There was no aura. The pain was sharp and severe, and the headaches would last between 5 and 15 minutes. The attacks would recur every 1 to 2 hours with a maximum of 24 attacks in a single day. The pain sometimes awakened her from sleep. Between headaches, she would experience a mild discomfort in the right periorbital distribution. Associated symptoms included nausea, right-sided nasal congestion, rare right-sided ptosis, and light-headedness, but no conjunctival injection, eyelid edema, or unilateral eye tearing. She denied suffering from photophobia, phonophobia, blurred or double vision, vertigo, stroke-like spells, or change in head pain with exertion. She could not function during the headache either at work or at home because of the severity of the pain. Triggers for the headache attack included chewing and stress. She could not lie quietly with a headache, although she denied pacing.

She had tried multiple abortive headache medications, including acetylsalicylic acid, naproxen sodium, codeine, acetaminophen/aspirin/caffeine tablets, ibuprofen, acetaminophen, dihydroergotamine, and sumatriptan, without relief. At one time she was taking as many as 60 200-mg ibuprofen tablets a day with no pain relief.

She had no significant past medical history except for a cesarean section. There was no history of tobacco use or excessive alcohol use. She had a strong family history of migraine in her mother, brother, and maternal uncle. Her general examination was normal and her neurologic examination was intact except for tenderness on palpation over the right greater occipital nerve. There was no evidence of a miotic pupil or ptosis. Magnetic resonance imaging (MRI) examination of the brain and cervical spine was normal.

Questions about This Case

- How does the duration of the headaches and the frequency of the attacks help formulate your differential diagnosis?
- Should a patient with this clinical scenario have neuroimaging studies such as a computed tomography (CT) or MRI scan of the brain?

- How would you best manage this patient's headache?
- What specific therapies would you suggest?

Case Discussion

In this patient's case, we are able to create a differential diagnosis once we carefully examine all aspects of the headache history. When taking a pain history, it is of the utmost importance to define the location of the pain, the quality, intensity, duration, and frequency of attacks, associated triggers, and alleviating factors, as well as response to past pain medications.

Let us dissect this patient's headache history piece by piece. It is important to recognize that the patient is a woman. Not all headache disorders have a gender preponderance but some do, for example, migraine is a female-dominant disorder, while cluster is a condition found mainly in men.

The patient's pain is strictly unilateral with no shifting from side to side during or between attacks. The head pain is sharp and so severe it stops her from completing the activities of daily living. Each headache is very short in duration, only lasting between 5 and 15 minutes. The attacks are very frequent, sometimes occurring as many as 24 times a day.

Autonomic phenomena marked the patient's associated symptoms, including nasal congestion and ptosis. The patient tried multiple abortive headache medicines that normally would yield benefit in migraine, cluster, and tension-type headaches, but none of these afforded her any relief.

There are very few primary headache disorders that are marked by strictly unilateral pain, short attack duration, high frequency of attacks, and associated autonomic symptoms.

At first glance, this patient may appear to have cluster headaches, a disorder that is marked by very severe headaches in an orbital or temporal location. They are strictly unilateral, with almost no shifting from side to side during attacks and rarely between attacks. Headache duration is between 15 and 180 minutes with a mean attack duration of 45 minutes. Normal attack frequency is between one and three a day, but some individuals have up to eight cluster headaches in a day. This headache disorder is marked by autonomic symptoms such as ptosis, conjunctival injection, and nasal rhinorrhea, ipsilateral to the painful side. Cluster headache can be chronic (fewer than 14 headache-free days a year) or episodic.

Our patient certainly has some characteristics of cluster headache, but she does not have cluster headache for several reasons that we determined via the headache history. First of all, our patient is a woman, and cluster is a male-dominant condition, with a male:female ratio of 6:1. Secondly, this patient's attack duration would be on the very short end of a cluster attack, and the frequency of attacks is higher than would be seen with cluster headache. Both the case-study patient and cluster patients have significant autonomic symptoms during an attack. This patient had some difficulty lying still with a headache. Unlike migraine patients who like to lie down during a headache, cluster patients normally pace or rock, sometimes actually needing to bang their heads. This patient's headache satisfies some criteria for cluster headache, but there are notable differences.

This patient also does not fit the criteria for migraine headaches. The strict unilaterality of pain, the very short attacks (IHS criteria for migraine needs more than 4 hours) and the high frequency of attacks preclude migraine as a diagnosis. The patient also lacks the recognized associated symptoms for migraine including photophobia, phonophobia, and worsening of head pain with movement.

Short-lasting, unilateral neuralgiform headache with conjunctival injection and tearing (SUNCT) is one of the rarest headache disorders. First described by Sjaastad et al. in 1989, SUNCT, as its name suggests, is a short-lasting headache syndrome with autonomic symptoms. There are very few reported cases in the literature, but SUNCT appears to be a male disorder, with a male:female ratio of 8:1. The SUNCT pain is moderate to severe in intensity, stabbing in quality, and is located in an orbital or temporal distribution. The typical duration of an attack is between 5 and 250 seconds, although two patients have had attacks lasting up to 2 hours. Attack frequency can vary from one a day up to 30 an hour. Mean attack frequency is about

28, but up to 77 a day have been reported. Attacks can be precipitated by neck movement. No successful treatment regimens for SUNCT have been discovered. Our patient could possibly have SUNCT based on attack frequency, but the duration of attacks, lack of conjunctival injection, which is the most prominent symptom in SUNCT, and female gender, would suggest that this diagnosis is unlikely, although it is still one of the better candidates in the differential diagnosis.

Hemicrania continua is a strictly unilateral headache disorder marked by constant pain that is mild to moderate in severity. About 60% of patients experience added attacks of more severe, short-lasting pain often associated with autonomic symptoms. The autonomic symptoms are never as dramatic as they are in cluster headache. Men and women have almost equal prevalence. The case-study patient has some features of hemicrania continua, but the lack of continuous pain, higher pain severity, and prominent autonomic symptoms suggest another diagnosis.

Trigeminal neuralgia is marked by paroxysms of lancinating or electric-shock-like pains, each lasting about 1 second but recurring so frequently that the patient may not be able to identify pain-free periods. Pain is normally confined to the second and third division of the trigeminal nerve. The pain can be triggered by chewing, touching the face, or brushing the teeth. Trigeminal neuralgia responds to carbamazepine, phenytoin, and baclofen. Although chewing could trigger an attack in our patient, the duration of her attacks was too long to be trigeminal neuralgia. In addition, our patient's pain quality differs from the pain of trigeminal neuralgia.

The case-study patient best fits the diagnosis of chronic paroxysmal hemicrania (CPH), a short-lasting, unilateral headache syndrome marked by a female predominance. Head pain is strictly unilateral and the same side of the head is always affected. Pollmann et al. in 1986 presented a possible case of bilateral CPH. The CPH pain location is normally orbital, temporal, and above or behind the ear. The pain is severe in intensity and may radiate to the neck or ipsilateral shoulder. The pain has been described as boring, claw-like, or pulsatile. Residual pain may remain in between attacks. Normal headache duration is between 2 and 45 minutes (Case patient: 5 to 15 minutes). Headache frequency is between 1 and 40 attacks a day, although IHS criteria (Appendix 24–1) demand more than five attacks a day for more than half the time (Case patient: one attack an hour). Unlike cluster headache, there is no predilection for nocturnal attacks in CPH, although attacks can certainly awaken a patient from sleep. Associated symptoms are marked by autonomic phenomena. The case patient had unilateral ptosis and nasal congestion. Most CPH patients exhibit lacrimation (62%), followed by nasal congestion (42%), conjunctival injection and rhinorrhea (36%), and ptosis (33%). Unlike cluster headache, a true Horner's syndrome is not seen in CPH. The CPH patients may have photophobia, but gastrointestinal disturbances are rare. The CPH patients can sometimes trigger attacks by rotating the neck, flexing the head, or applying external pressure to the transverse processes of C4 to C5 or the C2 nerve root on the symptomatic side. Alleviating factors include sitting still or lying in bed, unlike the cluster patient, who would need to "pace the floors." The above discussion has presented the differential diagnoses for the case patient, and provided the reasoning for selecting CPH as the correct diagnosis.

This patient had an MRI of the brain and cervical spine which was normal. In most instances, neuroimaging of CPH patients will not uncover an underlying lesion, but there are a number of CPH cases that have been apparently caused by hidden structural lesions, making imaging a mandatory part of the work-up of a CPH patient. Structural mimics of CPH have included a parasellar pituitary microadenoma, a maxillary cyst, an occipital infarction, a gangliocytoma growing from the sella turcica, an ophthalmic herpes zoster infection, an arteriovenous malformation, a cavernous sinus meningioma, a frontal lobe tumor, and a Pancoast's tumor. An MRI is suggested as the neuroimaging procedure of choice, because of its higher sensitivity than that of a CT scan for visualizing tumors and vascular malformations.

With regard to treatment strategies, CPH is one of the rare headache disorders that by definition is totally responsive to indomethacin. Headache specialists will expose a probable CPH patient to a short, therapeutic trial of indomethacin, looking for a response. The normal starting dosage of indomethacin is one 25-mg tablet three times a day for 3 days; this dosage can be increased to two tablets (50 mg) three times a day if there is no response. Most individuals will respond by 150 mg a day, and the response can be dramatic, with rapid dissipation of headache symptoms. A beneficial effect will normally be seen within 48 hours after the correct dosage has been found. Some individuals need a dosage as high as 300 mg of indomethacin a day. If there is no response at 150 mg a day, and the physician still suspects CPH, an extra 25-mg dose of indomethacin can be added every 3 days, to a total of 225 mg a day or until the onset of side effects. If the patient does not respond at 75 mg three times a day, one should consider an alternative diagnosis. This patient had complete headache relief with 200 mg a day of indomethacin.

The side effects of indomethacin therapy are mainly gastrointestinal disturbances with either dyspepsia or ulcer development. The gastrointestinal side effects can normally be controlled with histamine type 2 receptor antagonists, proton pump inhibitors, or prostaglandins. Misoprostol at a dose of 100 to 200 μg, four times a day, is very successful in preventing nonsteroidal-drug-induced ulcers. This agent is not well tolerated by patients, however, because of its side effects of diarrhea and abdominal pain. The author has a patient who developed renal papillary necrosis on indomethacin therapy for CPH.

Management Strategies

- Establish the correct diagnosis based on a comprehensive headache history.
- This form of headache is rare and may not be easily recognized by nonheadache specialists. When recognized correctly, headache treatment can be simple and successful.
- If the patient has not had neuroimaging, it should be completed, preferably an MRI of the brain.
- Make sure to push the indomethacin dose to at least 150 mg a day if tolerated by the patient, and even to 225 mg a day if the physician believes the patient has CPH.

- Monitor for indomethacin side effects such as gastrointestinal distress, and hematuria which may signify renal damage.

Case Summary

- The patient has chronic paroxysmal hemicrania, which was responsive to indomethacin
- Diagnosis can sometimes be difficult, but once the correct diagnosis is made, a dramatic response to indomethacin is achieved.

Overview of Chronic Paroxysmal Hemicrania

What follows is an overview of chronic paroxysmal hemicrania (CPH). This overview should help put the present case in perspective, and give the reader useful information on this unique headache syndrome.

Chronic paroxysmal hemicrania is a rare syndrome marked by headaches of short duration, high frequency, and associated autonomic symptoms. It was first described by Sjaastad and Dale in 1974 and has now been diagnosed all over the world. As of 1996, over 100 cases of CPH have been reported in the literature, new cases are no longer being actively published.

Chronic paroxysmal hemicrania appears to be a disorder found in women. The female to male ratio is about 3:1. There is no difference between women and men with CPH with regard to the duration or frequency of attacks, or age of onset. Men experiencing long-duration CPH attacks have a lower frequency of attacks than do men with short-duration attacks. This inverse correlation is not seen in women. Chronic paroxysmal hemicrania appears to occur in all races. The true prevalence of CPH is unknown.

Chronic paroxysmal hemicrania normally develops in the second or third decade of life, but it can occur at any age. The youngest reported patient in the literature is 6 years of age while the oldest is 81 years. No one knows the true natural history of CPH as to whether it is a self-limited syndrome or a lifelong condition. In a review of all reported cases as of 1989, Antonaci and Sjaastad found a mean duration of illness to be 13.3 ± 12.2 years.

There does not appear to be a genetic predisposition for CPH, as no familial cases have been reported. Patients with CPH do not have a higher familial incidence of cluster headache. About 20% of CPH patients will have a family history of migraine; this is about equal to the percentage of cluster patients with a familial experience of migraine.

Chronic paroxysmal hemicrania is a disorder found in women, so hormonal factors would appear to play a significant role in its pathogenesis. Like migraine, CPH is influenced by female sex hormones, but no specific pattern has been noted. Women with CPH may have improvement or worsening during menses. There can be improvement of symptoms during pregnancy, and there are reported cases of CPH induction just after delivery. Oral contraceptives do not appear to influence CPH and no studies are available on the effect of menopause on CPH.

Past medical history in CPH patients is usually unremarkable although head trauma has been reported in up to 15% of patients and neck trauma in about 10%. Chronic paroxysmal hemicrania has developed after surgery for uterine polyps, maxillary sinusitis, and fibromas. There appears to be no relationship between CPH and other primary medical disorders, although histories of diabetes mellitus, hyperthyroidism, malignant melanoma, epilepsy, and idiopathic thrombocytopenia have been noted in documented CPH patients.

Chronic paroxysmal hemicrania, by IHS definition, is an indomethacin-sensitive syndrome. Individuals normally require a continuous dosage until the CPH syndrome has completed its course (this can be lifetime dosage). Symptoms usually recur as soon as 12 hours or up to several days after discontinuing the indomethacin. Sjaastad et al. (1995) found that individuals requiring high doses of indomethacin (200 to 250 mg per day) are more apt to have underlying secondary causes of CPH.

The literature provides very little assistance when indomethacin is no longer a viable treatment option for CPH. In 1996 Evers et al. presented alternative drug treatments for CPH. Twenty-two other agents have been studied in CPH; the most successful alternative preventive drug is verapamil, 240 to 320 mg a day. Acetylsalicylic acid, naproxen, and a piroxicam derivative have shown some effect in a small number of cases. Acetazolamide was effective in a single case report. Prednisone is effective in high doses for controlling CPH but is not considered an adequate chronic therapy regimen because of its side-effect profile. Chronic paroxysmal hemicrania shows a poor response to carbamazepine and oxygen. Sumatriptan has been a good abortive agent in several case reports. If these agents fail to control CPH headaches, the physician could attempt to use agents that have been successful in treating cluster headache, such as lithium and valproic acid, although there is no literature to support this maneuver.

The pathophysiology of chronic paroxysmal hemicrania is not known, but its symptoms suggest autonomic nervous system abnormalities of parasympathetic activation (tearing, nasal congestion) and sympathetic dysfunction (ptosis).

Carvalho et al. (1998) have performed pupillary studies on CPH patients. These studies demonstrated a miotic pupil ipsilateral to the pain side, probably representing a partial Horner's syndrome and, thus, sympathetic dysfunction. Chronic paroxysmal hemicrania patients appear to have normal facial sweating patterns, unlike cluster patients, and there have been no consistent changes in salivation and nasal discharge in individuals with CPH.

Changes in heart rate such as bradycardia, bundle branch block, and atrial fibrillation have been associated with CPH and probably reflects a failure of the autonomic nervous system during attacks.

It has been postulated that stimulation of a trigeminal-autonomic reflex pathway causes the symptoms of CPH. This pathway is the result of a brainstem connection between the trigeminal nerve and the facial nerve parasympathetic outflow. Trigeminal activation would lead to pain in the distribution of the trigeminal nerve, as experienced by CPH patients, as well as concomitant stimulation of the facial nerve parasympathetic outflow, producing lacrimation, nasal congestion, and rhinorrhea.

In 1996, Goadsby and Edvinsson identified a CPH patient with elevated levels of calcitonin gene-related peptide (CGRP), a trigeminal nerve peptide, and vasoactive intestinal polypeptide (VIP), a parasympathetic peptide, in jugular venous blood during a CPH attack. The values normalized after treatment with indomethacin. Stimulation of the trigeminal ganglion in cats causes the same elevation in CGRP and VIP levels, giving credence to the hypothesis that trigeminal-autonomic pathway activation actually occurs during CPH attacks. The exact triggering mechanisms for the trigeminal-autonomic complex in CPH patients is unknown. Laboratory investigative studies have given us a much greater insight into the pathophysiology of CPH and have provided the impetus for future studies investigating both the true cause of this unique headache syndrome and the reason why indomethacin is the only effective treatment.

Selected Readings

Antonaci F, Sjaastad O. Chronic paroxysmal hemicrania (CPH): a review of the clinical manifestations. Headache 1989; 29:648–56.

Carvalho DSS, Salvesen R, Sand T, et al. Chronic paroxysmal hemicrania. XIII. The pupillometric pattern. Cephalalgia 1988;8:219–26.

Evers S, Husstedt I-W. Alternatives in drug treatment of chronic paroxysmal hemicrania. Headache 1996;36:429–32.

Goadsby PJ, Edvinsson L. Neuropeptide changes in a case of chronic paroxysmal hemicrania—evidence for trigeminal parasympathetic activation. Cephalalgia 1996;16:448–50.

Goadsby PJ, Lipton RB. A review of paroxysmal hemicranias, SUNCT syndrome and other short-lasting headache with autonomic features, including new cases. Brain 1997;120: 193–209.

Pollmann W, Pfaffenrath V. Chronic paroxysmal hemicrania: the first possible bilateral case. Cephalalgia 1986;6:55–7.

Sjaastad O, Dale I. Evidence for a new (?) treatable headache entity. Headache 1974;14:105–8.

Sjaastad O, Saunte C, Salvesen R, et al. Short-lasting unilateral neuralgiform headache attacks with conjunctival injection, tearing, sweating, and rhinorrhea. Cephalalgia 1989;9: 147–56.

Sjaastad O, Stovner LJ, Stolt-Nielsen A, et al. CPH and hemicrania continua: requirements of high indomethacin dosages —an ominous sign? Headache 1995;35:363–7.

Editorial Comments

Chronic paroxysmal hemicrania (CPH) is a rare disorder and can be difficult to diagnose but, when recognized, is absolutely responsive to indomethacin. Dr. Rozen's case is very instructive in teaching us the appropriate diagnostic "thinking" in arriving at a diagnosis of CPH. Further, and importantly, he emphasizes the need to consider other diagnoses including secondary etiologies for CPH, and the need for neuroimaging. Common things are common is the clinical aphorism; however, clinical disorders such as CPH do exist and should not be overlooked or overdiagnosed. Caution in the use of indomethacin in this headache disorder is also emphasized by the author.

Appendix 24–1
IHS Diagnostic Criteria for Chronic Paroxysmal Hemicrania (1988)

A. At least 50 attacks fulfilling B–E

B. Attacks of severe unilateral, orbital, supraorbital, and/or temporal pain, always on the same side, lasting 2 to 45 minutes

C. Attack frequency >5 per day for more than half the time (periods with lower frequency may occur)

D. Pain is associated with at least one of the following signs or symptoms on the pain side:
  1. Conjunctival injection
  2. Lacrimation
  3. Nasal congestion
  4. Rhinorrhea
  5. Ptosis
  6. Eyelid edema

E. Absolute effectiveness of indomethacin (150 mg/ day or less)

F. At least one of the following:
  1. History and/or physical and/or neurologic examinations do not suggest one of the disorders listed in groups 5–11, i.e., organic headaches, headaches associated with drug withdrawal, metabolic disorder, etc.
  2. History and/or physical and/or neurologic examinations do suggest such a disorder, but it is ruled out by appropriate investigations.
  3. Such a disorder is present, but chronic paroxysmal hemicrania does not occur for the first time in close temporal relation to the disorder.

SECONDARY, RARE, AND UNUSUAL HEADACHE DISORDERS

CHAPTER 25

THE PATIENT WITH THE CHANGING HEADACHE

JOHN S. WARNER, MD

Case History

A 31-year-old woman came to the headache clinic with a history of migraine that had started early in childhood. During the previous 10 years these headaches occurred three times each month and sometimes lasted for 24 hours. The headache might start at anytime during the day or night, and she stated that she might see spots for 2 days prior to these headaches. No other prodrome had been noted and she denied an aura. The pain started in the right temple, spread to the right half of the head and neck, sparing the face, and had a throbbing sensation when at its maximum. Nausea, vomiting, lightheadedness, phonophobia, and photophobia accompanied most headaches. The pain was accentuated by cough, strain, or movement. Prior to her hysterectomy, there had been no relationship of these headaches with menses. "Migraine" never occurred on the left side. A magnetic resonance imaging scan 2 years earlier was reported to be normal. Ergotamine/bellafoline/phenobarbital tablets and metoprolol failed to prevent these headaches.

A different headache began 2 months prior to her initial visit to the clinic. These headaches were daily and nocturnal during the first 2 weeks. Thereafter they occurred as often as four times each day or night without a true circadian pattern. She noted the sudden onset of intense pain in the right temple and face spreading rapidly into the neck. She described this as "a knife that is continuously being pushed deeper into the head," more intense than the previous migraine, and without the prodrome or throbbing sensation. This pain would last for 10 to 15 minutes, rapidly subside to become a minimal dull discomfort for the next 2 to 3 minutes, then suddenly return as the intense pain. These episodes of repeated intense 10- to 15-minute pains, interrupted by 2 to 3 minutes of discomfort, might last for 45 minutes or continue as long as 7 hours. Vomiting often accompanied these headaches and the patient noted unilateral photophobia and scalp tenderness on the right. Movement of the eyes increased the pain, and pressure on the right orbit would provide partial relief. The pain was unrelated to position and did not change with cough or strain. During each of these headaches, she experienced ipsilateral conjunctival injection, increased lacrimation, nasal obstruction, and swelling of the face. Frequently, she experienced the sensation of her heart having skipped a beat.

The past medical history was otherwise noncontributory. Two days earlier she had been started on verapamil 80 mg t.i.d. and prochlorperazine 25 mg p.r.n. which provided partial relief. The neurologic examination was performed when she was headache free, and it revealed no abnormalities.

Questions about This Case

- Were her earlier headaches migraine?
- How do you classify the more recent headaches?
- What neurodiagnostic studies would you request?
- What therapy would you prescribe?

Case Discussion

This case study addresses the problem of changing pattern of headache, an occurrence which frequently precedes a patient's initial visit to a primary care physician or referral to a headache specialist. Most often, the change in the headache presents no immediate or urgent risk to the patient's future health. Exceptions include the warning or sentinel headache of a bleeding intracranial aneurysm or the initial headache of bacterial meningitis, conditions that often escape appropriate or timely evaluation.

Changing pattern of headache occurs in three forms. The first consists of changes of features of one headache type over a period of time. These changes are common in migraine and are revealed by taking a careful history from the patient or by comparing the notes from recent office visits with the notes of previous visits. A migraine might originally begin in the temple and then in later years start with pain in the upper neck and, in both instances, spread to become a unilateral headache. It is not unusual for a person to have migraine without aura prior to menopause and to have auras without headache after menopause. These changes in pattern of a single headache usually do not disturb the patient or present a problem to the physician.

The other two forms of changing pattern of headache involve the development of an entirely different headache type. During their lifetime, most people will experience different types of headaches. Rarely is there a person with an alcoholic hangover who has not had at least one previous tension-type headache. That individual almost always recognizes the cause and method of avoiding the intense early morning headache and vomiting which follow the prior evening's overindulgence. Although they may experience repeated hangover headaches, they almost never seek medical attention for this combination of headache.

Changing pattern of headache might consist of changing from one type of primary headache to another primary headache disorder as occurred in the patient whose history was cited at the start of this case history. Many patients with migraine following puberty will have noted tension-type headache prior to puberty. At times they have difficulty recognizing the onset of each of these primary headaches, and some authors question whether tension-type headache and migraine represent two extremes of only one condition.

On the other hand, changing pattern of headache might occur in a patient having an initial primary headache disorder and later developing a "secondary headache" caused by toxic, metabolic, infectious, vascular, neoplastic, and other conditions. Further into this discussion, it will be shown that the patient whose history was presented went on to develop two different secondary headaches and later had two additional pain-in-the-head and face problems, a total of six distinct conditions.

At the end of the case history, four questions were raised and this is an appropriate place to discuss them. The patient's prior headaches were migraine, fulfilling the International Headache Society's rigid definition of migraine without aura. She had noted more than five headaches of greater than 4 hours' duration. The pain was pulsating, unilateral, and accentuated by movement. Nausea, vomiting, photophobia, and phonophobia accompanied these migraine attacks. There is no indication for neurodiagnostic studies for migraine attacks of this duration. In the past, the patient had seen numerous physicians who had given various medications to abort the migraine attacks, but she had never received satisfactory treatment to prevent the episodes.

Her more recent headaches were episodic, unilateral, and accompanied by ipsilateral changes of the autonomic nervous system. Three headache syndromes present with these features. The first is true cluster headache, a condition that usually occurs in males. The pain of cluster headaches is periorbital, excruciating, lasting from 15 to 120 minutes, and rarely occurring more than four times a day. This patient's headache duration was shorter, lasting only 10 to 15 minutes. The attacks occurred more frequently and were more widespread. There was no circadian pattern, a feature that is often noted with cluster. Thus, the more recent headaches which this patient was experiencing are not cluster headaches.

A second unilateral headache with ipsilateral autonomic features is the short-lasting neuralgiform headache with conjunctival injection and tearing (SUNCT) syndrome, an extremely uncommon condition which thus far has been described in less than 30 Europeans, mostly male, Scandinavian, and over the age of 47 years at the time of their initial attack. The pain in SUNCT syndrome lasts less than 120 seconds and is reported to occur as often as 30 times an hour. Interestingly, the SUNCT syndrome has never been recognized in North Americans of pure Norwegian or Swedish descent.

The third cause of paroxysmal headache with ipsilateral changes of autonomic nervous system function is the primary headache disorder initially described as chronic paroxysmal hemicrania (CPH) but later recognized as occurring in an episodic pattern. This condition occurs at less than 10% of the incidence of cluster headache and less than 1% of the incidence of migraine. The typical patient with CPH is a female with unilateral headache of 20 minute duration that occurs at least 11 times each day. The intensity and location of maximum discomfort of this unilateral pain varies from one patient to the next. This is in contrast to the more prolonged, less frequent, excruciating periorbital pain of a cluster headache, the latter sparing the parietal, occipital, and vertex area. Characteristically, the headache of CPH responds to indomethacin.

To date, there is no satisfactory explanation for the neurophysiologic changes of CPH nor any understanding of the neurochemical changes that probably are occurring. Isolated reports of somewhat similar headaches secondary to organic disease have been published in recent years. Therefore, it would be appropriate to order magnetic resonance imaging and a platelet count for patients suspected of having CPH.

This particular patient's headache pattern was unusual for CPH in that she had flurries of intense headaches each day, each 10 to 15 minute pain separated by brief episodes of minimal pain at the same site. These flurries occurred daily and would last for as long as 7 hours.

Her headaches were classified as CPH presenting in the episodic pattern. She was started on indomethacin 75 mg t.i.d. at the first visit and experienced almost immediate relief. She was pain-free the following 2 days. At noon on day 4, she noted the gradual onset of a generalized throbbing headache with subsequent vomiting, the pain accentuated as she flexed her neck. The headache and vomiting continued throughout the night and she returned to the clinic on the morning of day 5. The presumptive diagnosis at that time was a generalized headache secondary to indomethacin therapy. A lumbar puncture was performed to exclude meningeal infection. Acellular fluid with normal protein and sugar was obtained, the opening pressure being 120 mm. The indomethacin was stopped and the generalized headache ceased, only to be followed the next day by typical postspinal headache which required a blood patch on day 8. These latter two iatrogenic headaches appeared during a 1-week interval and represented an example of primary headache(s) changing to secondary headache(s). Fortunately, the etiology of each of these secondary headaches was immediately recognized and appropriately treated without prolonged suffering by the patient.

Her episodes of paroxysmal hemicrania returned 1 week after the indomethacin was terminated. Verapamil 120 mg t.i.d. provided relief and after 1 month was discontinued. During the following 18 months she had migraine headaches about once every 3 weeks lasting 2 to 3 days. She was not on prophylactic therapy and was using only simple analgesics. After having been quiescent for 18 months, the right sided headache of CPH returned. The area of pain enlarged; the pain spread into the tongue and throat. Initially, the episodes occurred daily but over the following 4 weeks these increased to three per day. The usual episode lasted 1 or 2 hours during which time she noted intense pain for 10 to 15 minutes followed by minimal pain for 10 or 15 minutes, then a return to the intense pain. Ipsilateral autonomic changes accompanied each intense pain. These attacks ceased when she restarted verapamil 80 mg t.i.d., a drug that she continued for only 3 weeks.

Eleven months later, she was injured in a motor vehicle accident. During the following 3 months, she had constant daily, dull, generalized headache and more intense generalized migraine-like attacks 3 days each week. She was taking various over-the-counter analgesics at least four times each day. When she returned to the clinic with this history of 3 months of constant post-traumatic headache, she was told that these were a typical pattern of analgesic-induced or analgesic-rebound daily headache following trauma. She was instructed to stop all analgesics and her daily continuous headaches ceased approximately 1 week later.

Four months later, she was seen at another medical center for right-sided jaw, ear, and temple pain of 6 months' duration, a complaint that she had not voiced at previous visits. Surgery was performed on the right temporomandibular joint following which she noted some relief of the right-sided facial pain.

When last seen at the headache clinic, she reported the resumption of the pattern of one to three migraine headaches each month. In addition, she was noting frequent episodes of paroxysmal hemicrania with autonomic changes lasting for 3 to 4 hours each. Interestingly, she insisted that these latest attacks had shifted to the left side. Verapamil was again prescribed and she again failed to return for follow-up visits.

Since her last visit, she has not returned to the headache clinic. Attempts to contact the patient by phone and mail have been unsuccessful. In reviewing her records from the last 3½ years, it is noted that she had experienced every form of changing headache pattern. Her migraine had changed from right to left. A second primary headache problem, namely, chronic paroxysmal hemicrania in its episodic presentation, had appeared and later shifted to the other side. She had experienced iatrogenic indomethacin-induced headache and lumbar puncture headache. Following a motor vehicle accident, she developed analgesic-induced headache. Lastly, she developed what another center diagnosed and treated as temporomandibular joint pain. There is no record of simple tension-type headaches.

The lesson to be learned from this case is that over time, there are usually changes in headache pattern in a given individual. The physician encountering the headache patient must always carefully inquire as to the different types of pain that the patient might be experiencing. This has to be followed by specific questioning regarding the date of initial onset, frequency, duration, character of pain, and the accompanying features of each headache type. The proper therapeutic approach to each headache type often differs.

Portions of this patient's history were included in Case Histories from The Vanderbilt Headache Clinic #15. Headache Q 1994;5:159–60. It is reprinted with permission of the editor.

Editorial Comments

All physicians caring for patients with headache will fully appreciate this case from Dr. Warner. Most patients with headache have more than one type, and it is well known that migraine presents with multiple subtypes in many patients. Variability is common in headache as are changing patterns. It may seem that this patient has a remarkable array of headaches, and she does, but with careful historical inquiry and appropriate therapy for each subtype or type of headache, she can be effectively managed, as outlined by Dr. Warner.

We should all be vigilant to detect the changing headache as it could represent a new organic problem, even an iatrogenic one.

CHAPTER 26

THE PATIENT WITH HEADACHE AND ABNORMAL MENSES

GENNARO BUSSONE, MD

FRANCA MOSCHIANO, MD

Case History

The patient was a 35-year-old working woman who did not drink or smoke and led a normal life. She had no history of significant illness, except that at the age of 16 she suffered a bout of weight increase (putting on 20 kg in a few months) associated with reduced menstrual cycle frequency and flow. She managed to regain her previous weight after about a year without dieting or therapy. However, the menstrual cycle alteration persisted and at the age of 30 she developed oligomenorrhea, which was treated with estrogen/progesterone. The patient discontinued the medication on her own initiative after 6 months, and amenorrhea and headache appeared within a month; there was no galactorrhea.

The headaches were mild, seemed like a weight on the head involving the entire cranium, were without autonomic signs, lasted 4 to 5 hours, and resolved without the use of analgesics. After about a year, they were occurring every day, with more or less the same characteristics but with periods of intense head pain resembling migraine attacks associated with nausea, photo- and phonophobia. The patient started taking analgesics (indomethacin and ibuprofen) for the intense episodes. Initially these reduced the pain but never completely resolved it. Eventually she was taking analgesics daily and at this point decided to consult a neurologist who advised hospital admission for further examination.

On admission, the patient's clinical examination was normal, her blood pressure was 135/85, and her heart rate was 68 beats per minute; routine blood tests and a neurologic examination were all normal. An eye examination revealed normal fundi and visual fields. A head radiograph revealed an enlarged sella turcica, prompting a sellar region computed tomography (CT) study with contrast, which revealed an area of hypodensity at the median-paramedian base of the hypophysis, compatible with microadenoma. Magnetic resonance imaging (MRI) with and without gadolinium-pentetic acid showed a rounded, hypodense (compared to the gland) lesion in the hypophysis of about 8 × 10 mm compatible with hypophyseal adenoma (Figure 26–1). Given the high prolactin (PRL) level (180 ng per milliliter; normal level is 5 to 20 ng per milliliter) and normal thyroid-stimulating hormone (TSH), free triiodothyronine (FT_3), free thyroxine (FT_4), adrenocorticotropic hormone, cortisol, growth hormone, follicle-stimulating hormone, and luteinizing hormone levels, the patient was started on cabergoline (a dopaminergic ergot) (500 mg per week) resulting in amelioration and eventual disappearance of the headache, with return of the menstrual cycle and prolactin levels to normal (15.6 ng per milliliter) after about a year. An MRI performed after a year of cabergoline revealed a modest reduction in the volume of the lesion and the absence of intralesional or intrasellar hemorrhage

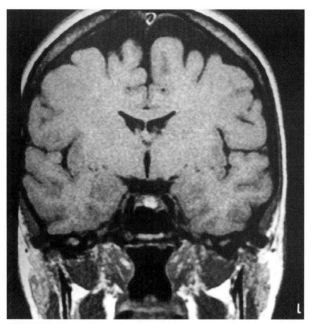

FIGURE 26–1. Coronal section of a T1-weighted MR image showing a dense pituitary microadenoma.

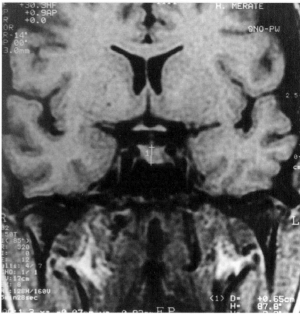

FIGURE 26–2. Coronal section of a T1-weighted MR image showing microadenoma after 12 months of cabergoline therapy.

(Figure 26–2). The patient remains asymptomatic and continues therapy with cabergoline.

Questions about This Case

- Is headache a prominent symptom of hypophyseal adenoma?
- What type of headache is typical of prolactinoma?
- What causes the headache—increased PRL levels or prolactinoma?
- What is the possible pathogenetic mechanism of this type of headache?
- What are the therapeutic possibilities for PRL-secreting hypophyseal tumors?
- Does headache improve in response to therapy?

Case Discussion

Our female patient presented with a history of worsening tension-type headache, interspersed with rare episodes of migrainous headache. There was an extended history of menstrual cycle alterations culminating in hyperprolactinemia-induced amenorrhea. Neuroradiologic investigations led to the diagnosis of PRL-secreting, hypophyseal microadenoma.

Headache is a symptom of 12 to 60% of women with PRL-secreting adenoma. Which is the primary cause of the headache, the hyperprolactinemia or the intracranial tumor with mass effect? The clinical impression is that the headaches resemble tension headaches, typically lacking prodromal signs and one-sidedness; they may last for hours and often require medication. In a study by Strebel et al. (1986) of a group of women with secondary amenorrhea, galactorrhea, or both, headache was four times more frequent in those with prolactinoma than in those without, and tended not to disappear when prolactin levels were restored to normal. The hyperprolactinemia was associated with headache only in the presence of a prolactinoma, and neither high nor intermediate levels of PRL were associated with headache after prolactinoma regression.

These findings seem to suggest that the mass effect of the prolactinoma is responsible for the headache in women with nonpuerperal hyperprolactinemia. Thus, in spite of its nonspecific nature, headache may indicate the presence of occult prolactinoma in women with secondary amenorrhea and/or galactorrhea. This is further supported by the fact that nonsecreting hypophyseal adenomas producing compressive signs are associated with headache in 70 to 80% of cases.

It is hypothesized that hypophyseal adenoma may give rise to headache through compression of the sella diaphragm or torsion of the cranial and dural blood vessels with activation of blood vessel nociceptors, and stimulation of the meningeal nociceptors. These events could trigger headaches in genetically predisposed patients characterized by a low pain threshold.

In conclusion, a strong association between persistent headaches of apparently tension type and prolactinoma suggests headache as an indicator of prolactinoma and not hyperprolactinemia. Prolactinoma is only rarely associated with migraine-like headache (without aura) and is extremely rare with a cluster headache-like syndrome.

Management Strategies

Administration of dopaminergic drugs is the current therapy of choice for both micro- and macroprolactinomas. Bromocriptine is the most used drug, but lisuride and cabergoline are effective alternatives. To reduce the side effects of bromocriptine (nausea, vomiting, and orthostatic hypotension) treatment should begin with low doses (e.g., 1.25 mg orally) in the evening, which are gradually increased until PRL levels return to normal. Typically 10 to 20 mg per day of bromocriptine is required.

The therapeutic efficacy is generally excellent: the headaches and galactorrhea disappear, the menstrual cycle returns to normal in women, and hypogonadism improves in men. In a high percentage of patients, the prolactinoma regresses and in some cases disappears altogether, apparently achieving a complete cure; 80% of microadenomas are cured. Adenomectomy is indicated only for patients who do not respond to or cannot tolerate dopaminergic medication.

It is important to distinguish microadenomas that do not produce visual disturbances from those which permanently compromise vision. In macroadenomas without disturbance of vision, surgery with or without subsequent bromocriptine, radiotherapy, or both, provide 10-year recurrence-free survival in 75 to 80% of cases and similar overall survival. This excellent prognosis worsens to 55 to 60% in macroadenomas when there is disturbance of vision (the most unfavorable prognostic factor). Following surgical excision of the tumor, vision recovers or returns to normal in 55 to 75% of cases and a similar proportion return to a normal life. In some operated cases, the patient's vision remains compromised and may even worsen. This usually occurs if visual damage is already extensive preoperatively (e.g., there is bitemporal hemianopsia) or when tumor removal involves extensive manipulation of the optic pathways.

Radical surgery associated with postoperative radiotherapy produces a definitive cure in the majority of cases. If carried out promptly, surgery for recurrences (which occur in 5 to 12% of cases) is not associated with higher mortality than for the treatment of primary disease, and a definitive cure can again be achieved. The probability of cure for prolactinoma declines if PRL levels exceed 2000 mU per liter, if the tumor is greater than 1 cm in diameter, if there is local invasion, and if the patient is more than 25 years old.

Recent studies indicate that in patients whose preoperative PRL levels exceed 1000 mU per liter, if the prolactinemia returns to normal within 6 weeks of the operation, the risk of recurrence is very low or zero over the succeeding 5 years.

Case Summary

We present the case of a 35-year-old woman who suffered chronic tension-type headache interspersed with occasional episodes of migraine without aura as defined by International Headache Society criteria. The patient had also suffered menstrual cycle alterations since the age of 16. At the age of 30, she developed amenorrhea with hyperprolactinemia. Computed tomography and MRI scans revealed a median-left intrasellar mass of about 8 × 10 mm.

Treatment with cabergoline resulted in complete resolution of both types of headache, and the menstrual cycle and PRL levels returned to normal. The therapy also reduced the volume of the tumor.

The clinical characteristics of the headache-hyperprolactinemia-hypophyseal-adenoma association are discussed, the various diagnostic and treatment possibilities are explored, and the etiology of the headache is considered in the light of several pathogenetic possibilities.

Overview of Headache Associated with Endocranial Tumors

For cerebral tumors in general, headache is the presenting symptom in around 20% of patients, and appears during the course of the disease in about 90% of cases. The head pain in brain tumor is generally deep, more diffuse than pulsating, and becomes progressively more intense. It may be exacerbated by coughing, effort, and sometimes by standing up. A slow-growing tumor may produce recurring headache over a period of months or even years, when the patient may otherwise be clinically normal.

Typically tumor headache presents at the beginning of the day in the early stages of the disease: the patient may wake with headache which passes after some minutes or perhaps an hour or so. As the tumor grows, the ventricles may be compressed leading to increased endocranial pressure, so that the headache becomes progressively more intense. At this stage, an attack often begins suddenly, increases rapidly in intensity, and disappears within a few minutes. At the height of the crisis, the patient often becomes confused. The increased pressure may provoke tonsillar herniation, which is evident as an intense neck-muscle spasm. There may be other, more specific characteristics of the headache, depending on the exact location of the tumor.

Overview of the Problem of Pituitary Tumors

Hypophyseal tumors are relatively common, constituting 6 to 18% of endocranial neoplasms. Small asymptomatic hypophyseal tumors are identified incidentally in 1.5 to 27% of autopsies or from MRI or CT scans and are called "incidentalomas." It is estimated that asymptomatic microhypophyseal adenomas are present in 10 to 20% of the adult population. These benign tumors can originate from any of the adenohypophyseal cells in the form of prolactinomas (52%), somatotropinomas (27%), or corticotropin-secreting tumors (20%); there are also the very rare TSH-omas and gonadotropinomas.

There are also nonfunctional or nonsecreting hypophyseal tumors which are classified according to their neuroradiologic characteristics: macroadenomas have a diameter greater than 10 mm, and the sella turcica is altered when viewed on a radiograph; they may cause neurologic manifestations due to expansion. Microadenomas have a diameter less than 10 mm and are visible only on MRI and high resolution CT with contrast.

Craniopharyngiomas must also be classified among the hypophyseal tumors. They constitute about 3% of all parasellar tumors, and are congenital neoplasms derived from remnants of Rathke's pouch. They take the form of encapsulated nodules that often contain cysts that arise from tissue degeneration and contain cholesterol crystals. They are located typically in the hypophyseal stalk and tend to expand toward the hypothalamus. They are nonsecreting but may give rise to delayed growth and hypogonadism, following disruption of hypothalamic-hypophyseal connections.

Although virtually all hypophyseal adenomas are histologically benign, some present histologic features (increased mitotic figures, cellular pleomorphism, nuclear hyperchromatism, and an increased nucleus-cytoplasm ratio) suggesting malignancy. Such cytologic features are not specific and only the presence of distant metastases (rare) can be accepted as a criterion of malignancy. However, hypophyseal tumors are more frequently "locally malignant" in the sense that they give rise to mass effects that seriously compromise vital structures such as the optic chiasm and the hypothalamus itself.

In addition to headache, the neurologic manifestations of prolactinomas include bilateral disturbances of vision and visual field defects in particular; the latter most commonly (60 to 70% of cases) takes the form of bitemporal hemianopsia. Typically this will begin in the upper quadrants (due to initial compression of the central part of the chiasm). It will extend to the inferior quadrants and eventually involve central vision. When the tumor develops unusually, visual field defects can take a very different course. While the fundus may appear normal initially, primary optic atrophy may develop (pallid disc with distinct margins) as the tumor expands. In around 5% of cases, eye motility is compromised.

The endocrine symptoms provoked by hypophyseal tumors may be of two types: the first is hyperfunction arising from the pathologically high secretory activity of the tumor cells, and the second is hypopituitarism following destruction of the tissue surrounding the tumor. The symptom of hyperprolactinemia is always to be considered pathologic except in pregnancy and lactation and when due to medications. It causes galactorrhea, oligomenorrhea, and lack of ovulation in 30 to 80% of women. Although prolactinomas, generally microprolactinomas, are the most frequent cause of hyperprolactinemia, it is important to remember that many other conditions can give rise to high circulating PRL levels, including tumors or lesions that disconnect the hypothalamus from the pituitary, systemic conditions such as chronic renal insufficiency, severe liver disease, primitive hypothyroidism, chest wall lesions, and a polycystic ovary. A mechanism for hyperprolactinemia may be obstruction of the capillaries of the hypophyseal stalk so that release of hypophyseal dopamine is blocked, in turn resulting in excess PRL secretion by the lactotrophic cells of the adenohypophysis. Also important are drug-induced prolactinemias, which are most frequently caused by phenothiazines, sulpiride, and neuroleptics in general but also cimetidine and other H_2 receptor antagonists, estrogenics, and opioids. The apparently idiopathic form called functional hyperprolactinemia is not rare. Prolactinomas are much less common in men than women. In men, the high PRL levels they produce result in depressed libido, impotence, and more rarely gynecomastia, and galactorrhea.

The diagnosis of prolactinoma is not difficult. It is suspected when there is hyperprolactinemia (more than 100 to 200 µg per liter) in patients with galactorrhea, amenorrhea/oligomenorrhea, gonadal disturbances, or any combination thereof. Other causes of hyperprolactinemia must, however, be excluded (Table 26–1).

It is important to emphasize that blood PRL levels in excess of 200 µg per liter are characteristic of prolactinomas (but also of chronic renal insufficiency and therapy with drugs that affect the dopaminergic pathways, for example, benzamides and neuroleptics). By contrast, voluminous sellar lesions (e.g., craniopharyngiomas, nonsecreting macroadenomas,

and meningiomas) typically induce only moderate prolactinemia (less than 200 µg per liter) by virtue of their interference with hypophyseal-stalk function. To distinguish prolactinoma-induced from drug-induced hyperprolactinemia, it is often useful to test the PRL response to thyrotropin-releasing hormone (TRH) challenge. There is usually no PRL response in the former but a strong PRL surge typically occurs in drug-induced hyperprolactinemias. High-resolution CT, with and without contrast, or MRI is necessary to visualize microprolactinomas (and other sellar lesions) and confirm the diagnosis. Computed tomography or MRI scan will also reveal the volume of the lesion and any expansion outside the sella turcica. For all hypophyseal adenomas, the key radiologic element is alteration of the sella turcica with asymmetry. Macroadenomas generally destroy the dorsum sellae and enlarge the sella craniocaudally; there may also be calcifications.

Recent studies in diagnostic neuroradiology have shown that MRI, particularly in association with gadolinium contrast, is superior to CT for identifying suspected microadenomas and for assessing the extent of hypophyseal and parahypophyseal lesions in general. An MRI has now become the first choice modality for the diagnosis and treatment planning of these lesions.

Macroadenomas compress the hypophysis, confining it, generally, to the cranioposterior periphery of the sella. Further growth modifies the form and structure of the bony walls of the sella; eventually the sella diaphragm yields and the tumor impinges on the chiasm and optic nerves. In the absence of thera-

TABLE 26–1. Main Causes of Hyperprolactinemia

- Hypophyseal conditions: prolactinomas, acromegaly, Cushing's disease, dissection of the pituitary stalk
- Hypothalamic conditions: craniopharyngiomas, meningiomas, dysgerminomas and other tumors, sarcoidosis, histiocytosis X, radiotherapy to neuraxis, vascular lesions
- Neurogenic causes: lesions of the thoracic wall or spinal cord, breast stimulation
- Drugs: neuroleptics such as phenothiazine, butyrophenones, MAO inhibitors, tricyclic antidepressants, reserpine, methyldopa, metoclopramide, verapamil, cocaine
- Other: pregnancy, hypothyroidism, renal insufficiency, liver cirrhosis
- Idiopathic

py, the tumor expands mainly in the direction of the hypothalamus, raising the floor of the third ventricle, occluding the foramen of Monro, thereby causing endocranial hypertension and hydrocephalus.

The various other complications that arise particularly when the tumor is not diagnosed or treated sufficiently early are as follows:

- Blindness if the tumor attains a large volume within the cranium (giant adenoma)
- Diabetes insipidus as a result of compression of the hypothalamus
- Jacksonian (partial) epilepsy if the tumor expands toward the temporal lobe
- Endocranial hypertension with papilledema following occlusion of the third ventricle
- Generalized epilepsy and psychiatric disturbances if the tumor expands frontally
- Intratumoral hemorrhage may occur with abrupt and violent headache, rapid deterioration of sight, ocular paralysis, confusional state, blunting of consciousness, and sometimes nuchal rigidity. In some patients the tumor can provoke hypophyseal apoplexy which is followed by death within hours or days.
- Invasion of the surrounding structures with rapid loss of sight and appearance of signs of invasion of the sinus cavernosus

Empty-Sella Syndrome

This is a condition in which an arachnoid diverticulum expands into the sellar cavity either because of a primary defect in the sellar diaphragm or as a result of alterations secondary to a hypophyseal tumor, or other pathologic or iatrogenic processes (surgery or radiotherapy) involving the hypothalamohypophyseal region. The presence of cerebrospinal fluid (CSF) within the sella results in remodeling of the walls and sometimes enlargement of the sellar cavity and compression of the hypophysis. The condition is associated with headache, obesity, and a variety of endocrine manifestations, including hyperprolactinemia, hypopituitarism, and diabetes insipidus.

In the absence of specific clinical indications or hormonal alterations, diagnosis depends on radiologic investigation. Radiography may reveal an enlarged sella, but only CT or MRI can demonstrate the presence of CSF within it.

Primary empty-sella is benign and does not require therapy. However, the patient should be followed to ensure the early treatment of any deficit arising in the various adenohypophyseal axes.

Selected Readings

Bonadonna G, Buraggi GL. Neoplasie delle ghiandole endocrine. In: Bonadonna G, Robustelli Della Cuna G, editors. Manuale di oncologia medica. Masson IV Ed. 1991;51:1057–66.

De Vita V, Hellman S, Rosenberg SA, editors. Cancer principles and practice of oncology. Philadelphia: Lippincott-Raven; 1997. p. 2066–8.

Domingue JN, Richmond IL, Wilson CB. Results of surgery in 114 patients with prolactin-secreting pituitary adenomas. Am J Obstet Gynecol 1980;137:102–8.

Hartman N, Voron SC, Hershman JM. Resolution of migraine following bromocriptine treatment of a prolactinoma (pituitary microadenoma). Headache 1995;35:430–1.

Headaches, diabetes insipidus, and hyperprolactinemia in a woman with an enlarged pituitary gland (clinicopathologic conference). Am J Med 1993;95 Suppl 3:332–9.

Hockaday JM, Peet KMS, Hockaday TDR. Bromocriptine in migraine. Headache 1976;16:109–14.

Jenkins JS. Clinical manifestations of pituitary tumours. In: Jenkins TS, editor. Pituitary tumours. London: Butterworths, 1973. p. 38–63.

Kemman E, Jones JR. Hyperprolactinemia and headaches. Am J Obstet Gynecol 1983;145:668–71.

Miller BJ, Boyd A, Molitch ME, et al. Galactorrhea syndromes. In: Post KD, Jackson IMD, Reichlin S, editors. The pituitary adenoma. New York: Plenum Medical Books Company; 1980. p. 65–90.

Milos P, Havelius HLF, Hindfelt B. Cluster-headache in a patient with a pituitary adenoma, with a review of the literature. Headache 1996;36:184–8.

Molitch ME. Nonsecreting adenomas. In: Post KD, Jackson IMD, Reichlin S, editors. The pituitary adenoma. New York: Plenum Medical Books Company; 1980. p. 151–8.

Molitch ME. Pathogenesis of pituitary tumors. Endocrinol Metab Clin North Am 1987;16:503–27.

Molitch ME. Management of prolactinomas. Ann Rev Med 1989;40:225–32.

Molitch ME, Russell EJ. The pituitary "incidentaloma." Ann Intern Med 1990;112:925–31.

Post KD. General considerations in the surgical treatment of pituitary tumors. In: Post KD, Jackson IMD, Reichlin S, editors. The pituitary adenoma. New York: Plenum Medical Books Company; 1980. p. 341–63.

Rush SC, Newall J. Pituitary adenoma: the efficacy of radiotherapy as the sole treatment. Int J Radiat Oncol Biol Phys 1989;17:165–9.

Sabbagh R, Kedar A. Increased prolactin level and pituitary adenoma as a cause of headache in two patients with sickle cell disease. Pediatr Hematol Oncol 1996;13:101–5.

Sherman B, Schlachte J, Halmi N. Pathogenesis of prolactin-secreting pituitary adenoma. Lancet 1978;2:1019–21.

Spaziante R, Irace C, De Divitiis E. Adenomi ipofisari prolattino-secernenti: il ruolo della chirurgia. Aggiornamento del medico 1989;13:471–85.

Stewart PM, Corrie J, Seckl JR, Edwards CRW, Padfield PL. A rational approach for assessing the hypothalamo-pituitary-adrenal axis. Lancet 1988;1:1208–10.

Strebel PM, Zacur HA, Gold EB. Headache hyperprolactinemia and prolactinomas. Obstet Gynecol 1986;68:195–9.

Tfelt-Hansen P, Paulson OB, Krabbe AA. Invasive adenoma of the pituitary gland and chronic migrainous neuralgia. A rare coincidence or a causal relationship? Cephalalgia 1982;2:25–8.

The pituitary adenoma study group. Pituitary adenomas and oral contraceptives: a multi-center case-control study. Fertil Steril 1983;39:753.

Wen B, Hussey DH, Staples J, et al. A comparison of the roles of surgery and radiotherapy in the management of craniopharyngiomas. Int J Radiat Oncol Biol Phys 1989;16:17–24.

Zarate A, Moran C, Miranda R, et al. Long-acting bromocriptine for the acute treatment of large macroprolactinomas. J Endocrinol Invest 1987;10:233–6.

Editorial Comments

Headache can be the presenting symptom in patients with pituitary neoplasms. Secondary irregularity of menses or amenorrhea is a signal to explore such headaches, even if they resemble primary headache disorders like migraine or tension-type headache. With modern imaging technology and sensitive hormone assays, the diagnosis should be relatively easy. Drs. Bussone and Moschiano present an excellent case with a good discussion of endocranial tumor headache, specifically pituitary tumor headache. They also carefully describe empty-sella syndrome. There is a lot to be learned here.

CHAPTER 27

THE MAN WITH EVOLVING HEADACHE

THOMAS N. WARD, MD

Case History

A 54-year-old male came to the office complaining of daily headaches. He was the president of the local hospital. He had a history of "migraine" for over 10 years. The headaches were usually left hemicranial pounding headaches. They were severe enough to make him curtail his customary activities and lie down. He experienced nausea, vomiting, and photophobia. There was no phonophobia. Sleep typically brought resolution of the headache.

Over the years, he had found ergotamine tartrate to be helpful and was using about 30 or more tablets per month. In fact, for the 2 months or so prior to his visit to the office, his headaches had evolved into a chronic daily pattern. His migraines never had an accompanying aura, and his headaches were still relieved with ergotamine tartrate and/or sleep.

In the past, he had been treated preventively with propranolol, which made him feel fatigued, so it was stopped. A computed tomography (CT) scan of the brain done 10 years before presentation was reportedly normal (with the films being no longer available for review). There was a family history of migraine in his father. His mother had a history of hypertension and apparently had suffered from a brain tumor, although he did not know which type. Perfume and certain brands of beer seemed to be triggers for his headaches. A complete neurologic examination was entirely normal.

The patient was placed on metoprolol with the dosage titrated up to 100 mg twice a day, and his ergotamine tartrate was stopped. There was significant improvement in his headaches (they became milder and intermittent), but over a period of some weeks he became slightly lethargic, and so the dosage of this drug was tapered off.

Diltiazem was substituted, which controlled his headaches but also gave him a sensation of fatigue, so this was discontinued. His headaches recurred, so a lower dose of metoprolol (50 mg twice a day) was initiated. He felt much better with occasional headaches he could control, but a confounding variable of stresses at work lead to a referral for behavioral medicine measures.

His headache pattern continued to wax and wane with intermittent headaches over the next few months. Eight months after his initial office visit, he complained of difficulty concentrating. He was using injectable sumatriptan to control his severe headaches, with good response. He was complaining again, however, of a low-grade constant headache and therefore his metoprolol was stopped and sertraline was begun. Five days later his wife called saying that he seemed even more depressed and was behaving oddly.

A CT scan of the brain was obtained which was abnormal. A magnetic resonance imaging (MRI) scan confirmed the existence of a large mass appearing to arise from the right frontal lobe and extending well into the right parietal lobe. Examination of the patient by neurology resident physicians after they had seen this scan still revealed only "possible papilledema" and a "possible" left pronator drift.

The patient was taken to the operating room. Stereotaxic biopsy revealed glioblastoma multiforme. Despite surgical debulking, radiotherapy, and chemotherapy, he had a progressive downhill course, and died approximately 1 year later.

Questions about This Case

- How many types of headache did this patient have?
- Why did this patient have episodes of both intermittent and chronic daily headache?
- When does a patient with a headache need a scan?
- What are the causes of daily headache?

Case Discussion

This case represents every physician's and patient's worst fear—having a secondary (threatening) rather than a primary (benign) headache syndrome. Actually, this patient had both; first a long history of migraine without aura, then a new headache (ergotamine-dependency) which resolved with the discontinuation of the offending medication, then yet another worsening presumably due to the intracranial tumor.

There is no doubt that the patient had migraine without aura. He had a long history of intermittent hemicranial severe pounding headaches, with nausea and vomiting, and photophobia. There was a family history of migraine, and the patient had triggers for his headaches. Between attacks, his health was normal. He had undergone a normal CT scan of his brain. He met the IHS criteria for migraine without aura.

Along the way, he developed a pattern of chronic daily headaches, in the setting of daily use of ergotamine. The ergotamine-dependency headaches are in many ways analogous to analgesic-rebound headaches. Increasing use of symptomatic medication results in a vicious cycle of more frequent refractory headaches and the consumption of increasing amounts of medication attempting to achieve relief. Abrupt cessation of the offending medication may result in a transient worsening of

the headaches, but cessation generally leads to improvement over a period of weeks to even months. This patient did return to an intermittent headache pattern after stopping ergotamine.

Medications can be a problem not only in that symptomatic remedies may worsen headache if overused but also because prophylactic options are limited both with regard to efficacy and side effects. Both beta-blockers and even a calcium channel drug provoked fatigue in this patient, although he achieved adequate relief of headache and amelioration of the side effects with a reduction of the dosage.

The recurrence of daily headache without the overuse of symptomatic medications was worrisome. There was the confounding variable of stress in his professional life—he had just had a very trying few months and a particularly difficult interaction with a staff physician who subsequently quit. The patient attributed the worsening headache pattern to his stress. Notably, his headaches (at least the severe ones) responded to sumatriptan. It is known that response to sumatriptan or other antimigraine drugs *is not* diagnostic of migraine.

Neuroimaging studies were carried out because of the patient's progressive headache pattern and the development of abulia. The presence of a malignant tumor was confirmed. The frontal lobe is notoriously a relatively "silent area" of the brain which may harbor lesions for a period of time before they are discovered, especially if the lesions are unilateral. Glioblastoma multiforme is an aggressive, infiltrative tumor, which is generally only diagnosed when incurable. These tumors cause progressive deterioration in most cases despite vigorous efforts at treatment, with the death of the patient generally within 1 year.

Management Strategies

- Establish the correct diagnosis in this case. This requires a complete history and examination.
- Follow the patient serially in the office, to assess their response to therapy, and make appropriate adjustments.
- Re-evaluate the patient by history and/or examination at the time of any significant negative change.
- Neuroimaging would generally be recommended for a patient with an abnormal examination, a

persistent refractory daily headache, or a worsening or changing headache pattern despite appropriate treatment. Laboratory work, and lumbar puncture (assuming neuroimaging shows no contraindication such as a mass lesion) may also be appropriate in some cases.

Case Summary

- The patient did have migraine without aura.
- The patient also had chronic daily headaches due to ergotamine overuse (ergotamine-dependency headaches).
- A brain tumor also occurred, presumably after the initial office visit (these tumors grow rapidly), and caused the reoccurrence of chronic daily headache.
- Patients may have multiple causes of headaches, and previous diagnoses of benign (primary) headaches do not mean that the patient cannot develop a threatening (secondary) headache.
- Flexibility in diagnosis and management implies assessing the patient's response to therapy and their changing symptoms over time.

Approach to the Patient with Frequent (Daily) Headaches

The assessment of the patient with daily or near-daily headaches can be difficult. Many patients who present with such headaches fear they harbor a brain tumor; fortunately, most do not. A thorough history and complete examination serve as the basis for deciding whether or not further testing is necessary and/or appropriate. Guidelines regarding neuroimaging procedures have been published (see *Selected Readings*).

In patients with a history of migraine and chronic daily headache, the inappropriate consumption of either analgesics or ergotamine is often the cause of the problem. The cessation of this overuse (either gradually as an outpatient under medical supervision or more rapidly in the hospital) usually leads to improvement over a number of weeks. Failure to improve should lead to further diagnostic considerations. Also, it is always possible that a chronic daily headache leads to the overuse of medications in an attempt to obtain relief.

Unrecognized medical conditions may lead to frequent headaches. Examples include thyroid disorders, polycythemia, malignant hyperthermia, and Lyme disease. In patients over 50 years of age (and occasionally younger), giant cell arteritis may be the cause of daily headaches. Appropriate physical examination (and an eye examination) plus laboratory evaluation is required.

Unrecognized psychiatric conditions may be associated with frequent headaches. Depressed patients frequently complain of unremitting headaches. There is a strong correlation, especially among women, between a history of abuse and refractory pain states, including headaches.

Unrecognized neurosurgical conditions may also be the source of refractory headache. Some patients with Chiari malformations (herniation of cerebellar tonsils below the level of the foramen magnum) will have headaches. These headaches are typically occipital/upper cervical and may be constant and/or worsened by Valsalva's maneuvers such as coughing. Surgical decompression may be curative.

Conditions that are being recognized with increasing frequency include various "cervicogenic headaches." Trapping of the dorsal C_2 nerve root may occur, for example, after trauma such as whiplash. There is typically a delay of a number of weeks, or months, between the injury and the development of head pain. Again, there may be unilateral (rarely bilateral) occipital/upper cervical aching with a tender occipital nerve, and pain which may radiate forward to above the ipsilateral eye. Pain sensation may be decreased on that side in the C_2 dermatome. A CT-guided anesthetic block of the C_2 ganglion may transiently relieve symptoms and suggest a response to surgery.

An intracranial neoplasm may present with headache although, surprisingly, about a half of patients with a brain tumor do not complain of headache. Headache is more likely to be present if there is raised intracranial pressure, shift/distortion of structures on neuroimaging, or if the patient had a previous history of headaches. In that case, the headaches associated with the brain tumor are always either more frequent or severe than their previous headaches *and* are accompanied by additional symptoms and/or physical signs.

The classic "brain tumor headache" written about so extensively (severe, awakening the patient at night with nausea/vomiting) turns out to be uncommon, reported only in 17% of brain tumor patients (as suggested by Forsyth). Patients with a long previous history of benign headache may develop a brain tumor and not even have a change in their headache pattern.

For intracranial masses above the tentorium cerebelli, a headache, when present, is usually bilateral, frontal, and somewhat worse ipsilateral to the mass. The headaches from intracranial mass lesions are nonspecific, may be mild (more like a tension-type headache in the majority unless the patient also has a history of migraine), and is usually detected by the presence of other signs or symptoms suggesting raised intracranial pressure or a focal lesion.

Patients with headaches should be considered for neuroimaging (I prefer MRI) when they develop new unexplained symptoms, abnormal signs on neurologic examination, or a different headache from their previous headache type. The lesson from this case is that a prior normal examination, a prior history of a benign (primary) headache such as migraine, the presence of other aggravating factors such as ergotamine-dependency headaches, and even previous normal neuroimaging do *not* prevent a patient from developing a brain tumor or other ominous lesion, and continuous vigilance in the assessment of headache patients is essential.

Selected Readings

Forsyth PA, Posner JB. Headaches in patients with brain tumors: a study of 111 patients. Neurology 1993;43:1678–83.

Frishberg BM. The utility of neuroimaging in the evaluation of headache in patients with normal neurologic examinations. Neurology 1994;44:1191–7.

Goldberg RT. Childhood abuse, depression, and chronic pain. Clin J Pain 1994;10:277–81.

Gross DW, Donat JR, Boyle CA, et al. Dihydroergotamine and metoclopramide in the treatment of organic headache. Headache 1995;35:637–8.

International Headache Society. Classification and diagnostic criteria for headache disorders, cranial neuralgias and facial pain. Cephalalgia 1988;8(Suppl 7):1–96.

Mathew NI, Kurman R, Perez F, et al. Drug induced refractory headache—clinical features and management. Headache 1990;30:634–8.

Pikus HJ, Phillips JM. Characteristics of patients successfully treated for cervicogenic headache by surgical decompression of the second cervical root. Headache 1995;35:621–9.

Report of the Quality Standards Subcommittee of the American Academy of Neurology. Practice parameter: the utility of neuroimaging in the evaluation of headache in patients with normal neurologic examinations. Neurology 1994;44:1353–4.

Editorial Comments

Dr. Ward presents and discusses a fascinating yet ominous case of a patient with three types of headache. Intrapatient variability of headache types is very common, yet most remain primary benign disorders. The evolving nature and behavioral changes seen in this patient are always easy to recognize in retrospect but may be overlooked during clinical care, especially when a prior neuroimaging procedure was "normal." All physicians caring for headache patients have cases similar to Dr. Ward's. We can hope that treatable reversible causes can be found in some cases.

So beware the changing headache, and do not hesitate to order a repeat scan if the clinical pattern has changed.

CHAPTER 28

THE PATIENT IN THE EMERGENCY ROOM: CASE 2

DAVID J. CAPOBIANCO, MD

Case History

This 49-year-old male with a history of migraine and hypertension presented to the emergency room with a severe headache. The headache began in the morning shortly after awakening. The pain was constant, with maximal intensity in the occipital region. However, the pain rapidly spread to include his entire head, neck, and interscapular region. Associated symptoms included nausea and "violent" vomiting. Indomethacin per rectum, which is generally quite effective, provided him no relief.

His migraine headaches began when he was 18. They have never been preceded by nor associated with any neurologic or ophthalmologic accompaniments. The headaches generally build in intensity over a period of 30 to 60 minutes. The migraine attacks are characterized primarily by right hemicranial throbbing pain associated with nausea, vomiting, photophobia, and phonophobia. The frequency is variable, approximately one every 2 to 3 months. He has been prescribed verapamil for his hypertension but is noncompliant.

The general and neurologic examination performed by the emergency room physician is reported to be normal, although he was noted to be in severe pain.

Questions about This Case

- What are your diagnostic considerations in this case?

- What additional history would be pertinent in this case?
- What would you like to know about the examination findings?
- Would you think that this patient requires any investigational procedures; if so, which, and how quickly should they be obtained?
- How would you manage this patient's headache?
- How would you evaluate a patient with the thunderclap headache profile?

Case Discussion

Headache is a common complaint. As such, it is necessary to distinguish the benign or so-called primary headaches from secondary or symptomatic etiologies. The vast majority of headaches are relatively benign. However, it is the occasional headache related to a sinister cause that the physician must urgently recognize and treat appropriately.

In evaluating the patient with headache, the three most important aspects of the evaluation are the history, the history, and the history. The evaluation is further supplemented by examination and appropriate laboratory as well as investigational studies when indicated. One must first determine why it is that the patient is now seeking the physician's opinion, in this case, in the emergency department. Is this the first or worst headache experienced by the patient? Alternatively, is the patient presenting now as a result of recurrent headaches?

There are several "red flags" which should alert the physician that the headache may be symptomatic of an organic disorder. These have been superbly summarized by Edmeads (1988) and include:

- The first or worst headache. The patient who has either never experienced a headache or is seldom prone to a headache and subsequently presents either to the outpatient or emergency department with a violent headache. Invariably, the patient and/or family will report the headache as being "different."

- Onset to peak pain. Migraine and even cluster headaches build up over a period of minutes, whereas the headache associated with a subarachnoid hemorrhage (SAH) begins apoplectically.

- Onset with exertion. It is true that migraine may be triggered by sustained physical exertion, so-called "exertional migraine." However, onset of a headache beginning abruptly during or immediately following exertion should be viewed with concern, suggesting the possibility of an SAH or alternatively, a lesional headache associated with or without increased intracranial pressure.

- Headache associated with meningismus. Painful limitation of forward flexion of the neck should suggest the presence of either blood or pus in the cerebrospinal fluid. However, the absence of meningismus does not imply a benign etiology. Meningeal irritation may not be present acutely. Meningeal signs may also be absent if the patient has sustained a mild SAH.

- Headache associated with posterior radiation of pain. Although migraine or tension-type headache may be associated with occipitonuchal musculoskeletal pain, the presence of interscapular pain is particularly worrisome. This can be suggestive of either subarachnoid blood or pus percolating down the neuroaxis.

- Headache associated with loss of consciousness, no matter how transient, should suggest the diagnosis of SAH.

- Headache accompanied by abnormal physical signs. Fever is not a feature of the primary headache syndromes, and its presence should suggest either a systemic or primary central nervous system infectious process. "Soft" neurologic signs such as a pronator drift, asymmetric nasolabial folds, clumsi-ness or equivocal plantar responses, particularly if asymmetric, may be suggestive of an organic cause for the headache. Headache associated with drowsiness or altered awareness is cause for concern and suggests the possibility of an organic etiology. Papilledema, if present, is consistent with increased intracranial pressure. Yet its absence does not imply normal intracranial pressure.

Additional danger signs include the failure of the headache to conform to a benign headache profile, onset in or after middle age, progressive course, associated immunocompromised state and lack of an obvious identifiable etiology.

It is important not to be lulled into a false sense of security in regard to the patient improving after treatment. The beneficial response to a symptomatic medication does not necessarily imply a benign mechanism.

To begin the discussion, we need additional history. Although it is clear that the patient has a prior history of migraine without aura, several key features of the present headache prompting this evaluation remain to be considered. First, he identified his present headache as the "worst ever," unlike any which he had experienced before. Second, headache onset to peak pain was apoplectic, that is, developing over a period of seconds. Third, onset of the headache occurred during intercourse. The patient did not inform the emergency room physician of this fact, as both he and his wife were "embarrassed." At times, in obtaining the headache history, direct questioning is necessary. This important point was obtained only when the patient was asked point blank if he was involved in any strenuous physical activity at the onset of his headache. In addition, the patient's wife noted that at the onset of the headache, her husband had briefly "passed out."

Sexual activity can be associated with three different types of headache. The most common beginning at or shortly before orgasm and has the same temporal profile as SAH, that is, the pain is severe and explosive in onset. The second pattern develops as sexual excitement increases and is characterized as a dull, aching pain. The third, and least common, is a postural headache, resembling the low-pressure headache which may follow a lumbar puncture (see Chapter 35).

The dilemma facing the physician is to distinguish the benign coital headache from that of a ruptured aneurysm. Fisher reported that in 3 of his 66 patients with a ruptured aneurysm, the rupture occurred during orgasm.

Although initially denying any recent change in his headache profile, the patient did recollect a severe headache occurring six weeks previously. Yet his wife was quick to point out that it "was because of the flu." Several family members had been diagnosed with the flu. Although in retrospect, the headache was not typical of his migraine headaches. Nonetheless, he was diagnosed with a "viral syndrome." He returned to work after being bedbound for 1 week.

This brings up the concept of the warning leak or minor SAH (sentinel bleed). Patients with a warning leak often either do not seek medical attention or, if seen, may be misdiagnosed. In my experience, the patient is typically misdiagnosed with either the "flu" or "sinusitis."

The patient's history is also notable for hypertension. A premorbid history of hypertension is not an uncommon finding in patients with an aneurysmal SAH. Whether this is a risk for SAH is up for debate. Other environmental factors such as cigarette smoking and heavy alcohol use (binge drinking) which may predispose the patient to aneurysmal SAH were not relevant in this case.

On examination, he was in obvious distress. The vital signs were notable for a slightly elevated systolic blood pressure. Pertinent findings in the neurologic examination included equivocal plantar responses, diffuse hyperreflexia, flattening of the right nasolabial fold, and meningismus. The disks were flat, although spontaneous venous pulsations were not present. No subhyaloid hemorrhage was present. He was otherwise alert and oriented to all spheres.

The general medical laboratory screening was normal. The electrocardiogram (ECG) demonstrated nonspecific ST changes. A prior ECG was unavailable for review.

Thus, the headache which prompted his emergency room visit is most consistent with an organic cause of headache. Based on the signs and symptoms, the working diagnosis was that of SAH.

Based on the examination findings, what can be said in terms of prognosis? Clearly, the major factor in determining prognosis is the neurologic status. The Hunt-Hess system is one of the commonly used scales based primarily on levels of consciousness and carries prognostic importance. The classification is as follows: Grade 0—unruptured aneurysm without symptoms; Grade I—minimal headache and slight nuchal rigidity; Grade II—moderate to severe headache, nuchal rigidity, and possible focal neurologic deficit; Grade III—severe headache, confused, drowsy with focal deficit; Grade IV—stupor, focal neurologic deficit; Grade V—coma with decerebrate rigidity. For grade I, the mortality rate is 10%, whereas for grade V SAH, the mortality rate is 100%.

The next question is how best to proceed. Computed tomography (CT) scan is the imaging modality of choice. A CT scan without contrast was obtained as a matter of urgency. A high-quality CT will identify the vast majority of structural diseases. In addition, the CT scan can not only detect blood in the subarachnoid space but also associated hemorrhage. When performed within 24 hours of the initial ictus, the CT will be positive in 90 to 95% of cases. The sensitivity of the CT drops off 24 hours after the bleed, and by 7 to 14 days following the ictus, it may be normal.

The differential diagnosis of SAH on CT includes meningeal carcinomatosis and leptomeningitis. In addition, I have encountered a patient who, after undergoing myelography to confirm lumbar spinal stenosis, developed low-pressure headaches within days of the procedure. A CT scan was requested by her primary physician. The radiologist interpreted the CT as being suggestive of an SAH. Do not forget the history! Iodinated contrast can cause increased density in the subarachnoid space.

What if the CT is normal even though performed within hours of the ictus? Should a magnetic resonance imaging (MRI) of the head be performed? The answer is no. The sensitivity of MRI in detecting acute hemorrhage is lower than that of CT. Blood from the acute bleed is isointense and, as such, may not be detected on an MRI done at the time of SAH.

If your clinical suspicion is that of SAH and yet the CT is normal, the next diagnostic step must then include a lumbar puncture (LP), looking for either xanthochromia or blood. Since Quinke first introduced the LP in 1891, this has remained an important procedure in the diagnosis of SAH. As superbly stated by Caplan, "in patients with sudden severe headache without focal neurologic signs, the only absolute contraindication to LP are no back and no needle." In this case, an LP was not required in that the CT demonstrated subarachnoid blood.

Yet what if, in this case, both the CT and LP done shortly after the ictus were normal? The literature suggests that an LP done within 2 to 4 hours of the SAH may be normal. For this reason, van Gijn advises deferring an LP in this situation for 12 hours, allowing for xanthochromia to develop. My own bias, however, has been to proceed with the LP once the result of the CT is known, that is, after a normal CT. The LP can be repeated in 12 hours if clinically warranted.

Unfortunately, a not uncommon scenario is that of the patient with a history of a severe, "different" headache beginning instantaneously several weeks prior to your evaluation. You are now evaluating them in the outpatient clinic. The headache has resolved and the neurologic examination is normal. Would a CT be helpful? Not likely. Would an LP be helpful? Perhaps, yet it will probably be normal in a minor SAH. In this situation, the decision comes down to MR angiography versus conventional catheter angiography. My bias in this situation would be to proceed with catheter angiography.

Now back to our case. An emergent neurosurgery consultation was obtained. The patient was stabilized and underwent a four-vessel cerebral angiogram. A left middle-cerebral-artery-bifurcation aneurysm was identified. On the day of admission, a left pterional craniotomy was performed with clipping of the aneurysm. The patient was immediately transferred to the intensive care unit. The initial medical management consisted of frequent assessments of the patient's neurologic status as well as frequent monitoring of the blood pressure and vital signs. He was placed on strict bed rest. A central line to monitor fluid status and an intra-arterial line for blood pressure monitoring were in place. Nimodipine was begun at a dose of 60 mg by mouth every 6 hours. The patient was also given phenytoin. He required parenteral codeine to con-

trol his pain. Aspirin must be avoided, given the resultant prolongation of bleeding time. In order to prevent excessive straining at stool, he was started on a stool softener.

The patient tolerated the surgery without complications, save for mild short-term memory impairment. He continues to experience infrequent migraine attacks which respond quite well to indomethacin PR. He is now taking verapamil as prescribed.

Case Summary

- The patient does indeed suffer from migraine without aura.
- The headache prompting this patient's evaluation in the emergency department was secondary to an aneurysmal SAH.
- A high index of suspicion is mandatory if timely diagnosis and treatment are to be instituted.
- The headache associated with SAH is severe and as such, patients should be given ample medication to provide relief. Aspirin should be avoided.
- The evaluation and treatment of a patient with a suspected aneurysmal SAH requires the close collaboration of the neurologist, neurosurgeon, neuroradiologist, and highly trained nurses.

Overview of Subarachnoid Hemorrhage

The majority of nontraumatic SAH are secondary to a rupture of an intracranial saccular aneurysm. Subarachnoid hemorrhage is the result of the extravasation of blood from the cerebral vessels into the subarachnoid space. Nearly 20% of strokes are hemorrhagic, with 10% being secondary to an SAH.

Saccular aneurysms are acquired lesions, typically occurring at the bifurcations of the large arteries located at the base of the skull. The vast majority of intracranial aneurysms in adults are located in the anterior circulation. Multiple aneurysms are seen in nearly 20 to 25% of patients.

Autopsy studies suggest that between 2 to 6% of adults harbor an intracranial aneurysm. These rates would imply that up to 12 million Americans have an intracranial aneurysm.

More than 25,000 Americans each year suffer from a ruptured intracranial aneurysm. Subarachnoid hemorrhage presents in all age groups, yet is uncommon under the age of 20, peaking between the ages of 40 to 60. Unlike other stroke types, women make up 60% of patients who sustain an SAH. Before the fourth decade, aneurysmal SAH occurs predominantly in men.

Risk factors for aneurysmal SAH remain to be fully identified. Cigarette smoking and alcohol use, particularly binge drinking, increase the risk of SAH. Hypertension may be an additional risk factor for aneurysmal SAH.

Familial cases of intracranial saccular aneurysms have been well documented. The risk of a ruptured intracranial aneurysm is nearly four times that of the general population among first-degree relatives of patients stricken by an SAH.

There are several connective-tissue disorders associated with intracranial aneurysms. These include autosomal dominant polycystic kidney disease, Ehlers-Danlos syndrome, Marfan syndrome, pseudoxanthoma elasticum, neurofibromatosis type 1, and fibromuscular dysplasia.

Despite our recent advances both in the diagnosis and treatment of aneurysmal SAH, the prognosis remains grim. Subarachnoid hemorrhage from aneurysmal rupture is a common cause of death in otherwise healthy young adults. The mortality rate from the initial rupture is nearly 50%. Those who survive often experience neurologic sequelae which may include memory impairment, behavioral disturbances, as well as focal neurologic deficits.

The clinical spectrum of patients harboring an intracranial saccular aneurysm can be divided into three major categories. These include prodromal symptoms resulting from either direct massive effect or a minor "warning leak," major SAH, and delayed neurologic sequelae.

Prodromal symptoms may on occasion include focal neurologic signs. The onset of a pupil-sparing third-nerve palsy is suggestive of a posterior communicating artery aneurysm. Aneurysms of the internal carotid artery, at the origin of the ophthalmic, may result in optic-nerve ischemia. Basilar bifurcation aneurysms may result in bulbar signs, memory impairment, and quadriparesis. New onset face pain, particularly in or about the eye may be suggestive of an enlarging aneurysm in the setting of an incomplete or partial third-nerve palsy.

The "warning leak" or sentinel headache may occur in up to 60% of patients prior to their major SAH. The headache, even in the headache-prone patient, is identified as being unlike any previous headache. The onset is instantaneous, with onset to peak pain occurring in seconds, and not 30 to 60 minutes as is typical with a migraine attack. The pain is severe, and often, yet not exclusively, occipitonuchal in location. It is important to note that there is no one typical location. The headache may last from 48 hours up to a week or perhaps longer. It is estimated that nearly 50% of patients with a warning or sentinel leak do not seek medical attention. Many of those who do may unfortunately be misdiagnosed as having migraine, viral syndrome, aseptic meningitis, sinusitis, or musculoskeletal neck pain.

The cardinal symptom of a major SAH is headache. Yet in up to 2% of patients, the headache may inexplicably be absent or mild. Like the headache associated with a warning leak, the pain is severe, different from previous headaches and apoplectic in onset. The headache is continuous, a throbbing quality being present in only 5% of cases. Nausea and vomiting are also prominent symptoms, typically occurring simultaneously with the abrupt onset headache. Meningismus is frequently seen, yet may be absent initially. On occasion, the neck pain may be more severe than the headache. A sudden brief loss of consciousness can occur in up to 45% of patients. Nearly 66% of patients have some depression in their level of consciousness.

The setting in which the headache occurs may provide a helpful clue as to the underlying mechanism. Any headache beginning instantaneously during strenuous physical activity, including intercourse, should suggest SAH. Admittedly, one-third of SAH occur during sleep and an additional one-third during routine physical activity. Thus, aneurysmal hemorrhage can occur at any time.

The physical examination, although important, may range from normal to coma. The patient is often in distress and can be agitated. A mild elevation in the blood pressure is not uncommon. There may be a low-grade fever; presence of a markedly elevated temperature would suggest an alternative diagnosis such as meningitis. Meningismus is typically present, yet may take several hours to develop. Thus, the absence of meningismus in the acute setting should not dissuade one from the diagnosis of SAH. Focal neurologic signs, if present, may suggest the site of the aneurysmal rupture. Aphasia and hemiparesis would be consistent with a middle-cerebral-artery aneurysm. The presence of abulia, leg weakness, and bilateral extensor plantar responses suggest an anterior-communicating-artery aneurysm.

A noncontrast CT scan of the head is the initial diagnostic study which must be performed in any patient with a suspected SAH. The CT is positive in 90 to 95% of patients with SAH if performed within 24 hours of the ictus. The CT may also demonstrate hydrocephalus as well as the presence of any associated intracerebral hemorrhage. The sensitivity of the CT decreases to 80% by 3 days, 50% at 1 week, and 30% by 2 weeks. The distribution of the hemorrhage on CT may also suggest the location of the ruptured aneurysm. A large amount of blood within the subfrontal or interhemispheric fissure is consistent with an anterior communicating artery aneurysm. A large amount of blood in the sylvian fissure is suggestive of a middle cerebral artery aneurysm.

Magnetic resonance imaging is less sensitive than CT in demonstrating subarachnoid blood in the acute setting. The acutely ill patient may also be agitated and will unlikely lie still to allow for adequate images. Lastly, MRI is not readily available in most emergency rooms. Nonetheless, MRI may be more sensitive than CT in the subacute phase (7 to 14 days), during which time blood may demonstrate high signal intensity representing methemoglobin.

A lumbar puncture is crucial in patients with suspected SAH and a normal CT. Yet, the LP itself may be normal if performed within 2 hours of the ictus. For this reason, some authors advise withholding the LP for a minimum of 12 hours if possible.

The appearance of blood in the cerebrospinal fluid (CSF) at the time of LP requires that one exclude a "traumatic" or "bloody tap" from an SAH. In SAH, the opening pressure may be increased or normal, whereas in a traumatic puncture, the opening pressure is normal. When blood is detected in the CSF, the fluid should be collected in serial tubes. In SAH, the blood is evenly distributed between tubes 1 and 4. In a "bloody tap," the CSF typically clears rapidly between tubes 1 and 4. If blood is present in the CSF, it must be immediately centrifuged and the supernatant examined for xanthochromia, if at all possible by spectrophotometry.

If the CSF is bloody after an atraumatic LP and/or xanthochromic staining of the CSF is present, then cerebral angiography is necessary. An angiogram is required to confirm the presence of an aneurysm and/or exclude an alternative cause for the hemorrhage. In nearly 20% of patients with a suspected SAH, the angiogram will be normal. If this situation should arise, then repeat angiography is generally performed in 1 to 2 weeks. Perimesencephalic SAH is the most common type of SAH associated with a negative cerebral angiogram, and repeat cerebral angiography is not felt to be necessary in this situation.

The major causes of delayed neurologic sequelae include vasospasm, rebleeding, and hydrocephalus. Vasospasm occurs in nearly 30% of patients, typically between days 4 and 14. Nimodipine, a calcium channel blocker, has been shown to be helpful in decreasing the incidence and severity of vasospasm. Rebleeding occurs in 20% of patients in the first 2 weeks, 40% by the end of 6 months. The mortality rate with rebleeding is approximately 40%. Hydrocephalus typically develops between 4 and 20 days after SAH.

A review of SAH must include the "thunderclap headache." In 1984, Fisher reported on a group of patients who developed the abrupt onset of an excruciating headache. This was termed, "crash" or "blitz" migraine. In 1986, Day and Raskin described the case of a 42-year-old woman who experienced three episodes of severe, abrupt headache and coined the term, "thunderclap headache." The CT and CSF were normal following the initial two attacks. Following the third headache, catheter angiography demonstrated a 1.5 cm internal carotid artery aneurysm associated with diffuse vasospasm. No hemorrhage was observed at the time of surgery. The aneurysm was clipped, and the patient has remained headache free. Nonetheless, several prospective studies suggest that thunderclap headache is, in general, a benign syndrome and that angiography is not necessary, particularly if the neurologic examination is normal. However, several case reports recently published would favor Raskin's contention that a normal CT and LP in the setting of a thunderclap headache does not necessarily imply a benign etiology. In a study by Raps et al., it was shown that 7 out of 111 patients with an unruptured aneurysm presented with a severe, acute thunderclap-like headache identical to SAH.

Thunderclap headache may also represent the first symptom of cerebral venous sinus thrombosis (CVST). Headache can occur in up to 80% of patients with CVST. Debruijn et al. reported on 10 patients who presented with thunderclap headache mimicking SAH, who were felt to have CVST.

My approach is to proceed with a full evaluation in any patient presenting with a thunderclap headache profile. If the emergent CT is normal, then a lumbar puncture with measurement of the opening pressure should be performed. If the CSF as well as the opening pressure are normal, I believe that a high-quality magnetic resonance angiography (MRA) is sufficient, particularly if the headache is of short duration and the examination is normal.

Selected Readings

Caplan LR. Subarachnoid hemorrhage. In: Caplan LR, editor. Stroke, a clinical approach. 2nd ed. Boston: Butterworth-Heinemann; 1993. p. 389–423.

Couch JR. Headache to worry about. Med Clin North Am 1993;77:141–65.

Day JW, Raskin NH. Thunderclap headache: a symptom of unruptured cerebral aneurysm. Lancet 1986;2:1247–8.

Debruijn SFTM, Stam J, Kappelle LJ. Thunderclap headache as first symptom of cerebral venous sinus thrombosis. Lancet 1996;348:1623–5.

Edmeads J. Emergency management of headache. Headache 1988;28:675–9.

Edmeads J. Challenges in the diagnosis of acute headache. Headache 1990;30:537–40.

Fisher CM. Headache in cerebrovascular disease. In: Vinken PJ, Bruyn GW, editors. Handbook of clinical neurology. Vol. 5. Amsterdam: North-Holland; 1968. p. 124–56.

Fisher CM. Painful states: a neurological commentary. Clin Neurosurg 1984;31:32–53.

Hughes RL. Identification and treatment of cerebral aneurysms after sentinel headache. Neurology 1992;42:118–9.

Kistler JP. Management of subarachnoid hemorrhage from ruptured saccular aneurysm. In: Ropper AH, Kennedy SK, Zervas NT, editors. Neurologic and neurosurgical intensive care. Baltimore: University Park Press; 1983. p. 175–87.

Lance JW. Mechanism and management of headache. 5th ed. Boston: Butterworth-Heinemann; 1993.

Ng PK, Pulst SM. Not so benign "thunderclap headache." Neurology 1992;260:42.

Ostergaard JR. Headache as a warning symptom of impending aneurysmal subarachnoid hemorrhage. Cephalalgia 1991; 11:53–5.

Rapoport AM, Silberstein SD. Emergency treatment of headache. Neurology 1992;42(Suppl 2):43–4.

Raps EC, Rogers JD, Galettra SL, et al. The clinical spectrum of unruptured intracranial aneurysms. Arch Neurol 1993; 50:265–8.

Raskin NH. Headaches caused by alterations of structure or hemostasis. In: Raskin NH, editor. Headache. 2nd ed. New York: Churchill Livingston; 1988. p. 296–9.

Schievink WI. Intracranial aneurysms. N Engl J Med 1997; 336:28–40.

Slivka A, Philbrook B. Clinical and angiographic features of thunderclap headache. Headache 1995;35:1–6.

Vermeulen M, van Gijn J. The diagnosis of subarachnoid hemorrhage. J Neurol Neurosurg Psychiatry 1990;53:365–72.

Weir B. Headaches from aneurysms. Cephalalgia 1994;14:79–87.

Wijdicks EFM, Kerkhoff H, van Gijn J. Long term follow up of 71 patients with thunderclap headaches mimicking subarachnoid hemorrhage. Lancet 1988;2:68–9.

Editorial Comments

This case of subarachnoid hemorrhage by Dr. Capobianco complements the previous case discussion by Dr. Dodick. As difficult as it may seem at times, given the general benign nature of most headaches, subarachnoid hemorrhage must be properly diagnosed. Careful attention to the history, as recommended, is paramount, as well as examination. Further, Dr. Capobianco's approach to investigation is entirely reasonable, with the caveat that as neuroimaging procedures improve, especially MRA, then new investigative options will be available.

CHAPTER 29

SEVEN PATIENTS, SEVEN HEADACHES

LOUIS R. CAPLAN, MD

The inter-relationships between headache and cerebrovascular disease are complex. Strokes are often accompanied by headache that can occur before, at, or after the onset of neurologic symptoms and signs. Migraine can also cause strokes. Some disorders cause both headaches and strokes. In this chapter I will present seven different case histories that illustrate the complex interplay between headaches and cerebrovascular disease.

Case 1 History

A 55-year-old business executive had been having throbbing headaches several times a week for a month. He had not been prone to headaches in the past. The headaches were rather diffuse and poorly localized. Occasionally he felt the headache more in the right forehead. One morning, after bending down to pick up a newspaper and rising quickly, he noted greying of vision in his right eye. This lasted less than 1 minute but recurred several days later.

His past history included 8 years of moderate hypertension that had been well controlled with medication. He had been unable to stop smoking cigarettes, a habit since his youth. He had angina pectoris and took cardiac vasodilators. These drugs did not give him headaches. He got a cramping feeling in his left calf when he walked more than two blocks.

He has consulted his physician because of the headaches. He has also made an appointment with his eye doctor to obtain new glasses since he has not been refracted in years.

Questions about Case 1

- What is the most likely cause of the headaches and the episodic monocular visual loss?
- How does the vascular lesion in this patient cause headache?
- How should he be managed?

Case 1 Discussion

The presence of angina pectoris and claudication of a lower extremity indicate that this man has large artery atherosclerosis. Hypertension and smoking are very important risk factors for atherosclerosis. Hypercholesterolemia is also often associated with coronary artery and peripheral vascular occlusive disease but this patient does not know his cholesterol level. In white men, the most common associated cerebrovascular lesion is occlusive disease of the internal carotid arteries (ICAs) in the neck.

Occlusive disease of the internal carotid artery often presents clinically with transient ischemic attacks (TIAs). The most common TIAs are transient monocular visual loss and transient spells that indicate brain hemispheric ischemia. The visual loss is usually brief; it often consists of greying or dimming of vision, or resembles a shade descending or a curtain crossing the vision, and occurs in the eye ipsilateral to the ICA disease. Sometimes the attacks of transient monocular visual loss are precipitated by circumstances that lower systemic blood pressure or blood volume, such as quickly rising from a stooped posture or sudden exposure to very bright light.

Patients with severe atherostenotic lesions of large extracranial or intracranial arteries sometimes develop headaches. Headaches in patients with severe arterial stenoses or occlusions have been explained as being due to distention of the involved artery and dilatation of collateral arterial channels in order to compensate for the reduced blood flow to the brain tissue supplied by the diseased artery(ies). Vasodilatation is a known mechanism of vascular headache. In my experience, the prodromal headaches of atherosclerotic occlusive disease have invariably been accompanied by TIAs although the headaches and transient ischemia do not usually occur together. About 20% of patients with TIAs were previously unaccustomed to having headaches.

Evaluation of this patient with Duplex ultrasonography showed a severe stenosis of his right ICA with a residual lumen of only 0.5 mm and moderate (50%) stenosis of the left ICA. A magnetic resonance imaging (MRI) scan showed a small infarct in the right frontal subcortical white matter and a magnetic resonance angiogram (MRA) confirmed the severe right ICA occlusive lesion but identified no intracranial stenosis. The patient had an uneventful right carotid endarterectomy after which his headaches disappeared.

Case 2 History

A 46-year-old woman sneezed vigorously while eating lunch with her elderly mother. The mother saw the patient immediately slump to the left. The patient's left limbs did not move, her face was twisted to the right, and her speech was slurred but the patient did not recognize any symptoms except headache, which she began to develop over the right side of her head.

Six years previously, the patient had had cardiac surgery to replace a mitral valve that was severely damaged by rheumatic heart disease. A prosthetic valve was inserted and since then she had been taking warfarin sodium, the dosage of which was closely supervised by her physician. She took no other medicines except prophylactic antibiotics before dental and other manipulations. She had no history of hypertension or hypercholesterolemia. She never used tobacco, seldom drank alcohol, and exercised

regularly. She rarely had headaches and could not recall a single very bad headache in the past, even during her three pregnancies. She considered herself to be quite fit.

An examination performed shortly after hospitalization revealed an alert woman who clutched her right head because of her headache. The headache throbbed. Her blood pressure was 125/80; her pulse was 80 beats per minute and regular. She had no fever. She was totally unaware of and unconcerned about any neurologic deficit. She had a severe left hemiplegia and hemisensory loss. Her eyes were conjugately deviated to the right. She ignored stimuli to her left and drew and copied very poorly. Her answers to queries were impulsive and her affect quite flat.

Questions about Case 2

- What are the most likely causes of her condition?
- How should she be evaluated?
- What is the mechanism of her headache?

Case 2 Discussion

The neurologic signs in this patient developed almost instantly while she was closely observed. Sneezing, coughing, sudden bending, and arising at night to urinate are well known to set off an embolism. It is postulated that the sudden activity shakes loose a thrombus from the heart, the aorta, or the proximal arterial system. Moreover this woman had a prosthetic heart valve, an important source of cardiac origin embolism. The alternative diagnosis to embolism in this patient is intracerebral hemorrhage (ICH). Although she was not hypertensive, she was taking anticoagulants. In any patient on anticoagulants, intracranial hemorrhage must always be considered and excluded. Intracerebral hemorrhage usually develops gradually during minutes and even hours and does not happen instantly in contrast to the neurologic deficit in patients with embolism which is most often at its maximum at onset.

This patient's neurologic deficit is severe and can be readily localized to the right cerebral hemisphere. Intracerebral hemorrhage often involves deeper brain structures in the hemisphere and can lead to such a severe deficit. However, when ICH causes a hemiplegia or other very severe neurologic deficits usually there is a considerable mass effect caused by the extra tissue (blood) within the brain parenchyma. A shift of intracranial contents occurs and vomiting and decreased consciousness ensue. It is unusual to see a patient with ICH with severe hemiplegia and conjugate gaze palsy who is completely alert and awake. Embolic infarcts usually do not produce much mass effect at or soon after onset. Brain edema develops later.

Both ICH and brain embolism cause headache. Mass effect with displacement of pial arteries and leakage of blood into the meningeal spaces is the presumed mechanism of headache in patients with ICH. Usually in ICH patients, the first symptoms and signs relate to the local hematoma within the brain parenchyma. As the hematoma grows, the mass effect develops and vomiting, headache, and decreased consciousness follow. In embolism, the onset is usually abrupt. The headache is postulated to be related to acute distention of the recipient artery and dilatation of collateral arteries. Later, headache can result from brain edema and mass effect. In contrast to the patient in case 1 who had a premonitory headache before the onset of a persistent neurologic deficit, headaches in patients with brain embolism most often develop at or shortly after the onset of neurologic signs. In ICH, headache develops later and mostly in patients with sizable hematomas.

In this patient, it was essential to obtain a brain imaging test quickly. Either a cranial computed tomography (CT) scan or a FLAIR MRI image would be acceptable. In this patient, CT showed poor definition of the basal ganglia and the insular cortex. A hyperdense middle cerebral artery (MCA) sign was present confirming the presence of embolism. Her international normalized ratio (INR) was 1.2 and she admitted later to poor compliance with her anticoagulant treatment because of depression. She was not a candidate for thrombolysis because she had a severe neurologic deficit and was on anticoagulants. She was heparinized and later switched to a regimen of half a tablet of aspirin (165 mg) and warfarin soduim (INR 2.4 to 3) for subsequent prophylaxis.

Had an ICH been present, or if her INR was high, I would have reversed her anticoagulation. If she had worsened and developed brain herniation or a prominent shift of brain contents, she would have become a candidate for surgical drainage of the hematoma.

Case 3 History

A 65-year-old, white man described a history of three separate transient attacks during the past month. The first attack consisted of weakness of the right hand and leg; during the second attack, he had numbness and weakness of the right hand; and during the third attack, he momentarily could not speak and the right side of his face felt numb. He had smoked a pack of cigarettes daily for 40 years and was being treated for hypertension.

An examination showed that his blood pressure was 155/95; pulse was 80 beats per minute and regular. A high-pitched, long focal bruit was heard over his left carotid artery in the neck. A neurologic examination was normal. A duplex scan of the neck arteries showed a very high grade (>95%) stenosis of the left ICA in the neck and 65% stenosis of the right ICA. A transcranial Doppler ultrasound (TCD) showed low blood flow velocities in the intracranial left ICA and the left MCA attributed to the neck stenosis. The severe left ICA stenosis was corroborated by MRI and MRA that showed no intracranial stenotic lesions and no brain infarcts. The patient had an uneventful left carotid endarterectomy.

On the day after surgery he reported a moderately severe left frontal headache. His blood pressure was 165/100. The next day, the headache was more severe and he reported numbness of his right arm and leg. In the evening, he became sleepy, the headache was more severe, and he had a seizure witnessed by the nurse which began with rhythmic jerking of his right hand and then became generalized. After the seizure, the right limbs were weak and he could not speak. His blood presure was 185/110.

Questions about Case 3

- What was the cause of the headache, seizures, and neurologic signs?
- What diagnostic tests should now be performed?
- How should he be treated?

Case 3 Discussion

In this patient, headache was the first important symptom after carotid artery surgery. The patient then developed more severe headaches, elevated blood pressure, focal neurologic signs in the territory of the operated artery, and a focal seizure. The differential diagnosis of his postoperative course is (1) left cerebral ischemia/ infarction related to a direct complication of the surgery such as reocclusion of the artery and/or embolism from the operated site to an intracranial artery; (2) intracerebral hemorrhage; (3) the hyperperfusion syndrome that can follow carotid endarterectomy, and (4) diffuse vasoconstriction that occasionally develops after carotid endarterectomy. The first steps are to determine if there is a local complication of the surgery within the left ICA and whether there is a brain infarct or hemorrhage. A duplex scan of the neck showed a normal left ICA. A TCD showed elevated blood-flow velocities in the left MCA. A CT scan showed hypodensity in the white matter of the left parietal lobe and some brain swelling of the left cerebrum but no midline shift.

The initial tests excluded brain hemorrhage, which is a known and feared complication of carotid surgery. Brain hemorrhage is usually attributed to a sudden or severe rise in blood pressure after surgery. Carotid surgery causes a loss of baroreceptor function since the carotid sinus is located at the operative site. Blood pressure often rises after carotid surgery especially in patients who have had hypertension before surgery, as was the case with this patient. The sudden rise in blood pressure can cause a hemorrhage. Having excluded hemorrhage, the surgeon and neurologists were concerned about the possibility of brain infarction. The surgeon was still insecure about the status of the left ICA even after the ultrasound results so he asked the neuroradiologist to perform an emergency angiogram that showed a normal left carotid artery and intracranial branches. The operated site looked fine, and there were no embolic occlusions or vasoconstriction of intracranial arteries. A review of the CT scan showed that there was no cortical imaging abnormality; the changes involved just the white matter and did not look like an infarction.

This patient's headache and neurologic findings were caused by the hyperperfusion syndrome that may follow carotid surgery. This syndrome occurs in some patients who have had severe ICA narrowing before surgery. It is more common in previously hypertensive patients. Findings known to occur in the hyperperfusion syndrome include headache, which is often severe and throbbing, elevated blood pressure, decreased alertness that sometimes progresses to stupor or coma, focal neurologic signs in the hemisphere ipsilateral to the surgery, and seizures. A CT scan may be normal or show a sometimes severe white matter edema. Carotid artery surgery in a patient with severe stenosis results in a dramatic increase in blood flow in the ipsilateral hemisphere. The brain is literally flooded with blood. A loss of baroreceptor function can lead to increased systemic blood pressure as it did in this patient. The prolonged decrease in hemispheric blood flow before surgery leads to defective autoregulation, so that the capillary bed cannot adequately handle the influx of blood under high pressure. The capillaries and arterioles become incompetent and leak fluid; brain edema develops. The pathogenesis of the brain edema is similar to that found in patients with hypertensive encephalopathy, except that in the hyperperfusion syndrome, the encephalopathy and brain edema are unilateral and limited to the side of the surgery. The increased flow of blood distends the arteries and causes headache. In fact, headache may be the major or sole symptom reflecting hyperperfusion. Increased blood-flow velocities as measured by TCD confirm the presence of hyperperfusion.

The most important treatment is control of the blood pressure. This patient was given labetalol that normalized the blood pressure. Within 1 day, the headache and the focal neurologic signs disappeared and his CT scan later became normal. It is imperative that blood pressure be followed very carefully after carotid artery surgery. Some patients have developed hyperperfusion syndrome or brain hemorrhage during days 3 to 8 after surgery. Most patients have already been discharged by this time. Blood pressure must be carefully monitored at home for the first 2 postoperative weeks. The hyperperfusion syndrome can lead to a fatal brain edema if not treated promptly and effectively. The hyperperfusion syndrome is not well known. It is an important cause of headache after carotid endarterectomy.

Case 4 History

An 18-year-old woman had a flurry of moderately severe headaches. The headaches were unilateral and throbbing. They began abruptly, rapidly reached maximum intensity, and were sometimes followed by nausea and vomiting. At first, she had headaches every other day but during the week before presentation, they occurred daily. Two days previously, she noted numbness of her left hand, and on the morning of her consultation, she had some difficulty speaking. She used some inappropriate words and had difficulty understanding the newspaper. She was brought to the hospital because of a seizure that began with twitching of her right hand and then became a generalized tonic-clonic convulsion.

On examination, the patient's blood pressure was 125/70; her pulse was 75 beats per minute and regular. She had no fever. Her cardiac and general physical examinations were normal. She was alert but made paraphasic errors and read, wrote, and spelled poorly. Her visual fields were normal. The optic fundi on both sides showed early disk swelling. Motor, sensory, and reflex examinations were normal but her left plantar response was extensor.

Questions about Case 4

- What is the most likely cause of her headaches?
- What explains the seizure, the focal neurologic signs, and the early papilledema? Are they somehow related to the headaches?
- How should the clinician proceed to investigate and treat this patient?

Case 4 Discussion

After a prodromal period of headaches, this patient developed multifocal neurologic findings, increased intracranial pressure, and a seizure. The first step was to clarify the nature of her focal brain lesions. A CT scan showed several small areas of hypodensity within the white matter of the left parietal lobe and the right frontal lobe. The brain looked swollen and the

ventricles were small. No subarachnoid or intracerebral hemorrhages were seen. The brain lesions resembled infarcts but an inflammatory process could not be excluded. An evaluation for vascular occlusive disease, embolism, and hypercoagulability was indicated. Concern about a possibility of multifocal brain embolism led to echocardiography (at first transthoracic and later transesophageal) that was completely normal. A complete blood count, coagulation studies, thyroid functions, sedimentation rate, antinuclear antibody, and antiphospholipin antibody testing were all normal. Urinalysis and renal functions were also normal.

The vascular-type headaches and the multifocal signs suggested a vascular etiology. An extracranial ultrasound was normal but TCD showed uniformly increased blood-flow velocities in the intracranial arteries. An MRI showed several regions of white-matter abnormalities and MRA showed several regions of arterial narrowing located within the middle and posterior cerebral arteries (PCAs). A lumbar puncture showed an opening pressure of 300; there were no cells and the cerebrospinal fluid (CSF) protein and sugar levels were normal. Catheter angiography was performed to clarify the nature of the vascular lesions. Angiography showed multiple localized regions of arterial narrowing with some dilatations. These regions involved the larger intracranial arteries, the MCAs, PCAs, and anterior cerebral arteries (ACAs) as well as small cortical branches of these arteries. The basilar artery was also focally narrowed.

A detailed history from the patient and her mother revealed that, at the age of 14, the patient had had a series of headaches characterized by transient visual abnormalities lasting about 20 minutes and followed by severe unilateral throbbing headaches. The patient's mother also had migraine with aura.

The lesions within the intracranial arteries were typical of a disorder first described by Call, Fleming, et al. (1988) as the *reversible cerebral segmental vasoconstriction syndrome*. This disorder is relatively common (I see two or three patients a year with this syndrome), yet I find that most neurologists and headache specialists are unaware of its existence. The symptoms and signs are caused by intense multifocal vasoconstriction of intracranial medium-sized and small arteries. Patients usually develop headaches as the first symptom. The headaches become progressively more frequent, and often more severe, and are usually present daily. Their character is typical of vascular headaches. Most patients in my experience have had a past personal history compatible with migraine with or without aura. Focal neurologic signs, seizures, and brain edema can develop. The condition can be fatal. In my experience, the symptoms and vascular changes respond well to the calcium channel blockers verapamil and nimodipine. Vascular changes can be monitored by TCD. With clinical improvement, the intracranial blood-flow velocities gradually return to normal.

The Call-Fleming syndrome is most common in adolescent girls but also occurs in the puerperium and during menopause. It has also been reported after carotid endarterectomy. I view the syndrome as a type of severe migraine status. Patients are often misdiagnosed as having cerebral vasculitis—the most overmade diagnosis in all of clinical medicine.

A similar important but clinically distinct syndrome of recurrent attacks of focal neurologic signs including aphasia and headache was described by Bartleson (1984). These patients are young, predominantly male, and have a CSF pleocytosis. Flurries of headaches and aphasia usually occur over weeks and then disappear, usually leaving no residual deficits. Calcium channel blockers may be effective. The nature of the inflammatory changes is unclear but a viral syndrome causing vasoconstriction has been postulated most often. The Bartleson and Call-Fleming syndromes are important because of their potential reversibility. These syndromes are seldom if ever recognized by non-neurologists.

Case 5 History

A 23-year-old woman reported a severe headache over her right eye which began 2 days previously. During the 2 days, she had noted several very brief attacks of transient loss of vision in the right eye, lasting for just seconds and precipitated by standing up quickly from a stooped position on one occasion. She had also had pain in her right jaw, face, and neck. She heard a pulsatile whistling noise periodically in her right ear. The morning of presentation, her left arm and leg became numb and weak. She also noted that her voice was hoarse and that she had difficulty swallowing liquids.

She was an athletic woman. Each day, despite a rigorous schedule in her law office, she worked out at a gym and often played basketball and volleyball. She remembered no recent severe incidents of head or neck trauma but did say that the basketball scrimmages could be rather rough and physical.

Her pulse and blood pressure were normal. An examination of her visual field was normal. The right eyelid was drooped. The right pupil was 2.5 mm and the left was 4 mm. Her right tongue, palate, sternocleidomastoid, and shoulder shrug were weak. The left hand, arm, face, and thigh were also weak and she could not localize touch well on her left hand. The left tendon reflexes were increased and she had a left Babinski sign. She had no neglect of the left side of pictures or reading matter and she drew and copied pictures normally. She was fully aware of her left limb deficits.

Questions about Case 5

- What was the cause of her headache, visual obscurations, and right-cerebral-hemisphere neurologic signs?
- What explains the weakness of the muscles innervated by the right-lower cranial nerves?
- How should she be evaluated and treated?

Case 5 Discussion

This was clearly an urgent situation which demanded rapid evaluation and treatment. The patient showed four characteristics that are typically found in patients with extracranial carotid artery dissection; these are (1) pain in the neck, face, and jaw; (2) pulsatile tinnitus; (3) Horner's syndrome; and (4) weakness of the muscles innervated by cranial nerves IX to XII. Moreover, she was young and had no risk factors for atherosclerotic disease. She was athletic and had numerous opportunities for stretching and tearing her extracranial arteries.

Extracranial dissections involve the pharyngeal portions of the carotid and vertebral arteries. These segments of the arteries are relatively mobile and can be stretched and torn by sudden movements. The cervical carotid and vertebral arteries are anchored at their origins when they pass within the foramena transversaria of the vertebral column and at their penetration intradurally into the cranial cavity. Dissections are most often precipitated by sudden turning or stretching motions and by neck manipulations. Some patients have an underlying abnormality of the connective and elastic tissue fibers within the media of their arteries that makes them more vulnerable to dissections. Edema of arteries during and after migraine attacks may also increase the likelihood of arterial dissections.

A tear within the arterial media leads to the development of an intramural hematoma. This hematoma dissects longitudinally within the artery and can rupture through the intima into the arterial lumen. Dissection through the adventitia often leads to a pseudoaneurysm since the extravasated blood remains tightly bound by muscle and fascia. The intramural hematoma compresses the lumen and leads to a sudden decrease in blood flow in the territory supplied by the dissected artery. This often causes a series of brief transient ischemic attacks. In patients with carotid artery dissection, transient monocular blindness or attacks of minor dysfunction of the ipsilateral cerebral hemisphere are common. The attacks are usually brief and multiple (dubbed "carotid allegro" by Miller Fisher, 1968) and may be precipitated by sudden standing or Valsalva's maneuvers. They are caused by hypoperfusion. These attacks nearly always stop spontaneously within days. Strokes, when they occur, are caused by embolism of a luminal thrombus into the intracranial arteries. The clot reaches the carotid lumen by dissecting through the intima, or by forming in situ within the lumen of the artery. By narrowing the lumen and irritating the endothelium, thus triggering activation of platelets and the coagulation cascade, the intramural dissection creates a milieu within the lumen that strongly promotes thrombus formation. The lumenal clot is at first poorly organized and nonadherent and so has a tendency to embolize.

In this patient, MRI showed a small striato-capsular infarct in the right cerebral hemisphere. The ICA in the neck was narrowed over a long segment and the MCA was occluded by an embolus. She was treated immediately with intravenous heparin. Within the anterior circulation, embolism goes most often to the MCA and its branches. Within the posterior circulation, emboli most often go to the ipsilateral intracranial vertebral artery causing cerebellar infarction in the territory of the ipsilateral posterior inferior cerebellar artery. Occasionally emboli reach the rostral basilar artery and its superior cerebellar and PCA branches.

The predominant symptom in patients with arterial dissections is pain. In ICA dissections, the pain is often in the anterior neck, face, or jaw locations that seldom are painful in atherosclerotic disease. Headache is common and may be generalized or ipsilateral to the dissection. In verterbal artery dissections, the pain is most often located in the neck, shoulders, mastoid, or occiput. In some patients, pain is the only major symptom. In patients with extracranial vertebral artery dissections, the pain can be radicular, simulating a herniated cervical disk. This pattern of pain radiation is explained by aneurysmal dilatation of regions of the dissected artery that compress nerve roots.

Dilatation of the ICA causes dysfunction of the cervical sympathetic fibers on the surface of the artery so Horner's syndrome is a common finding. When the dissection extends to the skull base, it can compress or render ischemic the adjacent lower cranial nerves that exit the skull through the jugular (IX, X, and XI) and hypoglossal (XII) foramina. The ICA is located near the middle ear and dissections that extend to the skull base often are accompanied by pulsatile tinnitus. I have now seen a number of patients with headache, Horner's syndrome, and pulsatile tinnitus caused by ICA dissections who have no transient or persistent brain ischemia.

Extracranial arterial dissections often can be recognized by ultrasound and magnetic resonance imaging. Cut sections of the neck using MRI can definitively show dissecting hematomas within arterial walls. Most observers believe that anticoagulation with heparin and then warfarin sodium is the preferred treatment although there are no randomized trials that confirm or deny the utility of this treatment. Heparin is used to prevent the formation, propagation, and embolization of intraluminal thrombi. The course of the dissection can be followed by serial vascular imaging including ultrasound, MRA, or computed tomographic angiography (CTA). I continue warfarin sodium until the arterial lumen is no longer severely narrowed (usually 2 to 4 months). In patients with total occlusions of the arteries that remain persistently occluded, I discontinue warfarin sodium after 3 months. By then, the thrombus is well organized and adherent and has little likelihood of embolizing. During that period, collateral circulation becomes firmly established and compensates well during circulatory stresses and changes in blood pressure and blood flow.

Case 6 History

A 35-year-old woman had a long history of migraine with aura. The attacks were relatively stereotyped. They usually began with bright spots or zigzag lines in one or the other visual field. The objects would scintillate and move in place and then become more numerous, gradually migrating across the visual field. Often they left a region of darkness in their wake. Occasionally, the patient noticed difficulty seeing to one side after the brightness disappeared but this always cleared and her vision would return to normal within half an hour. The visual symptoms would last on average 20 minutes but could last from 15 to 60 minutes. Often a throbbing, unilateral headache followed the visual symptoms, sometimes beginning an hour after the visual symptoms were gone.

The day before presentation, she had one of her usual attacks. After the zigzag lines passed, she could not see to her left. On this occasion, her visual deficit did not clear and she consulted a physician because of a residual left homonymous hemianopia, which was verified on examination. She had no headache, did not neglect the left visual field, had normal optokinetic nystagmus, and drew and copied normally. She was normotensive, did not smoke, and had no known risk factors for cerebrovascular disease.

Questions about Case 6

- What is the cause of the hemianopia?
- Does she have a disorder other than migraine?
- How should she be evaluated and treated?

Case 6 Discussion

Migraine patients occasionally have strokes. In Table 29–1, I have listed the postulated relationships between migraine and stroke in migraineurs. Some define "migrainous strokes" loosely to include virtually any stroke that occurs in a patient with migraine. Others use a strict definition that includes only neurologic ischemic deficits that are essentially persistent migrainous auras. Table 29–2 lists the criteria of the International Headache Society for migrainous brain infarction. This patient certainly had classic migraine (migraine with aura). In the circumstance presented, she had her usual migrainous aura but this time the visual deficit persisted. Sometimes a persistent deficit can clear even after days. During a migraine aura, there is brain ischemia. In at least some patients, diminished blood flow and vasoconstriction have been documented. Brain tissue can be infarcted if blood flow is sufficiently diminished for enough time. In other patients, there is insufficient blood flow and delivery of needed nutrients for the brain tissue to continue to function but the reduction in blood flow is not sufficient to cause cell death and brain infarction. This state that lies between normal and infarcted is sometimes called "stunned brain." Brain imaging can be helpful in predicting this circumstance. If CT or MRI show a definite infarct, the likelihood of good recovery is lower than if imaging is normal.

In this patient, an MRI scan showed a right calcarine infarct. Magnetic resonance angiography, performed at the same time, showed an occluded right PCA. The extracranial and intracranial vertebral arteries and the basilar artery were normal. Echocardiography showed a normal heart and aorta. There was no right-to-left cardiac shunt. The platelet count was normal, as were coagulation studies. She did not have anticardiolipin antibodies or lupus anticoagulant. Blood chemistries including serum calcium determinations were also completely normal. No condition other than migraine could be identified to account for the right PCA occlusion and occipital lobe infarction. This patient meets all of the International Headache Society criteria for migrainous brain infarction.

TABLE 29–1. Explanations for Strokes in Migraineurs

- The stroke has a well-recognized cause—migraine is merely incidental and unrelated.
- A systemic disorder causes both the stroke and migraine (e.g., CADASIL, MELAS, antiphospholipid antibody syndrome, mitral valve prolapse, systemic lupus erythematosus).
- Migraine predisposes to arterial dissection, which causes a stroke.
- Vascular disease, such as a vascular malformations, dissection, or a brain embolus, causes headaches which mimic migraine.
- Migraine promotes development of vascular abnormalities such as aneurysms and fibromuscular dysplasia that cause stroke.
- The prolonged vasoconstriction associated with migraine causes brain infarction.
- Migraine and vasoconstriction activate platelets promoting thrombus formation.
- Vascular endothelial damage related to migrainous vasoconstriction activates the coagulation cascade leading to thrombus formation.
- Dehydration and vomiting during a migraine attack can cause thrombosis and stroke.
- Treatment of a migraine attack with a vasoconstrictive drug can cause a worsening of vasoconstriction with resultant prolonged brain ischemia.
- Reperfusion of brain regions containing arterioles and capillaries damaged during a migraine attack causes brain hemorrhage.

Vasoconstriction is a known phenomenon in migraine. Theorists argue that vasoconstriction may be secondary to a brain event and may not be the primary pathogenesis of migraine. Nevertheless, if vasoconstriction continues long enough, it alone can cause infarction. Vasoconstriction also causes edema of the endothelium and the vessel wall. Irritation of the endothelium activates both platelets and the coagulation cascade. Narrowing of the arterial lumen also promotes thrombosis in situ. Among a series of 35 consecutive patients with unilateral occipital lobe infarcts in PCA territory studied by Pessin et al. (1987), there were 5 patients with migraine. All had PCA occlusions, 3 of the main trunk and 2 of the branches. Because of the occurrence of thrombosis, I usually suggest that patients who have migraine with aura take an anticoagulant (usually aspirin). In patients with frequent, severe, or prolonged auras, I usually prescribe prophylactic calcium channel blockers to prevent vasoconstriction. Adequate hydration during a migraine attack is also important to maintain blood volume and blood flow.

Other vascular diseases can probably cause migraine, especially in individuals with a genetic predisposition. Brain embolism can cause vasocon-striction in the recipient artery. Hypercalcemia can also cause vasoconstriction and migraine-like disturbances. Patients with the antiphospholipid antibody syndrome and mitral valve prolapse have a higher than normal frequency of migraine and of strokes. Hyperthyroidism and an increase in very low density lipoproteins can also trigger migraine and vasoconstriction. I advocate full evaluations of patients with migraine strokes to ensure that other predisposing causes are not present.

Some patients with migraine develop intracerebral hemorrhages (ICH) after a prolonged headache subsides. Delayed ICH after prolonged migraine has been described by Cole and Aube (1990) and is usually explained by a reperfusion hemorrhage. Prolonged vasoconstriction causes injury to blood vessels that then leak when the vasoconstriction abates and the ischemic zone is reperfused. These delayed hemorrhages are rare but should be recognized.

Case 7 History

A 32-year-old woman had frequent headaches since her teens. The headaches were unilateral and throbbing and developed quickly. They occurred most often before her menstrual periods but also could be precipitated by red wine. On one occasion, she had a hemianopic visual experience that lasted 20 minutes preceding one of her usual headaches. She had seen a neurologist who diagnosed her condition as migraine. Recently, she had been using sumatriptan to successfully stop her headaches.

She came to the emergency ward because of an unusually severe headache that she could not abort with an injection of sumatriptan. The headache developed very suddenly during intercourse with her

TABLE 29–2. International Headache Society Criteria for Migrainous Brain Infarction (IHS 1.6.2)

One or more migrainous aura symptoms not fully reversible within 7 days and/or neuroimaging confirmation of ischemic infarction *and*

1. the patient has met criteria for migraine with neurologic aura.
2. the present attack is typical of past attacks but neurologic deficits are not reversible within 7 days and/or neuroimaging shows an infarct in a region appropriate to the neurologic symptoms.
3. other causes of infarction are excluded by appropriate testing.

boyfriend. The headache reached its maximum intensity almost immediately. She thought that she had passed out for a moment at the onset of the headache, and she soon needed to vomit. The headache was the "worst migraine that she had ever had." She denied ever using cocaine, amphetamines, or any other drugs.

On examination, her blood pressure was 125/80. Her pulse was 80 beats per minute. She seemed restless and had difficulty lying still for an examination. On several occasions, she excused herself to go to the bathroom. She was oriented. Her neck was not stiff. The neurologic examination was normal except for her restlessness. She repeatedly requested more sumatriptan and insisted on going home.

Questions about Case 7

- What are the major differential diagnostic considerations?
- How should this patient be evaluated and treated?

Case 7 Discussion

This patient undoubtedly had migraine. Several features, however, separated this latest headache from her usual migraines. These aspects included (1) the precipitation of headache during coition; (2) the suddenness of onset and severity of the headache; (3) the possible loss of consciousness at or near onset; and (4) vomiting soon after onset. All of these features suggested that she had had a subarachnoid hemorrhage (SAH) and not a migrainous attack.

Subarachnoid hemorrhage is most often caused by the sudden release of blood under arterial pressure into the subarachnoid space. Rupture of an arterial aneurysm or an arteriovenous malformation on the surface of the brain or within the subarachnoid space causes a sudden influx of blood under high pressure. This sudden change in intracranial pressure causes a lapse in alertness and activities, as well as headache and vomiting. The loss of alertness is a very important diagnostic point since it does not occur at the onset of migraine attacks. At the onset of SAH, the legs may buckle if the patient is standing and, in some patients, there is momentary amnesia or confusion. If enough blood is released, there may be an alteration in the state of consciousness. Drowsiness or restless agitation (as in this patient) are most common but frank

stupor or coma may occur. Restlessness—an inabliity to lie or sit quietly—is especially common and is often misinterpreted as being psychologically mediated. The headache of SAH is usually at its maximum at or near onset. The sudden increase in intracranial pressure causes vomiting. Vomiting is common during migraine attacks but usually not at the onset of the headache; vomiting occurs only after the migraine headache is well developed. Subarachnoid hemorrhage can be precipitated by vigorous physical activity or straining, e.g., during sexual intercourse.

Patients such as this one should have an emergency CT scan. If the scan does not show blood, they need a lumbar puncture. Computed tomography scans can be negative if the amount of bleeding is small or if the scan is taken more than 48 hours after onset. Because blood in the subarachnoid space disseminates quickly around the brain and spinal cord, lumbar puncture always shows blood in a patient with a recent SAH. The pressure of the fluid is also elevated. This patient had an equivocal CT scan but a spinal tap showed bloody spinal fluid under increased pressure. Arteriography showed a right-posterior communicating artery aneurysm which was repaired satisfactorily.

Subarachnoid hemorrhage is an extremely serious condition. Between one-fourth and one-half of patients with SAH die despite treatment. Many patients who later develop fatal hemorrhages have promonitory smaller "warning leaks" before the larger hemorrhages. A small disruption in the apex of an aneurysm weakens the wall and often precedes a larger rupture. Unfortunately, many patients with warning leaks are sent home from emergency rooms and doctors' offices without a definitive diagnosis only to return moribund days or weeks later. When there is a suspicion of SAH, a lumbar puncture is imperative unless brain imaging studies show SAH or intracerebral blood.

The past history of migraine should not dissuade clinicians from a diagnosis of SAH since the two conditions often coexist. Some have postulated an increased incidence of aneurysms in migraineurs. Since up to one in four individuals in the community has migraine, by chance alone a significant number of migraineurs will have aneurysms or vascular malformations.

Suggested Readings

Adams HP, Jergenson DD, Kassell NF, Sahs AL. Pitfalls in the recognition of subarachnoid hemorrhage. JAMA 1980; 244:794–6.

Bartleson JD, Swanson JW, Whisnant JP. A migrainous syndrome with cerebrospinal fluid pleocytosis. Neurology 1981;31:1257–62.

Bartleson JD. Transient and persistent neurological manifestations of migraine. Stroke 1984;15:383–6.

Breen JC, Caplan LR, De Witt LD, et al. Brain edema after carotid surgery. Neurology 1996;46:175–81.

Call GK, Fleming MC, Sealfon S, et al. Reversible cerebral segmental vasoconstriction. Stroke 1988;19:1159–70.

Caplan LR. Migraine and vertebrobasilar ischemia. Neurology 1991;41:55–61.

Caplan LR. Stroke: a clinical approach. 2nd ed. Boston: Butterworth-Heinemann; 1993.

Caplan LR. Posterior circulation disease. Clinical findings, diagnosis, and management. Boston: Blackwell Science; 1996.

Cole AJ, Aube M. Migraine with vasospasm and delayed intracerebral hemorrhage. Arch Neurol 1990;47:53–6.

Fisher CM. Headache in cerebrovascular disease. In: Vinken PJ, Bruyn GW, editors. Handbook of clinical neurology. Vol. 5. Headaches and cranial neuralgias. Amsterdam: North-Holland Publ. Co.; 1968. p. 124–56.

Gomez-Aranda F, Canadillas F, Marti-Masso JF, et al. Pseudomigraine with temporary neurological symptoms and lymphocytic pleocytosis. A report of 50 cases. Brain 1997;120: 1105–13.

Gorelick PB, Hier DB, Caplan LR. Headache in acute cerebrovascular disease. Neurology 1986;36:1445–50.

Hauerberg J, Andersen BB, Eskesen V, et al. Importance of the recognition of a warning leak as a sign of a ruptured cerebral aneurysm. Acta Neurol Scand 1971;83:61–4.

Kase CS, Caplan LR. Intracerebral hemorrhage. Boston: Butterworth-Heinemann;1994.

Lopez-Valdes E, Chang H-M, Pessin MS, Caplan LR. Cerebral vasoconstriction after carotid surgery. Neurology 1997; 49:303–4.

Mokri B, Houser OW, Sandok BA, Piepgras DG. Spontaneous dissection of the vertebral arteries. Neurology 1988;38:880–5.

Ojemann RG, Fisher CM, Rich JC. Spontaneous dissecting aneurysms of the internal carotid artery. Stroke 1972;3: 434–40.

Pessin MS, Lathi E, Cohen MB, et al. Clinical features and mechanisms of occipital infarction. Ann Neurol 1987;21:290–9.

Sturzenegger M. Ultrasound findings in spontaneous carotid artery dissection: the value of Duplex sonography. Arch Neurol 1991;48:1057–63.

Welch KMA, Levine SR. Migraine-related stroke in the context of the International Headache Society Classification of head pain. Arch Neurol 1990;47:458–62.

Editorial Comments

The relationships of headache with cerebrovascular disease are intriguing and deserve more attention from all clinicians managing headaches. Dr. Caplan provides seven such scenarios in which he outlines pertinent diagnostic strategies and management suggestions from the literature and his own clinical experience. Interestingly, he discusses the entities of Bartleson's and Call-Fleming syndromes and emphasizes that they are underdiagnosed because they are under-recognized. Migraine, arterial dissection, subarachnoid bleed, and atherothombotic disease are discussed here in relationship to headache. As well, the headache following carotid endarterectomy is described, which is an entity that also deserves more attention. Much is to be learned from this excellent chapter.

Chapter 30

The Woman with Postpartum Headache

Valérie Biousse, MD

Marie-Germaine Bousser, MD

Case History

A 35-year-old woman was seen in the emergency room 2 weeks after the delivery of her baby for an unusual recent constant headache. Her past medical history was remarkable only for migraine without aura since childhood. Her migraine attacks usually occurred once a week and resolved with aspirin. She did not have any migraine attacks during her pregnancy.

The pregnancy was uneventful, and she had a normal vaginal delivery with epidural anesthesia. A few days after delivery, she started to complain of daily headache. The headache was moderate and nonthrobbing but increased gradually and was associated with nausea. She did not present with tinnitus, diplopia, or other neurologic symptoms. Her neurologic and general examinations were unremarkable. Her blood pressure was 145/80.

She was diagnosed as having lumbar puncture headache related to the epidural anesthesia. It was also emphasized that her present headache could be partly related to the recurrence of migraine after delivery. She was placed on acetaminophen, and an epidural blood patch was performed. She was sent home but she still complained of a persistent headache. Two days later, she had a grand mal seizure and was taken back to the emergency room. Except for a persistent headache and a slight loss of alert-

ness atributed to the seizure, her neurologic examination was normal. A funduscopic examination showed a bilateral disk edema. Her blood pressure was 165/100. A computed tomography (CT) scan of the head, with and without contrast, was performed and was normal. She was then diagnosed as having "postpartum eclampsia," and received magnesium sulfate. After 24 hours in the hospital, she recovered completely, her blood pressure was 145/80, and she was sent back home.

One week later, she was re-admitted because of worsening of her headache and progressive alteration of consciousness in the absence of recurrent seizures. On examination, she was somnolent and agitated but had no focal deficits. A funduscopy showed worsening of the bilateral disk edema. Her general examination was normal, and her blood pressure was 135/75.

Questions about This Case

- What are your diagnostic considerations in this case?
- Would you perform other investigations?
- What is your final diagnosis?
- What specific therapy would you suggest?
- What are the relationships of this disease to pregnancy or puerperium?
- What should be the long-term management of the patient and the prognosis for this disease?

Case Discussion

This case is interesting in that it illustrates the diagnosis and appropriate management of headache occurring during pregnancy and/or puerperium. This patient has a history of migraine without aura that spontaneously resolved during pregnancy. This occurs in two-thirds of cases and is a highly characteristic feature of migraine. Postnatal headaches are common during the first postpartum week, occurring in 30 to 40% of women. Most often, these headaches are benign headaches that spontaneously resolve after 1 or 2 weeks. They are usually mild, bifrontal, and always isolated. Migraine attacks with or without aura can also occur during puerperium; they have the usual characteristics of migraine attacks except that they are sometimes particularly severe. Other "classic" conditions include lumbar puncture headache that can occur after epidural anesthesia. This headache is characterized by its appearance or worsening in an upright position and disappearance after resumption of the recumbent position. Eclampsia or pre-eclampsia can occur up to 2 weeks after delivery and can be a cause of persistent headache. Hypertension and proteinuria are constant features of this disease. Visual disturbances, seizures, coma, and disseminated intravascular coagulation develop if the patient is not treated. Other conditions that are classic in pregnancy and postpartum include pituitary and other intracranial tumors, cerebral venous thrombosis (CVT), subarachnoid hemorrhage, and meningitis. They must be ruled out before the diagnosis of chronic tension headache related to stress or postpartum depression is considered.

In our patient, migraine, lumbar puncture headache, and eclampsia were successively envisaged. Migraine should have been easily ruled out in the absence of well-defined attacks. Lumbar puncture headache should not have been envisaged in the absence of any postural worsening. Eclampsia could have been ruled out because of the absence of severe hypertension and proteinuria.

Our patient has a rapidly worsening headache with nausea and papilledema that is typical of raised intracranial pressure. This should have been considered when the patient was seen in the emergency room the first time. In this patient with recent headache, a funduscopic examination could have been easily performed in the emergency room to look for disk edema. Indeed, when the patient came back with persistent headache, she had bilateral disk edema, confirming intracranial hypertension. Investigations are urgently needed in such cases, particularly when, as in our patient, seizures occur. Numerous lesions can cause intracranial hypertension. In our patient, the normal CT scan, with and without contrast, ruled out the possibility of tumors, abscesses, or hemorrhage. However, it did not rule out CVT and meningitis. Thus, the diagnosis at this point is that of intracranial hypertension but other investigations are needed to determine the cause.

Management of raised intracranial pressure with a normal CT scan is now standard (Figure 30–1). Chronic meningitis (infections such as syphilitic meningitis or carcinomatous meningitis), CVT, dural fistula, or idiopathic intracranial hypertension (pseudotumor cerebri) are possible causes of isolated raised intracranial pressure. Therefore, after a normal CT scan, a lumbar puncture with cerebrospinal fluid (CSF) analysis and careful measurement of the opening pressure should be performed in order to confirm raised intracranial pressure, to rule out meningitis, and to rapidly improve vision. In our patient, the opening pressure was 350 mm H_2O, proteins were normal, and there were no cells, thus ruling out meningitis. The patient's headache improved rapidly after lumbar puncture. Despite this improvement, other investigations were needed, in particular magnetic resonance imaging (MRI) and angiography. Magnetic resonance imaging disclosed, in T1- and T2-weighted images, an increased signal in the superior sagittal sinus, which is diagnostic of CVT, without any parenchymal lesion (Figure 30–2). Had MRI been equivocal, which is the case in the very first days of sinus thrombosis, angiography (magnetic resonance angiography [MRA] or intra-arterial angiography) would have been required. It is also important to do an ophthalmologic examination in order to evaluate the severity of the disk edema and its complications. Therefore, visual-acuity measurement and formal visual field testing should be performed in addition to funduscopy, initially and during follow-up.

The initial presentation of this patient was already suggestive of CVT. Indeed, progressive headache associated with disk edema is one of the most frequent presentations of CVT (40% in our series). Puerperium (much more than pregnancy) is such a classic cause of CVT that any progressive headache or seizure occurring during postpartum should immediately prompt investigations to confirm or rule out this condition.

In our patient, the diagnosis of CVT was not considered initially, and rapid worsening occurred leading to a decreased level of consciousness. The patient was then at risk of focal deficits, repeated seizures, and coma that can occur at any time in the course of CVT and can sometimes be rapidly lethal. She was also at risk of deep vein thrombosis and pulmonary embolism, which is a well-established cause of death in patients with CVT. Thus, as soon as the diagnosis of CVT is established, an urgent treatment is required.

After MRI confirmed the diagnosis of CVT, our patient was treated with intravenous heparin (activated partial thromboplastin [aPTT]) and with valproate to prevent the recurrence of seizures. She rapidly improved so that it was not felt necessary to prescribe drugs to lower the intracranial pressure, such as mannitol, glycerol, or steroids. After 5 days, heparin was replaced with warfarin (INR 2.5 to 3.5). The headache resolved within 2 weeks, and repeated funduscopy after 1 month showed disappearance of the disk edema. There were no further seizures.

Puerperium and, to a much lesser extent, pregnancy are among the causative factors most commonly identified in CVT and are present in about 20% of patients. The proportion seems to be higher in the developing countries. Third trimester and puerperium can be considered as naturally occurring prothrombotic states characterized by increased levels of procoagulant proteins, suppression of fibrinolysis by raised levels of plasminogen activator inhibitors, and diminished anticoagulant substances such as protein S. The prevalence of thrombosis in any site

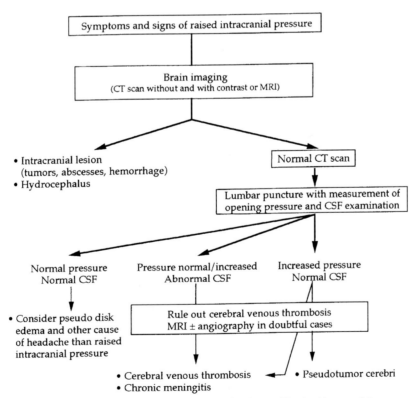

FIGURE 30–1. Algorithm for the management of patients with raised intracranial pressure and a normal CT scan.

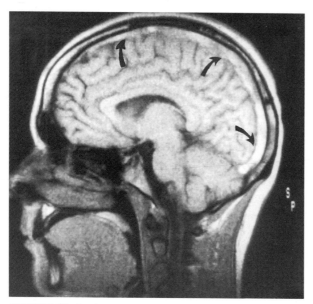

FIGURE 30–2. Sagittal view of T1-weighted-image MRI showing an increased signal in the thrombosed superior sagittal sinus (*arrows*).

TABLE 30–1. Main Neurologic Symptoms and Signs in CVT

Symptom/Sign	Incidence (n=135)	
Headache	105	(78%)
Papilledema	67	(49%)
Seizures	56	(41%)
Focal deficit (motor, sensory, aphasia)	55	(40%)
Disorder of consciousness	38	(28%)
Multiple cranial nerve palsies	16	(12%)
Bilateral or alternating cortical signs	5	(4%)
Cerebellar Incoordination	4	(3%)

(most often veins of the leg) is approximately 1 per 1000 during pregnancy and 4 per 1000 in the puerperium. The clinical features of pregnancy-related CVT conform to the classic description. The superior sagittal sinus is most commonly affected. The onset is usually acute from 1 to 20 days after delivery and, in a smaller number of patients, during the second or third trimester of pregnancy. The risk of puerperium- or pregnancy-related CVT is higher in women with thrombophilia but there is no association with toxemia or hypertension. Therefore, a systematic work-up should include tests for inherited thrombophilia, such as activated protein C resistance (factor V Leiden), antithrombin III, and protein C and S deficiencies. These investigations were negative in our patient.

Since the etiologic work-up was negative, warfarin was stopped after 3 months, while valproate was prolonged for 6 months. The patient did not have any subsequent seizure or any other neurologic problem.

The long-term prognosis for CVT is usually good and is mainly related to the underlying disease. The risk of recurrence is not well known; it was about 11% in our series, and most reccurrences took place within the first year.

There is no contraindication to subsequent pregnancies but particularly close follow-up is then required. We also advocate low-molecular-weight heparin post partum, in order to prevent any recurrent venous thrombosis.

Management Strategies

- The occurrence of progressive daily headache should raise the possibility of raised intracranial pressure. Immediate funduscopic examination should be performed to detect papilledema, which confirms the presence of intracranial hypertension.
- After ruling out intracranial tumors, abscesses, hemorrhages, and hydrocephalus by CT scan, the physician should know how to manage a patient with raised intracranial pressure and normal CT scan (see Figure 30–2). A lumbar puncture is crucial to rule out meningitis, to confirm the raised pressure, and to improve vision.
- An MRI is then mandatory to rule out CVT in a patient with isolated raised intracranial pressure. Be aware that the diagnosis of CVT on MRI, based on the hypersignal of the thrombosed vessel, is not so easy. There are false negative results, particularly in the very first days, when the thrombosed vein can present as a hypo- or isosignal and, after the first month, when the signal becomes isointense again or even hypointense if the vessel has recanalized. Angiography is still helpful in doubtful cases.
- Angiography needs to be performed in a patient with intracranial hypertension, when a CT scan, MRI, and CSF composition are all normal. Magnetic resonance angiography (venography) is

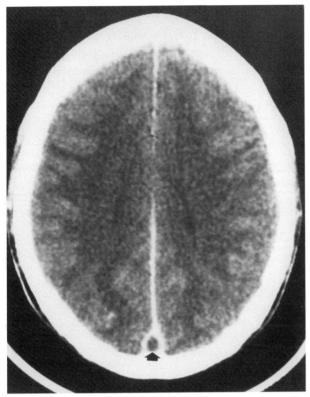

FIGURE 30-3. A CT scan of the brain with contrast showing the empty delta sign (*arrow*).

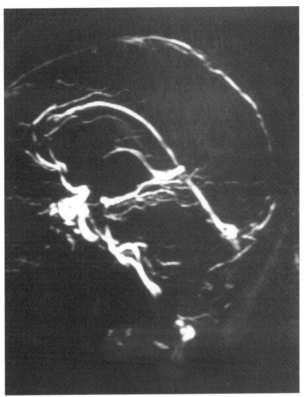

FIGURE 30-4. Two-dimensional time of flight MRA: thrombosis of the superior sagittal sinus.

preferable because of its noninvasiveness. If it is not possible, or if MRI cannot be performed at all, then intra-arterial angiography is still required.

- The short-term outcome of and the long-term prognosis for CVT are usually good provided that appropriate treatment is started.

Case Summary

- This patient has a postpartum superior sagittal sinus thrombosis that occurred in the absence of other underlying diseases.
- She presented with raised intracranial pressure (headache and disk edema) and a grand mal seizure, which is one of the most common patterns of presentation of CVT.
- She had a normal CT scan which does not rule out CVT.
- Headache and seizures post partum should be diagnosed as CVT until proved otherwise.

- Unfortunately, our patient's story is not unique and, despite increasing awareness, CVT is still a disease in which the correct diagnosis is frequently overlooked or delayed.
- Management strategies are outlined and serve as a guide to all patients presenting with "isolated intracranial hypertension and a normal CT scan." It is recommended that the reader consult Chapter 33.

Overview of Cerebral Venous Thrombosis

Cerebral venous thrombosis (CVT) has for many years been diagnosed mainly at autopsy. This has led to the description of a very rare and lethal disease characterized clinically by papilledema, seizures, focal deficits, coma, and death and pathologically by hemorrhagic infarction contraindicating the use of anticoagulants. The introduction and widespread use of cerebral angiography, CT, and, more recently, MRI has made the early diagnosis of CVT possible and has completely modified our knowledge of this condition. However, CVT remains a diagnostic and therapeutic challenge for the clinician because of its often misleading presentation and sometimes difficult treatment.

Although CVT presents with a remarkably wide spectrum of signs (Table 30–1), headache is the most frequent symptom (75% of cases) and often the initial one. Although it is mainly described in superior sagittal sinus thrombosis, which is the most common variety of CVT, headache has no topographic value and is common in other situations such as lateral sinus thrombosis or cerebral vein thrombosis. The headache is most often diffuse but can be unilateral, localized to any region of the head, or even limited to the neck. The severity is again highly variable, ranging from a mild sensation of heaviness to a severe "thunderclap" headache. The mode of onset also varies from patient to patient. Most frequently, the onset of headache is subacute over a few days but it can also be sudden, acute (lasting fewer than 48 hours) or chronic (lasting more than 30 days). In the vast majority of cases, headache is persistent but it can be intermittent, particularly initially, and can sometimes occur in attacks. It is typically present on waking and is aggravated by a short-term rise in venous pressure, as in stooping or coughing. Headache in CVT thus has no typical clinical characteristic or specific temporal profile. The only suggestive features are its progressive worsening and the presence, in more than 95% of cases, of associated symptoms and signs.

Headache can be associated with any of the symptoms and signs listed in Table 30–1, either in isolation or in combination. Taking into account all the varieties of associated symptoms and signs and the different modes of onset, five groups can be distinguished.

Headache with Isolated Intracranial Hypertension

This is the most homogeneous pattern of presentation, particularly when thrombosis is limited to the dural sinuses. It is mainly characterized by progressive headache and bilateral papilledema, which are almost invariably present, usually in combination. Less frequently, horizontal diplopia from sixth-nerve palsy, tinnitus, and transient visual obscurations are also present. Such a presentation is that of benign intracranial hypertension (pseudotumor cerebri)

TABLE 30–2. Main Causes or Predisposing Conditions Associated with CVT

Infective causes
  Local
  - Direct septic trauma
  - Intracranial infection: abscess, subdural empyema, meningitis
  - Regional infection: otitis, sinusitis, orbital cellulitis, tonsillitis, of the teeth, stomatitis, cutaneous cellulitis
  General
  - Bacterial: septicemia, endocarditis, typhoid, tuberculosis
  - Viral: measles, hepatitis, herpes, CMV, HIV, encephalitis
  - Parasitic: malaria, trichinosis, toxoplasmosis
  - Fungal: aspergillosis, cryptococcosis
Noninfective causes
  Local
  - Head injury (open or closed, with or without fracture)
  - Post neurosurgery
  - Tumors (cholesteatoma, meningioma, metastasis, jugular chemodectoma)
  - Occlusion of the internal jugular vein (e.g.,infusion, compression)
  General
  - Any surgery with or without deep vein thrombosis
  - Gyneco-obstetric
      Pregnancy and puerperium
      Oral contraceptives
  - Cardiac insufficiency
  - Nephrotic syndrome
  - Severe dehydration of any cause
  - Malignancies: any visceral carcinoma, lymphoma, leukemia
  - RBC disorders: polycythemia, sickle cell disease, posthemorrhagic anemia, paroxysmal nocturnal hemoglobinuria
  - Thrombocythemia (primary or secondary)
  - Coagulation disorders: ATIII, protein C, and protein S deficiencies, activated protein C resistance, disseminated intravascular coagulation (DIC), antiphospholipid antibodies, hyperhomocystinemia, heparin-induced thrombocytopenia
  - Hyperviscosity (monoclonal gammopathy)
  - Digestive: cirrhosis, Crohn's disease, ulcerative colitis
  - Vasculitis: systemic lupus erythematosus, Behçet's disease, Wegener's granulomatosis, giant cell arteritis, sarcoidosis
"Idiopathic"

CMV = cytomegalovirus; HIV = human immunodeficiency virus; RBC = red blood cell count.

and in some series, accounts for up to 40% of cases with CVT. This stresses the need to perform MRI and/or angiography systematically in all patients with so-called "benign intracranial hypertension" to rule out CVT. Indeed, patients with CVT and isolated intracranial hypertension can later develop focal neurologic signs, seizures, and coma due to the extension of thrombosis to the cortical veins.

Headache with Focal Signs

This is the most frequent presentation accounting for about 75% of published cases, particularly when thrombosis involves the dural sinuses and dural veins. It is a heterogeneous group depending on the mode of onset of focal signs, their nature (deficits, seizures, or both), and their possible association with altered consciousness and signs of raised intracranial pressure. Acute cases simulate an arterial stroke, chronic ones simulate tumors, and subacute cases mimic encephalitis or abscess.

Cavernous Sinus Thrombosis

Cavernous sinus thrombosis has a distinctive clinical picture that includes, in classic acute cases, chemosis, proptosis, and painful ophthalmoplegia that is initially unilateral but frequently becomes bilateral.

Subacute Encephalopathy

Less commonly, CVT can present as a generalized encephalopathic illness without localizing signs or recognizable features of raised intracranial pressure. This occurs more often in very old or very young patients suffering from cachexia and malignant or cardiac disease.

Unusual Presentations

Cerebral venous thrombosis can mimic a ruptured intracranial aneurysm with a severe headache of sudden onset, neck stiffness, and a CT scan or lumbar puncture with evidence of subarachnoid hemorrhage. Finally, isolated headache (without papilledema) may be the only manifestion of CVT that might be suspected only when there is a suggestive underlying condition.

In a patient with headache of recent onset, the presence of any of the symptoms/signs mentioned in Table 30–1 should prompt appropriate investigations. A CT scan, with and without contrast, should be performed first. Its main purpose is to rule out other conditions but it can detect CVT in some 20% of cases, showing the delta sign that is diagnostic of thrombosis of the posterior part of the superior sagittal sinus. The empty delta sign appears after contrast injection and reflects the opacification of collateral veins in the sinus wall, contrasting with the noninjection of the clot inside the sinus (Figure 30–3). Nevertheless, because a CT scan may be normal or show nonspecific changes, MRI with or without angiographic confirmation should be obtained in all cases. At present MRI is the method of choice for the diagnosis and follow-up of CVT because of its noninvasiveness and its ability to visualize the thrombus itself (Figure 30–4). Angiography has been the key procedure in the diagnosis of CVT for many years but it is now performed only when MRI is contraindicated or in doubtful cases (see Figure 30–4). Indeed, interpretation of MRI can be difficult for the diagnosis of thrombosis of the cortical veins and at a very early or very late stage, when the occluded vessel appears isointense or hypointense.

Cerebrospinal fluid examination can still be useful because it is often abnormal in composition (increased protein, presence of red blood cells, and pleocytosis) or in pressure. Although CSF investigation has become obsolete in most cases of nonseptic CVT presenting with focal signs, it remains necessary in patients presenting with intracranial hypertension and a normal CT scan to rule out meningitis, to confirm the increase in CSF pressure, and to remove CSF when vision is threatened.

Once the diagnosis of CVT is established, an extensive work-up is needed to try to find one of the numerous causative and predisposing conditions (Table 30–2). They include all surgical, gynecoobstetric, and medical causes of deep vein thrombosis as well as a number of local or regional causes, infective or noninfective, such as head trauma and brain tumors. The most frequent medical causes include infections, malignancies, inflammatory diseases such as Behçet's disease, connective tissue diseases, and hereditary thrombotic disorders. In young women, CVT is still frequent during puerperium and pregnancy in the developing countries whereas in the developed countries the role of oral contraceptives is more important as a cause of CVT. Hereditary resistance to activated protein C should be systematically looked for, since it is now considered to be one of the first causes of venous thrombosis, particularly in combination with other factors such as oral contraceptives. In neonates and children, regional infections (otitis, mastoiditis) are very frequent causes of CVT; other causes include severe dehydration, head trauma, and congenital heart disease. Despite the continuous description of new causes, the proportion of cases of unknown etiology remains around 20%.

The prognosis for CVT is much better than classically thought, with a rapid disappearance of headache and a complete recovery in the majority of cases (77% in our series). Nevertheless, death still occurs in 5 to 30% of cases due to an extensive thrombosis, a malignant etiology, or pulmonary embolism. The natural history of CVT is highly variable, and spontaneous recovery is common; however, a massive hemorrhagic infarction with focal deficit and coma can occur at any time, and its prognosis remains unpredictable for any given patient. The two main prognostic factors are the topography of the thrombosis (deep cerebral vein thrombosis and cerebellar vein thrombosis carrying a much higher risk than cortical vein thrombosis) and the underlying cause (septic CVT still has a high mortality rate). Other factors classically considered to indicate a poor prognosis are the rate of evolution of thrombosis, the presence of coma, the age of the patient (with a high mortality in infancy and in the aged), the presence of focal symptoms, and the presence of a hemorrhagic infarct. Therefore, it is important to recognize CVT before the occurrence of complications, in order to start appropriate treatment immediately.

Treatment is based on an individualized combination of symptomatic medications (anticonvulsants, methods to reduce intracranial pressure) antithrombotic treatments, and etiologic treatment such as antibiotics in infectious thrombosis.

In patients with isolated intracranial hypertension, threatened vision and a normal CT scan, a lumbar puncture should be performed (before starting heparin) to measure the CSF pressure and to rapidly lower it. The efficacy of this treatment on headache and tinnitus is immediate in most cases. If intracranial hypertension is not controlled, other treatments should be used such as steroids, acetazolamide, mannitol, glycerol, or even lumboperitoneal shunting.

The best antithrombotic treatment in CVT is heparin. Its use has long remained controversial because of the risk of further bleeding into an already hemorrhagic infarct. However, the risk of increasing intracranial hemorrhage has been vastly overestimated. There are several reports of patients with hemorrhagic infarcts who did improve on anticoagulants, and in a recent randomized study, heparin was found beneficial even in such patients. Patients with CVT should thus be anticoagulated as soon as possible, provided that there is no general contraindication to the use of heparin. The duration of anticoagulation is not standardized. By analogy with deep vein thrombosis, we have been using heparin for the first few days and oral anticoagulants for the next 2 to 3 months, except when there is a known thrombotic tendency, for which prolonged treatment is usually necessary. Thrombolytics have recently been used in patients with extensive CVT, persistent coma, and no improvement despite symptomatic and heparin treatment. However, their benefit/risk ratio in CVT is unknown.

In summary, headache is the most frequent sign of CVT. It has no specific feature but it is almost invariably associated with other neurologic symptoms and signs (focal deficits, seizures, or disorder of consciousness) and/or papilledema. The best diagnostic tool for CVT is MRI. The etiologies are numerous. Therapy is based on symptomatic measures, heparin, and etiologic treatment. The outcome is excellent in most cases provided that the appropriate treatment is started as early as possible in the course of the disease.

Selected Readings

Ameri A, Bousser MG. Cerebral venous thrombosis. Neurol Clin 1992;10:87–111.

Ameri A, Bousser MG. Cerebral venous thrombosis. In: Oleson J, Tfelt-Hansen P, Welch KMA, editors. The headaches. New York: Raven Press; 1993. p. 671–3.

Bousser MG, Ross Russell R. Cerebral venous thrombosis. London: WB Saunders; 1997.

Cantu C, Barinagarrementeria F. Cerebral venous thrombosis associated with pregnancy and puerperium: a review of 67 cases. Stroke 1993;24:1880–4.

Daif A, Awada A, Al-Rajeh S, et al. Cerebral venous thrombosis in adults. A study of 40 cases from Saudi Arabia. Stroke 1995;26:1193–5.

Einhaupl KM, Villringer A, Meister W, et al. Heparin treatment in sinus venous thrombosis. Lancet 1991;338:597–600.

Preter M, Tzourio C, Ameri A, Bousser MG. Long-term prognosis in cerebral venous thrombosis. Follow-up of 77 patients. Stroke 1996;27:243–6.

Tehindrazanarivelo A, Evrard S, Schaison M, et al. Prospective study of cerebral sinus venous thrombosis in patients presenting with benign intracranial hypertension. Cerebrovasc Dis 1992;2:22–7.

Editorial Comments

Headache during pregnancy and the puerperium can be problematic for the patient and her doctor. In an excellent, detailed overview of headaches in the puerperium, the authors have choosen to illustrate one diagnostic entity, cerebral venous thrombosis (CVT), through their case. It is a potentially fatal disorder with many symptoms and signs reflecting the neurologic diversity of this condition. Nevertheless, postpartum headache with papilledema is CVT until proved otherwise. Prompt investigation with MRI and intervention should ensure a favorable outcome. Read this case carefully as it is most instructive.

THE WOMAN WITH ACUTE SEVERE HEADACHE

JOHN F. ROTHROCK, MD

Case History

A 25-year-old woman presented with a 3-day history of uncharacteristic, severe, and unremitting headache. The headache initially was present upon awakening, was moderate in intensity at that time, and subsequently worsened. The pain was largely nonpulsatile but became "throbbing" and more severe when she attempted to walk. The pain was nonlateralized and centered at the vertex. There was no significant positional component. She described associated photophobia and some sonophobia but no nausea, vomiting, or aura. She described eye pain with eye movement in all directions of gaze. She denied fever, neck stiffness, recent trauma, or symptoms consistent with recent systemic illness.

Her past medical history was unremarkable, and she specifically denied any prior history of headaches sufficiently severe to inhibit or prohibit daily activity. She took no medication chronically, and she specifically denied recent use of an antibiotic.

Her physical examination was normal except for an oral temperature of 37.8°C. There was no evidence of neck pain or stiffness with anterior flexion.

She was treated with sumatriptan 6 mg subcutaneously, and within 30 minutes her headache declined in intensity from severe to mild. Lumbar puncture was performed, and the opening pressure was normal; cerebrospinal fluid (CSF) analysis yielded 257 white blood cells per cubic mm (98% lymphocytes), no red blood cells, protein concentration 58 mg/dL and glucose 62 mg/dL; Gram's stain was negative for organisms.

Questions about This Case

- Given the patient's history, what diagnoses should have been considered prior to lumbar puncture?
- What do the cerebrospinal findings suggest, and what do they rule out?
- How should this patient be managed?

Case Discussion

This previously healthy and headache-free woman presented with a severe headache. The most common stimulus for this clinical presentation is new onset migraine, but that diagnosis must be considered suspect for three reasons. First, the International Headache Society (IHS) diagnostic criteria for migraine headache stipulate that an individual must have experienced at least five attacks of characteristic headache in order for that diagnosis to be made with a reasonable degree of certainty. Second, and regardless of whether or not the patient has an established history of migraine, the "worst headache of my life" invariably requires careful diagnostic intervention and exclusion of conditions which may mimic migraine. Lastly, the patient is febrile, and when fever accompanies headache as the primary presenting complaint, infection involving the central nervous system must be excluded.

The most important condition to consider here is subarachnoid hemorrhage from a ruptured berry aneurysm. Clinically devastating aneurysmal rupture often is heralded by a low-volume "sentinel" leak, and it is imperative that the correct diagnosis be made at this earlier point. The incidence of mortality or major neurologic morbidity from high volume aneurysmal hemorrhage is distressingly high, and little satisfaction can be taken from establishing the diagnosis after this cataclysmic event has occurred. On the other hand, if the sentinel bleed is diagnosed without delay, and if the aneurysm is then secured surgically, disaster can be averted.

Many other conditions may mimic new onset migraine, and a number of these are potentially dangerous. Patients with infectious meningitis may present with acute, severe headache, and fever and neck stiffness are not always present. Although tuberculous meningitis typically is more subacute in onset, patients with bacterial or viral meningitis become ill quickly, and it is virtually impossible to distinguish between the two without CSF analysis. Patients with viral encephalitis often complain of headache; if there is alteration of consciousness, focal neurologic deficit, seizure activity, or some combination thereof, this diagnosis should be considered. [*Editors' note: Lyme disease from* Borrelia burgdorferi *should be considered in some parts of the world. A history of tick bite, bull's-eye rash, or residence in an area with a large deer or mouse population is usually present.*]

There are noninfectious conditions which may mimic new onset migraine. Patients with primary intracerebral hemorrhage from hypertensive arteriopathy, recreational drug abuse, or other causes frequently complain of headache which may possess migrainous features, but parenchymal hemorrhage is with few exceptions accompanied by focal neurologic signs. Patients with extra-axial (subdural or epidural) hematoma from recent head injury may present with headache as the chief complaint, and focal neurologic signs may be subtle or absent. Patients with low intracranial pressure from a dural tear and associated CSF leak may present with acute headache, but during the first few days to weeks that headache typically has a strong positional component (much worse while the individual is upright and relieved by lying flat); a history of an inciting traumatic event is not always elicited.

This patient's positive response to treatment with sumatriptan did not assist in establishing a diagnosis. Sumatriptan is nonspecific therapy and has been reported to be effective in patients with postictal headache or headaches from aneurysmal subarachnoid hemorrhage. The same can be said for any medication used to treat acute migraine headache. A variety of stimuli will activate the peripheral trigeminovascular system and central pathways which generate and modulate head pain, and any agent which exerts its pharmacologic effect within those areas may work to oppose pain, regardless of the stimulus involved.

Taken along with her clinical presentation, the results of this patient's CSF analysis indicate that the correct diagnosis is viral meningitis. The normal glucose level, lymphocytic pleocytosis, and elevated protein concentration are characteristic of aseptic meningitis of viral origin. There was no evidence of recent subarachnoid hemorrhage; no fresh red cells were present, and the protein concentration was not elevated to the level one would expect from recent crenation of a high volume of red cells. Results of the Gram's stain and the lack of history of recent antibiotic use exclude untreated or partially treated bacterial meningitis. The CSF profile is consistent with viral encephalitis, but the patient did not express symptoms or exhibit signs referable to the brain itself.

Management Strategies

Management of this patient should hinge primarily on the question: is hospitalization for general support required? If the patient is able to maintain oral hydration, her head pain can be managed with oral or subcutaneous medication, and there can be someone at home who will observe her and confirm that her course is consistent with resolving viral meningitis, then hospitalization makes little sense. On the other hand, dehydration will aggravate and prolong the symptoms of meningitis, and intravenous fluids may be required to avoid this.

To the author's embarrassment, this patient was admitted by his department's service despite near total resolution of her headache following administration of sumatriptan, her ability to maintain oral hydration, and the availability of concerned and informed family members at home. She was placed in an isolation room, and antibacterial and antiviral medications were administered intravenously. A brain imaging study was performed and was normal. Electroencephalography was requested.

None of this makes very good sense. Medical resources were needlessly used, and worse, the patient suffered unnecessary discomfort and some risk exposure. Such aggressive diagnostic and therapeutic intervention should be reserved for patients with presumed viral meningitis whose presentations are more atypical (examples include antibiotic treatment prior to lumbar puncture, atypical CSF profile, or depression of consciousness). Straight-forward viral meningitis should be managed in a straight-forward fashion.

Case Summary

- Patients presenting with uncharacteristically severe acute head pain require meticulous diagnostic evaluation.
- In such circumstances, aneurysmal subarachnoid hemorrhage must be excluded.
- Viral meningitis is a common, temporarily disabling but typically benign condition which most often can be managed with simple supportive therapy only.

Overview of Aseptic Meningitis

"Aseptic meningitis" implies inflammation of the meninges in the absence of bacterial or fungal infection and without symptoms or signs referable to the brain, brain stem, or spinal cord. Afflicted patients present with fever, headache, signs of meningeal irritation, and characteristic CSF findings. Many have come to regard aseptic meningitis and viral meningitis as being synonymous, and although it is true that viral infection is the leading cause of this syndrome, the CSF profile associated with aseptic meningitis may be produced by conditions as widely varied as treponemal infection, Behçet's disease, and exposure to certain medications or contrast agents (e.g., nonsteroidal anti-inflammatory drugs, gamma globulin, iohexol). Aside from viruses, infections which may produce aseptic meningitis include leptospirosis, Lyme disease, syphilis, mycoplasma, and chlamydia. Parainfectious causes include partially treated bacterial meningitis, parameningeal infection, and endocarditis. Among the noninfectious causes not already mentioned are sarcoidosis, collagen vascular diseases, and migraine. If the term is employed in its broadest sense, encompassing both acute and more chronic processes, the list of causative conditions expands significantly, and there can be said to be no single characteristic clinical presentation. For example, a patient with acute aseptic meningitis of viral origin or from exposure to contrast material used in myelography may present rapidly and with prominent symptoms, in contrast to a patient with human immunodeficiency virus (HIV)-related syphilitic meningitis who may express no symptoms whatsoever.

The CSF profile in aseptic meningitis generally demonstrates a white cell pleocytosis which numbers in the tens to hundreds, and the cells are chiefly lymphocytes. The glucose concentration is normal, and the protein concentration is moderately elevated. The degree of abnormality present in the CSF tends to parallel the severity of the patient's symptoms. In a minority of cases, and especially when the meningeal inflammatory response is intense and lumbar puncture is performed early in the course, the white cell count may be higher, a greater proportion of neutrophils may be present, and the glucose concentration may be decreased. In that event, bacterial or tuberculous meningitis becomes of greater concern, and it may be safer to initiate appropriate antibiotic therapy and to continue such treatment until cultures initially obtained return as negative and repeat lumbar puncture demonstrates findings consistent with evolving aseptic meningitis.

As indicated previously, most acute aseptic meningitis is viral in origin, and patients presenting with viral meningitis may appear quite ill, exhibiting fever, headache, lethargy, irritability, and varying degrees of neck stiffness; the last is variable and may be absent. Photophobia may be prominent, and patients often complain of pain with eye movement. On rare occasions the examiner will find evidence of early papilledema, but alteration of consciousness, focal neurologic signs, or seizure activity are typically inconsistent with the diagnosis of aseptic meningitis and demand that encephalitis or other conditions which involve the brain itself be considered.

Viral meningitis is evanescent; the patient rapidly becomes sick and miserable and almost as rapidly improves to his or her normal state of health. Long-term sequelae are very rare. The viral agents incriminated most commonly in cases of aseptic meningitis are enteroviruses (echovirus and coxsackievirus), but the mumps virus, herpesviruses (notably, type 2), lymphocytic choriomeningitis virus, and Epstein-Barr virus may be culpable as well. Benign recurrent aseptic meningitis (Mollaret's meningitis) may result from reactivation of a herpesvirus. Human immunodeficiency virus may cause aseptic meningitis early in its course, and the meningitis may coincide with or predate seroconversion.

The peculiar intersection of migraine and aseptic meningitis deserves a brief mention. Both are common clinical conditions, and it is inevitable that a certain percentage of individuals with established migraine will contract viral meningitis. Beyond the coincidental relationship, however, there is some evidence to suggest that migraine itself may induce a meningeal response similar to that observed with aseptic meningitis and that in this situation efforts to establish an infectious or other noninfectious source for the meningitis will be fruitless. Compounding the potential for diagnostic confusion, patients with migraine-associated aseptic meningitis may exhibit progressive obtundation or express sensorimotor symptoms. Suffice it to say that the incidence and biogenesis of "migraine meningitis" remain obscure and that the diagnosis of this condition should be considered tenuous at best.

Selected Readings

Beghi E, Nicolosi A, Kurland LT, et al. Encephalitis and aseptic meningitis, Olmstead County, Minnesota, 1950–1981: epidemiology. Ann Neurol 1984;16:283–94.

Ratzan KR. Viral meningitis. Med Clin North Am 1985;69:399–413.

Editorial Comments

Aseptic meningitis is usually a self-limiting disorder without sequelae. However, the diagnosis is not always easy or straightforward, and the differential diagnoses include several serious and life-threatening disorders. Dr. Rothrock leads us through an erudite overview and discussion of this entity. He points out the pitfalls in diagnosis and provides sensible management strategies. He even mentions the entity of "migraine meningitis," an obscure disorder, somewhat familiar to neurologists and physicians dealing with acute headache.

CHAPTER 32

THE MAN WITH HEADACHE AND FEVER

RUTH ANN MARRIE, MD

THOMAS J. MARRIE, MD, FRCPC, FACP

Case History

This 72-year-old man had an abrupt onset of rigors followed by fever late one evening. When seen by his family physician the next day he also complained of myalgia. Apart from the fever, his physical examination was unremarkable. Acetaminophen was prescribed for the fever and the myalgia.

Three days later at about 8 AM, he complained of severe headache and stiffness of the neck. Over the next 2 to 3 hours he became progressively confused and was brought to the emergency room (ER) by his family.

On examination he was acutely ill; his oral temperature was 39°C, he was arousable but did not respond to most questions. There was nuchal rigidity and crackles were heard on auscultation over the right side of his chest anteriorly and laterally.

Ceftriaxone, 2 g every 12 hours intravenously, and ampicillin, 2 g every 6 hours intravenously, were administered. A lumbar puncture (LP) revealed an opening pressure of greater than 500 mm H_2O. The cerebrospinal fluid (CSF) was cloudy and had a protein concentration of 2827 mg per deciliter, and a glucose concentration of 0 mg per deciliter; the white blood cell count was 425 cells per cubic millimeter, of which 81% were polymorphonuclear leukocytes. A Gram's stain of a centrifuged specimen of CSF showed many polymorphonuclear leukocytes and gram-positive diplococci. At this point, ampicillin was discontinued and vancomycin, 1 g every 12 hours intravenously, was added to the ceftriaxone.

A computed tomography (CT) scan of his head showed atrophy consistent with his age, left mastoidectomy, and opacification of the mastoid air cells on the right.

The next day both blood and cerebrospinal fluid cultures were positive for *Streptococcus pneumoniae*. The pneumococcus was susceptible to penicillin with a minimal inhibitory concentration (MIC) of 0.016 µg per milliliter.

Over the first 48 hours in hospital he became afebrile. When the results of the susceptibility tests were known, antibiotic therapy was changed to penicillin, 4 million units every 4 hours intravenously.

By day 5 he was responding to comments and indicated that he still had a headache. He slowly improved and by day 11 he was headache free; antibiotics were discontinued on day 14 and he was transferred to a rehabilitation facility on day 21.

Questions about This Case

- Why are the characteristics of the headache so poorly described in this case?
- What is the differential diagnosis?
- What other approach to care might be taken?
- Should a neurologist evaluate this patient?

Case Discussion

The characteristics of the headache are poorly described in this patient for several reasons.

It was evident that the patient was seriously ill with a life-threatening disease. His physicians quickly decided that the headache was not the problem and they focused (as they should) on immediate therapeutic and diagnostic procedures since it was evident that the most likely diagnosis was bacterial meningitis. Time is of the essence in the management of bacterial meningitis. The median time from arrival in the emergency room until the administration of antibiotics was 2 hours (interquartile range 1.25 to 3.33 hours) for 93 children with bacterial meningitis who were studied from 1987 to 1989. Indeed only one child received antibiotics within 30 minutes of presentation.

The second reason for the poor description of the characteristics of the headache was the mental status of our patient. He was confused and not able to provide detailed answers to any questions. A review of 493 episodes of acute bacterial meningitis in adults found that 51% were confused or lethargic on presentation, 22% were responsive only to pain, and 6% were unresponsive to all stimuli. Only 22% were alert.

The third reason is the age of our patient. In one study, only 46% of 48 patients over 60 years of age with bacterial meningitis complained of headache; other studies quote figures as low as 21%. Comparisons of the features of meningitis in the elderly with those in younger patients have shown that older patients are more likely (statistically significantly so) to have a higher incidence of severe mental status abnormalities and to have concurrent pneumonia than younger adults.

The final reason for the poor description of this patient's headache was that the physicians involved in his management included an emergency room physician, an intensivist, and an infectious diseases physician. A neurologist surely would have described this headache much better!

Characteristics of the Headache Caused by Bacterial Meningitis

Maybe a neurologist would not have done much better with our patient. A review of the literature on bacterial meningitis in adults reveals that headache due to bacterial meningitis is poorly described. In most instances, only the percentage of patients with headache is given. Some authors state that a distinctive feature of headache seen in bacterial and viral meningitis is the retro-orbital component which is markedly exacerbated by the slightest motion of the eyes. In the experience of one of us, this occurs in aseptic meningitis and is uncommon in bacterial meningitis. Furthermore this phenomenon is also seen in optic neuritis and with idiopathic vascular headaches.

Our patient's presentation is instructive in dissecting the features of headache due to meningitis—especially if it is combined with an overview of the presentation of other patients with meningitis. This 72-year-old man developed pneumococcal pneumonia and then his meninges and right mastoid air cells were infected as a result of pneumococcal bacteremia. The initial fever and myalgia represent his response to the pneumonia. Interestingly, in our study of 2287 adults with community-acquired pneumonia, we found that 64.1% of the 944 outpatients and 44.1% of the 1343 inpatients had headache as one of their symptoms. Thus, many patients with meningitis will initially have a headache as part of the nonspecific manifestations of the infection that led to the meningitis, be it pneumonia, sinusitis, mastoiditis, or endocarditis. At this stage myalgia accompanied by a dull throbbing generalized headache of moderate intensity is common. For those patients in whom the sinus, ear, or mastoid is the focus of infection leading to meningitis, headache due to inflammation of these structures is also present. Only 25% of 225 adults with community-acquired meningitis had no predisposing factors that could lead to this infection. The most common predisposing factors were acute otitis media 19%, pneumonia 15%, sinusitis 12%, endocarditis 7%, chronic otitis media 7%, recent head injury 5%, previous head injury 4%, diabetes mellitus 10%, alcoholism 18%, altered immune state 19%, cerebrospinal fluid leak 8%, and an implanted neurosurgical device 1%.

Perhaps the best setting in which to gain an understanding of the features of headache in bacterial meningitis is in the setting of *Neisseria meningitidis* infection in a young adult. Even here there are two distinct presentations, that of fulminant meningococcemia and the other which is dominated by meningitis. In the former, a previously healthy young adult (often 16 to 25 years of age) has a sudden onset of chills, fever, myalgia, and headache. The headache is usually dull and not the dominant feature. Within 4 to 12 hours this "flu-like" illness has evolved so that the individual is now hypotensive, has multiple petechial hemorrhages, and may be stuporous. In these patients the picture is that of fulminant sepsis and clinical meningitis may not be present. However, if therapy is successful in prolonging or saving life, it is evident that the meninges have been infected. In patients with meningococcal disease in whom the meningitis predominates, headache is a dominant feature. In our study of 51 patients with group C meningococcal meningitis, whose mean age was 13.6 ± 12.9 years, 51% had headache. However, 49% had purpura and fell into the fulminant meningococcemia category—thus most of those with the meningitis presentation had headache (10% had photophobia). This headache starts as part of the infection prodrome as a dull headache but over 2 to 24 hours it becomes intense and changes its character to that of a throbbing generalized headache made worse by head movements, coughing, and straining.

Management of Headache Associated with Bacterial Meningitis

This is the simplest form of headache to deal with; treat the meningitis. The major (and frequent mistake) is delay in administering antibiotics. During an outbreak of meningitis in the U.K., children who were suspected to have meningitis when seen in the physician's office and who were given intramuscular penicillin and sent to hospital had a much better outcome than those who were sent to hospital without antibiotic therapy.

For the optimal treatment of (headache associated with) meningitis do the following:

1. Blood cultures
2. Intravenous antibiotics should be administered within 30 minutes of arrival in the ER (choice of antibiotics depends on the age of the patient and the local epidemiology, e.g., the presence of penicillin-resistant *Streptococcus pneumoniae*). In most instances of meningitis in adults, ampicillin and ceftriaxone represent reasonable empiric therapy. Remember cephalosporins are not effective against *Listeria monocytogenes* which is the third or fourth most common cause of meningitis in this age group. In a review of 253 adults with community-acquired meningitis, *Streptococcus pneumoniae* accounted for 38%, *Neisseria meningitidis* 14%, *Listeria monocytogenes* 11%, streptococci 7%, *Staphylococcus aureus* 5%, *Haemophilus influenzae* 4%, mixed bacterial species 2%, and 13% were culture negative. Once a pathogen is isolated, therapy can be changed to more specific antibiotics based upon susceptibility studies. This is not a chapter on the treatment of meningitis but remember to give antibiotics intravenously for at least 10 days—never switch to oral therapy—most antibiotics are not sufficiently absorbed through the gastrointestinal tract to achieve high enough blood levels to attain 10 times the MIC of the infecting organisms (the concentration of antibiotic that is necessary for cure) in the CSF. Furthermore, as inflammation settles with therapy, the permeability of the blood-brain barrier decreases so that high blood levels are even more important.
3. Lumbar puncture—if you suspect bacterial meningitis, do not wait for an LP before giving antibiotics. The CSF will not be sterile by the time you do the LP (unless you are very slow).
4. A CT scan of the head does not have to be done immediately but it should be done since it provides evidence of focal disease. Never delay antibiotic therapy while awaiting a CT scan. The LP can be delayed if you feel there is likely to be a contraindication to it based on the CT results.
5. Search for a source for the meningitis. This includes a chest radiograph and a careful physical examination to rule out endocarditis; the CT scan will reveal a mastoid or sinus infection.
6. Supportive care—many patients will require initial management in an intensive care unit. Attention to their fluid and electrolyte balance is critical.
7. Patients who are alert may require analgesia for relief of headache.
8. Monitor carefully for both central nervous system (CNS) and systemic complications. The former include cerebral edema, hydrocephalus, brain abscess, subdural empyema or effusion, and

cerebrovascular involvement (arterial and venous thrombosis). Systemic complications include septic shock, disseminated intravascular coagulation, adult respiratory distress syndrome, septic or reactive arthritis, and therapy-associated complications.

In most patients, treatment of the meningitis results in total resolution of the headache within 7 to 10 days. Some patients suffer from lumbar puncture headache. This is more common in patients with aseptic meningitis in our experience but this most likely represents an ascertainment bias since the former group of patients are not nearly as ill as those with bacterial meningitis and hence are more likely to complain about ongoing headache.

Some patients have daily headaches following bacterial meningitis, which are usually associated with a normal neurologic examination. Patients who are headache free or who have only occasional headaches prior to the onset of meningitis are unlikely to have this pattern altered by the meningitis. In all likelihood the meningitis has served as a trigger to turn recurrent headaches into daily headaches. Since up to 17% of males and 20% of females have recurrent headaches, it is surprising that more patients do not have daily headaches following meningitis.

Pathophysiology of Headache Due to Bacterial Meningitis

The pathogenesis of meningitis is as follows—bacteria colonize and penetrate the nasopharyngeal membrane and enter the bloodstream. Invasion of the central nervous system then occurs. Bacteria multiply in the subarachnoid space leading to increased permeability of the blood-brain barrier. The bacteria and bacterial products induce transendothelial migration of granulocytes and monocytes with the release of cytokines and prostaglandins. The end result is cerebral edema, increased intracranial pressure, and impaired circulation.

It is evident from this overview of the pathogenesis of meningitis that headache in meningitis is due to vascular dilatation mechanisms early in the illness, and that later in the course of the infection, it is as a result of increased intracranial pressure. [*Editors' note: Meningeal neurogenic inflammation probably adds to the head pain. Once the infection is effectively treated, some headache experts treat the pain with IV or IM DHE. The triptans may also be effective.*]

Selected Readings

Bonadis WA. The cerebrospinal fluid: physiologic aspects and alterations associated with bacterial meningitis. Pediatr Infect Dis J 1992;11:423–32.

Durand ML, Calderwood SB, Weber DJ, et al. Acute bacterial meningitis in adults. A review of 493 episodes. N Engl J Med 1993;328:21–8.

Meadow WL, Lantos J, Tanz RR, et al. Ought 'standard' care be the 'standard of care'? A study of the time to administration of antibiotics in children with meningitis. Am J Dis Child 1993;147:40–4.

Pfister H-W, Feiden W, Einhaupl K-M. Spectrum of complications during bacterial meningitis in adults. Results of a prospective clinical study. Arch Neurol 1993;50:575–81.

Rasmussen HH, Sorensen HT, Moller-Petersen J, et al. Bacterial meningitis in elderly patients: clinical picture and course. Age Ageing 1992;21:216–20.

van Furth AM, Roord JJ, van Furth R. Roles of proinflammatory and antiinflammatory cytokines in pathophysiology of bacterial meningitis and effect of adjunctive therapy. Infect Immun 1996;64:4883–90.

Editorial Comments

Bacterial meningitis is truly a life-threatening disorder, requiring early diagnosis, appropriate investigation, and effective management with parenteral antibiotics. Headache along with nuchal rigidity and fever are the major symptoms, but as the authors of this chapter point out, the patients' descriptions of their headache symptoms may be poor for many reasons, especially because they are so sick. A high index of suspicion is needed in cases with bacterial meningitis which is treatable and curable. They say, somewhat tongue-in-cheek, that neurologists may have described the headache better. This is possible, but unlikely since most patients with bacterial meningitis are more often managed by non-neurologists!

CHAPTER 33

The Woman with Generalized Headache and Transient Visual Obscurations

STEPHEN D. SILBERSTEIN, MD, FACP

Case History

A 42-year-old obese woman developed, over the last year, a constant holocranial headache associated with intermittent nausea, pulsatile tinnitus, and transient visual obscurations (TVOs). She had been consuming acetylsalicylic acid on a daily basis for her headaches. Her menses were often irregular. She had a prior history of migraine without aura which was usually triggered by menstruation and relieved with each of her pregnancies. A neurologic examination was normal except for the presence of bilateral papilledema.

Questions about This Case

- What is your diagnosis and differential diagnosis?
- What diagnostic procedures would you perform and why?
- How would you manage the patient's headaches?
- What is the major morbidity associated with this disorder?

Case Discussion

This 42-year-old woman with a prior history of migraine developed a chronic daily headache associated with papilledema due to intracranial hypertension. A mass lesion must be ruled out by neuroimaging, preferably magnetic resonance imaging (MRI). The MRI was done and was normal except for an empty sella, which is often associated with increased intracranial pressure. A magnetic resonance venogram showed no evidence of venous obstruction. A lumbar puncture (LP) was next performed. This is obligatory as chronic meningitis can mimic the syndrome of idiopathic intracranial hypertension (IIH). The opening pressure was 300 mm of cerebrospinal fluid (CSF). The cell count, protein, and glucose were normal. Fungal cultures and cryptoccocal antigens were negative. The patient had no acquired immunodeficiency syndrome (AIDS) risk factors and no evidence of hypoparathyroidism or systemic lupus erythematosus (SLE), and she did not take any of the drugs associated with increased intracranial pressure.

Intracranial hypertension may be either (1) idiopathic, with no clear identifiable cause, or (2) symptomatic, as a result of systemic lupus, renal disease, hypoparathyroidism, venous sinus occlusion, radical neck dissection, vitamin A intoxication, or drug side effects (nalidixic acid, danocrine, steroid withdrawal) (Table 33–1). Symptomatic intracranial hypertension can be secondary to changes in cranial venous outflow, which may influence intracranial pressure by increasing cerebral blood volume, producing brain edema, and impairing CSF absorption. Intracranial venous outflow obstruction can be caused by tumors, head trauma, chronic otitis, and hypercoagulable states.

TABLE 33–1. Syndromes of Increased Intracranial Pressure

Primary
  A. Idiopathic intracranial hypertension with papilledema
  B. Idiopathic intracranial hypertension without papilledema
Secondary
  A. Hydrocephalus
  B. Mass lesion, neoplasm, stroke—hematoma
  C. Meningitis/encephalitis
  D. Trauma
  E. Major intracranial and extracranial venous obstruction
  F. Drugs: vitamin A, nalidixic acid, anabolic steroids, steroid withdrawal
  G. Systemic disease: renal disease, hypoparathyroidism, SLE

Idiopathic intracranial hypertension (pseudotumor cerebri) is a disorder of increased intracranial pressure of unknown cause which occurs predominantly in obese women of childbearing age. Its major morbidity, visual loss, occurs in 80% of patients; blindness occurs in 10%. Headache occurs in most, but not all, patients. Transient visual obscuration, an episode of visual clouding in one or both eyes, usually lasting seconds, is common and occurred in this patient. Transient visual obscuration is seen in all forms of increased intracranial pressure with papilledema but is not a specific symptom. Transient visual obscuration can occur even in patients without increased intracranial pressure who have elevated optic disks (not papilledema) from other causes (drusen, coloboma, disk edema, and optic nerve sheath tumors). Other common symptoms of IIH include diplopia, visual loss, and pulsatile tinnitus. Some patients have shoulder and arm pain (perhaps secondary to nerve root dilation) and retro-orbital pain. Signs include papilledema and sixth nerve palsy.

Idiopathic intracranial hypertension occurs with a frequency of about 1 case per 100,000 per year, rising to 19.3 cases in obese women between the ages of 20 and 44. The patient with IIH is commonly a young, obese woman with chronic daily headache (CDH), normal laboratory studies, normal neurologic examination (except for papilledema), and empty sella (Table 33–2). Idiopathic intracranial hypertension is not associated with pregnancy, hypertension, diabetes, thyroid disease, iron deficiency anemia, or the use of tetracycline or oral contraceptives.

The pathophysiology of IIH is unknown. Postulated mechanisms include (1) increased rate of CSF formation; (2) increased intracranial venous pressure; (3) decreased rate of CSF absorption; and (4) increased interstitial fluid in the brain (edema). Recent studies suggest that a decreased rate of CSF absorption at the arachnoid villi and interstitial brain edema are the major contributors.

Most patients describe their headache as their most severe ever. Common features include daily headache present upon awakening and pulsating in character, retro-ocular pain with eye movement, and nausea, vomiting, and pulsatile tinnitus.

In one series of patients, the mean age was 31 years and headache was reported by 92% (73% had CDH, 93% said it was the most severe ever, and 83% said it was pulsatile). Nausea occurred in 57%, vomiting in 38%, and orbital pain in 43%. Transient visual obscuration was present in 71%, diplopia in 38%, and visual loss in 31%.

Occasionally patients with IIH are incidentally found to have papilledema while being examined for another purpose. Five to 10% of patients are essentially asymptomatic. Loss of visual field and visual acuity are the only significant complications of IIH with papilledema.

An ophthalmologic examination should include intraocular pressure, visual fields (Goldmann or Humphrey), optic disk photos, visual acuity, and search for a relative afferent pupil.

TABLE 33–2. Features of Idiopathic Intracranial Hypertension

1. Headache: chronic tension-type headache with migrainous features, may be present upon awakening; can be intermittent or absent
2. Associated features: pulsatile tinnitus, transient visual obscurations, diplopia, visual loss, shoulder and arm pain
3. Patients: predominantly obese women aged 20 to 50
4. Physical and neurologic examination: within normal limits except for papilledema, visual loss, obesity, and a sixth nerve palsy (occasionally bilateral)
5. Neuroradiology: CT or MRI show no evidence of intracranial mass, hydrocephalus, or venous sinus thrombosis. (Empty sella may be present.)
6. Lumbar puncture: demonstrates increased CSF pressure with a normal composition. (May show decreased protein.)
7. No other causes of increased CSF pressure present.

TABLE 33–3. Treatment of Idiopathic Intracranial Hypertension

1. Eliminate symptomatic causes
2. Weight loss, if obese
3. Standard headache treatment
4. Carbonic anhydrase inhibitors and loop diuretics
5. Short course of high-dose corticosteroids
6. Serial lumbar punctures
7. Lumboperitoneal or ventriculoperitoneal shunt
8. Optic nerve sheath fenestration

In some patients, intracranial hypertension without papilledema has been described. Patients, particularly obese women, with CDH and symptoms of increased intracranial pressure, i.e., pulsatile tinnitus, history of head trauma or meningitis, an empty sella on neuroimaging studies, or a headache that is not relieved by standard therapy, should have a diagnostic LP. The clinical, historic, radiographic, and demographic characteristics are identical to those of patients with papilledema except for (1) possible association with prior head trauma or meningitis; (2) extended delay in diagnosis, which requires an LP in the absence of papilledema; and (3) no evidence of the visual loss seen in patients with IIH.

The reason there is no papilledema in these cases of intracranial hypertension is not known. Congenital or acquired optic nerve sheath defects, "chronic IIH" with resolution of papilledema, or early IIH are alternative explanations.

In patients with suspected intracranial hypertension (with or without papilledema), the diagnosis is based on an LP following neuroimaging. If the LP is unremarkable and intracranial pressure is elevated to greater than 200 mm of water (in nonobese subjects), then IIH is the likely diagnosis. Routine blood chemistries, prothrombin time (PT), partial thromboplastin time (PTT), antinuclear antibodies (ANA), venereal disease research laboratory (VDRL), chemistry profile, thyroxine (T_4), and thyroid-stimulating hormone (TSH) are helpful.

Management Strategies

Once the diagnosis of IIH is made, secondary causes should be sought and eliminated. Over 50 diseases, conditions, toxins, or pharmaceuticals have been associated with IIH. Obese patients should be encouraged to lose weight. If the patient is asymptomatic and has no visual loss, then no treatment is indicated. Careful ophthalmologic follow-up is needed. If there is no papilledema, or papilledema with no visual loss, and the only complaint is headache, then the headache should be treated aggressively. Headache associated with IIH and papilledema has been reported to frequently respond to standard headache treatment (Table 33–3).

If rigorous headache therapy is unsuccessful, or if there is visual loss, then a 4- to 6-week trial of furosemide or a potent carbonic anhydrase inhibitor (acetazolamide) should be given. These drugs decrease elevated intracranial pressure. The use of high-dose steroids (prednisone or dexamethasone) is controversial but may be effective in IIH. Headache commonly recurs when steroids are withdrawn.

Lumbar puncture typically relieves headache in IIH. Since CSF is rapidly replaced, prolonged symptomatic relief may reflect a persistent CSF leak. Alternatively, transient reduction of CSF pressure may allow decompression of the arachnoid villi, allowing for prolonged enhanced CSF absorption. Patients with IIH who have visual loss or severe incapacitating headache that does not respond to medical therapy or repeated LP may need surgical management.

Some suggest treating IIH with a lumboperitoneal shunt, but this often has to be repeated and has the potential for development of hindbrain herniation and a new headache. For others a ventriculoperitoneal shunt is the preferred shunting procedure.

Optic nerve sheath fenestration (ONSF) entails surgical incision of the dura mater covering the intraorbital optic nerve. The proposed mechanism is improved optic nerve axoplasmic flow and continuous intraorbital CSF drainage. Sixty-five to 76% of patients get relief of medically uncontrolled headache with ONSF. Although ONSF has been performed on patients with unilateral papilledema, to our knowledge it is untried in patients with IIH without papilledema. Without the threat of loss of vision, the small risk of visual loss due to the surgery probably outweighs the potential benefits.

Selected Readings

Corbett JJ, Thompson HS. The rational management of idiopathic intracranial hypertension. Arch Neurol 1989;46: 1049–51.

Fishman RA. Cerebrospinal fluid in diseases of the nervous system. 2nd ed. Philadelphia: W.B. Saunders Company.

Marcelis J, Silberstein SD. Idiopathic intracranial hypertension without papilledema. Arch Neurol 1991;48:392–9.

Silberstein SD, Marcelis J. Headache associated with changes in intracranial pressure. Headache 1992;32:84–94.

Wall M. The headache profile of idiopathic intracranial hypertension. Cephalalgia 1990;10:331–5.

Editorial Comments

The finding of papilledema in a patient with headache usually suggests an ominous etiology; however, when initial imaging procedures are normal, the diagnosis of "idiopathic intracranial hypertension" or what used to be called "pseudotumor cerebri" is entertained. In its idiopathic form, this disorder almost approaches a syndromic status. Dr. Silberstein clearly overviews this disorder in this case, along with differential diagnostic concerns and management strategies. Although Dr. Silberstein states that IIH is not associated with tetracycline use, the editors have treated such cases.

It is wise to exclude "secondary," treatable etiologies in all cases. As outlined by Dr. Silberstein, careful attention to visual symptoms and their progression is a high priority in such cases, as other symptoms frequently abate and resolve themselves over time.

CHAPTER 34

Two Patients with Posterior Head and Cervical Pain

Joseph M. Phillips MD, PhD

Case 1 History

This 27-year-old woman was well until the past 2 years, during which she has suffered from insidiously developing worsening headaches. She rarely had headaches as an adolescent, but her mother had been diagnosed as having "migraine." At first her headaches were infrequent, experienced once or twice a week, and generally located in the back of her head. Her neck was not involved. There was no history of trauma. She attributed her headaches to tension and controlled them with over-the-counter analgesics.

As time passed, the headaches progressed both in intensity and frequency. The headaches remained localized in the occipital region unless they were at their greatest intensity, at which time they seemed to involve all of the head in a fashion she vaguely described as a "head rush." Sometimes the pain was frontotemporal in location. The headaches throbbed and could be present for a whole day at a time. Sometimes the headache made her nauseated. When her head did not hurt, she was constantly aware of "pressure" in the back of her head.

Most of the time, but especially when her headaches were severe, she felt "dizzy." She denied having true vertigo but noted a giddiness that seemed to affect her walking. While she was afraid that she appeared unsteady in her gait, this was never noticed by her acquaintances. She experienced no visual symptoms but noticed it was difficult to read when having a headache, and she attributed this to problems with concentration. As time went by, she found aerobic exercise and jogging could bring on a headache. Coughing, laughing, and yawning could also provoke a headache out of the blue. Her very worst "head rush" followed blowing up balloons for her daughter's birthday.

She sought medical attention because she was afraid she had a brain tumor, but a computed tomography (CT) scan of the head obtained by her primary care provider, with and without contrast, showed no abnormalities. She was referred to a neurologist.

Her neurologic examination was entirely normal, except for borderline difficulty with tandem gait. In the course of her evaluation, a lumbar puncture was performed. Opening pressures as well as protein, glucose, and cell counts were normal but she developed a characteristic severe headache which lasted for several days afterward. While the headache was considered to be a lumbar puncture headache, she was adamant that the symptoms were in many respects identical to her headache syndrome.

Efforts to treat her with standard migraine medications failed. Beta-blockers seemed to be effective at first but lost their benefit. Tricyclics enhanced her subjective gait instability. She claimed she felt even more "drugged." Opioid analgesics allowed her to sleep during her worst headache.

Because of the predominantly occipital location of the headache, both a greater occipital nerve block and C2 root blocks were performed; all blocks produced analgesia of the scalp but not even transient relief of pain or symptoms.

She was finding it harder to put in a full day of work, so in desperation a magnetic resonance imaging (MRI) scan was obtained. It showed a normal brain and ventricular system, but the cerebellar tonsils were "beaked" and descended 5 mm below the foramen magnum to the posterior arch of the C1 lamina. There was no evident cisterna magna.

Questions about Case 1

- What is the most likely diagnosis? What is its natural history?
- Is it surprising that a CT scan of the head was normal?
- Is it surprising that the patient's neurologic examination was normal?
- Is there a medical management for her symptoms? Is there a surgical management?

Case 1 Discussion

Formerly known as the "Arnold-Chiari malformation," cerebellar tonsillar herniation beyond the foramen magnum with elongation of the medulla and downward displacement of the cerebellum is now referred to as a "Chiari I malformation." This is distinct from the "Chiari type II malformation," that is associated with myelomeningocele, a kinked and elongated medulla, and a more formidable extension of the cerebellar tonsils into the spinal canal. The Chiari type I malformation can be completely asymptomatic, or associated with myriad neurologic dysfunctions. Symptoms and neurologic conditions associated with type I malformations include pyramidal tract compression with spasticity and extensor plantar responses, posterior column dysfunction with impaired proprioception and vibration sense, and lower cranial nerve disorders including tongue atrophy, swallowing impairment, and hearing loss. Cerebellar function can be compromised, producing ataxia and downbeat nystagmus, the latter most apparent when the patient attempts to read.

However, the spectrum of problems associated with this congenital condition can be entirely subjective and thus the neurologic examination may be totally unrevealing. Headache, head pain and pressure in the occiput and neck, and subjective gait instability are among the most common of the subjective symptoms. These symptoms are so nonspecific, that in this case, for instance, there was no reason to jump to the diagnosis right away, and to some degree the diagnosis was discovered through my obtaining an MRI in desperation!

In a child, the Chiari I malformation may or may not be associated with syringomyelia and is frequently associated with scoliosis but not with headaches. However, in adolescence, and extending into the next two decades, a previously asymptomatic Chiari I malformation, for unknown reasons, can become symptomatic as a progressive source of headaches.

The patient in case 1 is quite typical, with a constellation of typical subjective symptoms such as headache, head pressure, and perceived gait dysfunction out of proportion to the neurologic examination. In such a patient, without neurologic findings, the diagnosis cannot really be made with clinical certainty, but the above triad of complaints (posterior headache, posterior head pressure, and subjective gait instability), especially the patient's perception of head "pressure" when not in the throes of a headache, makes the syndrome atypical for most migraine diagnoses. Triggering of headache by coughing, yawning, and Valsalva's maneuvers is classic for Chiari I headaches, and ought to make someone with neurologic training at least consider the diagnosis.

A CT scan rarely reliably reveals a Chiari I malformation because of bony interference at the foramen magnum. Consequently, it is MRI that has made the greatest contribution toward identifying this entity. In the pre-MRI era, a diagnosis could only be made with cisternography or high myelography, so cases associated with a normal neurologic examination were rarely identified, for they simply did not justify invasive procedures and uncomfortable examinations. The ease with which MRI identifies the anatomy of the craniocervical junction has put a totally new perspective on the Chiari I malformation, showing it to be a source of headache without neurologic dysfunction. However, since the malformation is frequently seen on MRI without any symptoms in the patient, the association of headaches without neurologic disturbance and the malformation is always far from certain and must be entertained only when the complaints are particularly suggestive.

Even though the Chiari I malformation does not produce symptoms in many patients who possess it, when symptoms of headache do emerge they are usually progressive, although there is practically no evidence that the patient without syringomyelia is at special risk of neurologic injury, except in instances of severe head and neck trauma, even when the headaches are worsening. The headaches may be related to cerebrospinal fluid (CSF) pressure discontinuities between the head and the spinal canal, and evidence of this in Case 1 is the worsening of symptoms with a spinal tap, which would enhance the pressure differential between the two compartments.

The various medical therapies for migraine and its prophylaxis have, according to anecdotal evidence, helped with Chiari I malformation headaches, although there is no specific preferred medical treatment. Patients with mild symptoms can get relief with mild analgesics, as did the patient in Case 1 at first. For the patient with intractable symptoms of an unacceptable nature, surgery is appropriate.

The surgical therapy for Chiari I malformation requires the creation of a new cisterna magna—the making of an open space that allows easy CSF flow across the craniocervical junction. This is achieved by suboccipital craniectomy, C1 laminotomy, and dural opening and widening with a tissue graft. While the neurologic morbidity of this procedure is small in experienced hands, it represents a substantial operation with respect to the patient's pain and suffering, involving several days of hospitalization and over a month of recovery. The patient in Case 1 underwent such a procedure resulting in a reversal of her symptoms.

Case 1 Management Strategies

- Low threshold for MRI scanning in the patient with the triad of symmetric posterior headache, head pressure, and subjective gait instability, or symptoms provoked by Valsalva's maneuvers, coughing, or straining.

- The patient without syrinx is generally not at risk of permanent neurologic injury, so conservative approaches are justified.
- Definitive treatment is surgical.

Case 2 History

This 70-year-old man has a 1-year history of right-sided, predominantly occipital headache following a mild whiplash injury when his car was rear-ended. The pain began within 2 days of his accident. It was sharp, originating at the base of the right occiput, and, by his account, extraordinarily intense, projecting to the vertex of the right side of the head, with a component jabbing into the right fronto-orbital region. At first the pain was occasional, experienced as a darting sensation two or three times a day, dissappearing as rapidly as it came. However, by the end of a year, it was present more often than not and was particularly painful when he extended his neck or rotated it to the right. It could persist for hours at a time.

Because neck movement could provoke a headache, he was given a hard collar, which helped but did not eliminate his symptoms. A diagnosis of "post-traumatic migraine" and "occipital neuralgia" was advanced. Migraine medications of a prophylactic nature did not help. Potent analgesics in increasing doses were used, which he stated "masked the pain and made it bearable" but did not eliminate the symptoms.

On neurologic examination there was hypalgesia to pin prick over the right occiput. He was mildly hyperreflexic in all extremities, but symmetrically. Palpation and manipulation of the spinous process of C2 partially reproduced some of his pain.

A CT scan of the head showed some cerebral atrophy but no lesion. A plain cervical spine radiograph showed multilevel spondylosis. An MRI of the neck was performed showing moderate cervical spinal stenosis.

A lidocaine injection at the level of the right greater occipital nerve produced analgesia of the right posterior scalp but no pain relief. However, a similar block at the level of the right dorsal root ganglion of C2 produced both analgesia and pain relief for the duration of the anesthetic, but ultimately a return of the patient's symptoms.

Questions about Case 2

- What are the diagnostic possibilities?
- Could this be "occipital neuralgia?"
- Should this be considered a headache syndrome or a radiculopathy?
- What is the natural history of the condition?
- Can a more immediate treatment be offered?

Case 2 Discussion

This is actually a rather common problem consisting of unilateral headache and upper neck pain that frequently, but not always, follows a mild neck injury. Other than scalp hypalgesia, there is no aura or prodrome, and characteristically head and neck movement, particularly extension and rotation, not only exacerbates the pain but triggers it. Naturally, the headache must be distinguished by its history from true, post-traumatic migraine, and a migrainous quality is certainly absent from this patient's description. With a darting, jabbing component, it certainly is not migrainous in quality but is reminiscent of neuralgia, raising the question of greater occipital neuralgia. However, the fact that a lidocaine block of the greater occipital nerve was not effective makes that diagnosis unlikely.

Cervical spondylosis makes pain of radicular origin more likely, and a block of the right C2 dorsal root ganglion where it rests between the lamina of C1 and C2 completely abolishes all the patient's pain, confirming at least that the C2 ganglion mediates the head pain. This diagnostic procedure is best performed with some form of radiographic guidance and with experienced hands present. For all practical purposes, therefore, the problem is one of "radiculopathy"; that is, the headache is secondary to the nociceptive activity of a cervical nerve root and ganglion, one which happens to innervate the right posterior half of the scalp.

The patient's headache is, technically speaking, "cervicogenic," in that it originates from neck structures. In this case, however, that vague term would more appropriately be replaced with "C2 radiculopathy."

C2 radiculopathy is probably a frequent accompaniment to whiplash injury and, consequently, in most cases, has a benign and self-limited natural history. Most whiplash symptoms improve spontaneously. However, cases where symptoms persist for more than 6 months usually go on for another 6 months, and then the improvement rate is only about 20% per year. The long duration, therefore, of these symptoms in some patients makes aggressive, and occasionally surgical treatment, reasonable. A greater occipital neurectomy would be expected to be useless in this case given the lack of efficacy of a direct anesthetization of the nerve. Even when there is benefit from a greater occipital nerve block, surgical division of the greater occipital nerve has a high, nearly 100% recurrence rate due to regeneration of the peripheral nerve.

More recently, in cases of intractable pain with the failure of empirical medical therapy, a provocative block of the C2 root with abolition of pain is a very good predictor that decompressive exploration of the C2 root could relieve the symptoms. Most patients have soft tissue or bony irritation of the root, particularly at the even more sensitive dorsal root ganglion level. Sometimes the compression of the root is caused by local engorged vascular structures. In the case of this patient, hypertrophy of the C1/C2 joint and facet was producing compression of the root, and the symptoms were relieved completely by surgical decompression of the bony structures.

Case Summaries

- Cases 1 and 2 present patients with posterior or predominantly occipital headaches, the first associated with the Chiari I malformation, and the second with the C2 root.
- Both syndromes are "anatomic," that is, identifiable as related to a distinct neuroanatomic structure, either the cerebellar tonsils at the craniocervical junction or the dorsal root and ganglion of C2.
- The headache associated with the Chiari I malformation is spontaneous and bioccipital but is sometimes global and symmetrical and is associated with pressure and gait instability, while the C2 syndrome is usually unilateral, most often seen following neck trauma and is transiently abolished by a chemical block of the root.
- Both syndromes can be managed medically, but surgical options do exist in the form of decom-

pressive craniectomy for the Chiari I malformation and decompression or ablation of the C2 dorsal root ganglion for the latter.

Selected Readings

Dyste GN, Menezes AH, Van Gilder JC. Symptomatic Chiari malformations: an analysis of presentation, management, and long-term outcome. J Neurosurg 1989;71:159–68.

Elster AD, Chen MYM. Chiari I malformations: clinical and radiologic reappraisal. Radiology 1992;183:347–53.

Nohria V, Oakes WJ. Chiari I malformation: a review of 43 patients. Pediatr Neurosci 1990–1991;16:222–7.

Pikus HJ, Phillips JM. Characteristics of patients successfully treated for cervicogenic headache by surgical decompression of the second cervical root. Headache 1995;35:621–9.

Pikus HJ, Phillips JM. Outcome of decompression of the second cervical root for cervicogenic headache. Neurosurgery 1996; 33:63–71.

Pillay PK, Awad IA, Little JR, Hahn JF. Symptomatic Chiari malformation in adults: a new classification based on magnetic resonance imaging with clinical and prognostic significance. Neurosurgery 1991;28:639–645.

Editorial Comments

Sooner or later, every diagnostician dealing with headache patients will experience a sense of humility when the diagnosis turns out to be a Chiari I malformation and the patient's symptoms, including predominant occipital nuchal pain, disappear with neurosurgical intervention. Such cases as the first one described here by Dr. Phillips are not rare and deserve our attention and definitive diagnosis by way of MR imaging. Case 2 is more problematic in terms of conceptualization and management but successful outcomes have been recorded elsewhere by Drs. Phillips and Pikus. The C2 radiculopathy is an interesting entity, which if correctly diagnosed, can lead to effective therapy in some patients. Cervicogenic headache is a controversial entity.

Chapter 35

The Woman with Headache Following Lumbar Puncture

Marek J. Gawel, MD

Anne Maggisano

Case History

The patient is a 43-year-old female who suffered from migraine on an intermittent basis. Her headaches were described as being preceded about 50% of the time by scintillations in her right visual field. Twenty minutes later, this was followed by a throbbing headache which was on the right side of the head associated with nausea, occasional vomiting, light sensitivity, and sound sensitivity. These attacks would come once or twice a month and would often be associated with her menses although they did not, however, have a fixed-time relationship, sometimes coming 3 days before or 3 days afterwards. She had two children aged 14 and 15. Note that her headaches had improved during the second and third trimester of both pregnancies only to return after she had finished breast feeding. Her menses were still regular but her mother had gone into menopause at the age of 46.

She had noted that her headaches had gotten slightly worse and were more frequent but did not think too much about it. They usually responded to oral administration of a serotonin agonist such as sumatriptan. She did not use prophylactic medication although 3 years ago she had tried propranolol for about 2 months to little effect. She woke up one morning with the worst headache she had ever had. She had a slight headache on going to bed the previ-

ous night but by the time she woke at 5 in the morning, she was vomiting, could hardly see, could hardly stand, was dizzy, and unable to keep any medication down.

She did have subcutaneous sumatriptan and one injection of this seemed to help the headache slightly after about 2 hours, then it came back with more force until she could not tolerate it any more.

At this stage she was taken to the emergency room where the physician examined her fundi and did not find any abnormality. He found her to be photophobic, coherent, able to give a good account of herself but in a lot of distress. Her neck was slightly stiff although she could touch her chin to her chest. Her reflexes were symmetrical, plantars were downgoing and her blood pressure was 150/100. Because of the combination of findings and the severe nature of the headache she underwent an emergency computerized tomography scan which was negative. The lumbar puncture was negative; it ended with some difficulty in that several attempts had to be made to enter the subarachnoid space.

She was given intravenous saline for rehydration with intravenous meperidine 100 mg and dimenhydrinate 50 mg. This seemed to help the headache significantly and by the next morning she was feeling a lot better and able to be discharged. Following arrival at home, she noticed that when she stood up she would get a headache which was extremely severe, although different in nature from her previous headache. This headache would become unbearable after about half an hour of standing and could be relieved by lying down again. She called her family doctor who advised her to take a lot of fluid and to rest.

For the next week these symptoms persisted and she was forced to seek further consultation. She was advised by the neurologist who saw her and examined her that she was suffering from a lumbar puncture headache. He advised further bed rest, fluids, and caffeine in high dosage. After 2 weeks she was still having the symptoms although now the headache was more persistent and would even persist when she was lying down.

During this time she had one of her usual migraines which came and went within 8 hours. It had all the usual characteristics and was relieved by oral sumatriptan. By now she was getting extremely worried and distressed. She saw the neurologist who diagnosed a lumbar puncture headache caused by low cerebrospinal fluid (CSF) pressure. He ordered a magnetic resonance imaging (MRI) with gadolinium enhancement which was done the following day. The MRI showed normal images of the brain; however, the post-gadolinium films demonstrated intense diffuse meningeal enhancement and thickening. This finding suggested that she indeed had low CSF pressure headaches and she was referred to an anesthetist who performed an epidural autologous blood patch. This involved the injection of 15 mL of autologous blood into the epidural space in the vicinity of the lumbar puncture. Within 2 days her headaches had settled and she no longer had the intense constant headache which was exacerbated by postural changes. She still had the episodic migraines as before.

Questions about This Case

- What was the diagnosis of the first headache sign suffered by the patient?
- Why are these headaches sometimes related to menses?
- What are the MRI findings of a low-CSF-pressure headache?
- What is the definitive treatment for a persistent low-pressure headache?

Case Discussion

This patient exemplifies a typical scenario for a lumbar puncture headache. There was ample justification for doing a lumbar puncture and, as is sometimes the case in emergency rooms, some difficulties were encountered possibly because of the patient's state of distress. Lumbar puncture headaches are caused by low CSF pressure. The pain is associated with headache, neck ache, stiffness, shoulder pain, backache, nausea, vomiting, blurred vision, and tinnitus. Typically the headaches were worse when the patient was standing and were relieved by her lying down.

A recent review of the literature by McSwiney and Phillips quotes a frequency of lumbar puncture headaches following 36.5% of cases of lumbar puncture and states that there is a high incidence in young females with a low body mass index. According to this review, the frequency of the headache is directly related to the gauge of the needle used. The cause of the headache is thought to be due to two factors. The first is traction on pain-sensitive structures with downward displacement of the brain and, in particular, traction of cranial nerves 5, 9, and 10 and the upper three cervical nerves. The second cause is thought to be due to vascular dilatation and venous engorgement. According to this review these headaches have been produced experimentally by draining about 20 mL of CSF in a standing patient.

Another frequent scenario for the induction of lumbar puncture headaches is myelography. Myelograms are usually done electively and hence there is the opportunity for minimizing the incidence of lumbar puncture headaches. A number of studies have confirmed that using small needles reduces the incidence of side effects including headache. Thus a study by Tourtellotte et al. compared the 22- versus the 26-gauge needle in volunteers. The use of the 22-gauge needle resulted in 36% of the subjects developing postural headaches compared to 12% with the 26-gauge needle. The difference was significant at $p = .005$.

Another study by McConaha, Bastiani, and Kaye compared the use of a 22-gauge needle with that of a 29-gauge needle. In this case the 29-gauge needle was inserted down the lumen of the 22-gauge needle once the ligament had been penetrated by the former. Results showed convincingly that the use of a 29-gauge needle dramatically reduced the incidence of lumbar puncture headache. The authors discuss the use of the introducer in order to reduce the problem of needle flex which can occur using the 29-gauge needle.

A study by Lenaerts et al. showed that there was no difference in the incidence of lumbar puncture headache in patients who were punctured using a circular atraumatic needle (Sprottes) or relatively with the frequency of traumatic taps. The atraumatic needle is widely used by anesthetists for spinal and epidural anesthesia but is not routinely used by neurologists for diagnostic lumbar punctures. One reason for this is that the Sprottes needle is much more expensive than a standard needle. In this study, therefore, no advantage was found in using the atraumatic needle in lumbar puncture but this is not to say that the atraumatic needle is not more useful in epidural anesthesia.

Traditionally, patients who have had a lumbar puncture have been asked to keep still and recumbent for at least 4 hours following the lumbar puncture although this period varies. Early recommendations were for bed rest for 24 hours. Carbaat and Van Crevel compared the effect of keeping 50 patients recumbent and the other 50 patients ambulant. The two groups were comparable in age, sex, and neurotic traits. There was no difference in the incidence of lumbar puncture headaches between the two groups suggesting that at least 24 hours of recumbency offers no advantage.

A study by Smith, Perkin, and Rose assessing 50 patients suggested that there was a significant advantage in keeping the patient for 30 minutes at a 30° head-down tilt followed by 3¾ hours of supine bed rest compared to a then standard 4 hours' supine bed rest.

Spinal anesthesia is another situation where lumbar puncture or postural puncture headache occurs. Lybecker et al. found that postural puncture headache occurred within 2 days in 96% of the 75 cases noted in the large study that they performed. A quarter of those with postural pressure headaches were classified as severe. Transient headaches were common following dural puncture. The incidence of postural puncture headaches was 7.35% of the overall sample of spinal anesthetics performed. This is clearly a small percentage but becomes relevant when seen in the context of patients with a previous history of headaches, including those with migraine.

There are no studies of the effect of prior migraine on the onset of lumbar puncture headaches. Low CSF pressure headaches can also appear spontaneously presumably as a result of minor trauma or straining. Such headaches are recognized by the postural nature of the headaches and by the relatively sudden onset of headache. In some cases the patients have felt a sharp pain between the shoulders and this is followed by the headache which may come on suddenly or within several days. If the headache becomes chronic, the postural nature may become less clear and a more diffuse chronic headache may occur.

Investigations

There have been various attempts made at investigating the presence of dural leak. Probably the most promising approach is the use of MRI with gadolinium enhancement. This technique shows significant dural enhancement following the injection of gadolinium. Other methods of investigation include myelography which demonstrates a rapid clearance of the contrast medium but this is probably not so useful. Frequently, investigations are unnecessary or difficult to obtain and in this case the history should point to the diagnosis. There have been a number of treatment modalities tried including the use of bed rest, high intake of fluid, caffeine in high doses, desmopressin acetate, steroids, and epidural autologous blood patches.

The epidural autologous blood patch should be considered if there has been no resolution of symptoms within 2 weeks following the lumbar puncture. Blood patching has been done for over 30 years; it has been shown to be effective. The first report by Gormely showed that by using 2 to 3 mL of autologous blood, a 100% cure was obtained in a series of 8 subjects, one of whom was himself. Currently, an average of 15 to 20 mL of blood is being used. What happens to the blood has been a matter of some speculation although a recent study by Beards et al. carried out MR imaging in five patients at intervals of 30 minutes, 3, 7, 9, and 18 hours after blood patching. At 30 minutes and at 3 hours the clot was shown to have a mass effect compressing the dural sac and displacing the conus medullaris and cauda equina. There was also compression or displacement of nerve roots nearby. The main bulk of the clot occupied four or five vertebral levels with thinner spread cephalad and caudad several vertebrae further.

By 3 hours, the blood had concentrated into a focal clot within the dural sac adherent to the dura, and from 7 hours onward, the mass effect had disappeared with a thinning layer of blood adherent to the dural sac but extending much further cephalad than caudad. It was assumed by the authors in the editorial of that same journal that this was probably a generalizable phenomenon as it occurred in all five patients.

A recent paper by Carp et al. reviews the effects of the serotonin receptor agonist sumatriptan on postdural-puncture headache in six patients. All of the six subjects had lasting relief after a single injection of subcutaneous sumatriptan 6 mg. One case required a second injection after 21 hours and one case received transient relief and requested an epidural blood patch for recurrent headaches after 24 hours. Further studies confirming these findings in a double-blind manner are not available but they certainly offer a scope for further investigation and may be considered prior to using an epidural blood patch.

Currently, epidural blood patching is the treatment of choice in lumbar puncture and postmyelography headaches.

Selected Readings

Beards SC, Jackson A, Griffiths AG, Horsman EL. Magnetic resonance imaging of extradural blood patches: appearances from 30 min to 18h. Br J Anaesth 1993;71:182–8.

Carbaat PAT, Van Crevel H. Lumbar puncture headache: controlled study on the preventive effect of 24 hours' bed rest. Lancet 1981;1133–5.

Carp H, Singh PJ, Vadhera R, Jayaram A. Effects of the serotonin-receptor agonist sumatriptan on postdural puncture headache: report of six cases. Anesth Analg 1994;79:180–2.

Gormely JB. Treatment of post spinal headache. Anesthesiology 1960;21:565–6.

Lenaerts M, Pepin JL, Tombu S, Schoenen J. No significant effect of an "atraumatic" needle on incidence of post-lumbar puncture headache or traumatic tap. Cephalalgia 1993;13:296–7.

Lybecker H, Dejernes M, Schmidt JF. Postdural puncture headache (PDPH): onset, duration, severity, and associated symptoms. Acta Anaesthesiol Scand 1995;39:605–12.

McConaha C, Bastiani AM, Kaye WH. Significant reduction of post-lumbar puncture headaches by the use of a 29 gauge spinal needle. Biol Psychiatry 1996;39:1058–60.

McSwiney M, Philips J. Post dural puncture headache. Acta Anaesthesiol Scand 1995;39:990–5.

Smith FR, Perkin GD, Rose FC. Posture and headache after lumbar puncture. Lancet 1980 June 7;1:1245.

Tourtellotte WW, Henderson WG, Tucker RP, et al. A randomized, double-blind clinical trial comparing the 22 versus 26 gauge needle in the production of the post-lumbar puncture syndrome in normal individuals. Headache 1972; 12:73–8.

Editorial Comments

When standing tends to worsen a headache and produce nausea, and lying down helps, suspect a low-CSF-pressure syndrome, such as a lumbar puncture headache. It is of some interest that low-pressure, lumbar puncture headaches occur as frequently as they do, given the significant number of patients who undergo this procedure. Obviously, most resolve without intervention but for those occasions when this does not occur, Dr. Gawel and Ms. Magissano have provided a detailed overview of the diagnosis, pathogenetic considerations, and treatment of this particular headache. A definitive diagnosis and favorable outcome can be expected and, as well, a smaller lumbar puncture needle may prove preventive.

CHAPTER 36

THE MAN WITH HEADACHE FOLLOWING A FALL

WILLIAM G. SPEED III, MD

Case History

A married, 47-year-old male was referred for a headache evaluation. He had a lifetime history of headaches occurring two to three times a year, each lasting 1 to 2 hours. No further details about these headaches could be recalled.

Five years earlier, he had slipped on a wet spot on the floor in the kitchen of the seafood restaurant which he owned and had fallen backwards, striking his head on the concrete floor. He was hospitalized for 1 week. A brain scan and a radiograph of his skull were within normal limits and an electroencephalogram (EEG) revealed only "minor changes" about which there are no further details. His headaches involved the bilateral occipital and suboccipital areas and persisted for 2 weeks after which there were none. He went back to work and there were no residual symptoms.

Five months prior to assessment, the patient slipped on a piece of lettuce on the floor of his restaurant kitchen, fell backwards, and again struck the back of his head on the concrete floor. He became semiconscious and was admitted to a local hospital where he was kept in the intensive care unit for 2 days and in the hospital for a total of 30 days because of the severe headache that was present as soon as he returned to full consciousness. A radiograph of his skull, a computed tomography (CT)

scan with contrast of his head, and a lumbar puncture (LP) were within normal limits.

He was referred by his internist because of difficulty in the management of his headaches. Immediately following the fall, the headaches were constant for the first 2 weeks, after which they occurred two to three times a day lasting from 30 minutes to 4 hours each time. A month before his referral he had tried going back to work in the restaurant he owned and managed but the intensity of the headache increased even though the frequency did not change. If he stayed home and did nothing, the headaches would gradually reduce in frequency to three to four times a week, and lasted up to an hour. The location of these headaches was generalized but it was most intense in the bilateral occipital, frontal, and temporal regions. All of the headaches were described as severe and 80% of the time they reached the incapacitating level.

Other pertinent findings in the history were impaired memory and concentration, insomnia, vertigo, depression without suicidal thoughts, decreased sexual interest, anger outbursts, and easy fatigability. These symptoms all developed immediately after the last fall and had never been present prior to that.

He had always been an active, full-of-energy, happy workaholic. He was reduced to total disability because of postinjury headaches that would become severe and incapacitating with increased activity. He suffered from short-term memory loss and the inability to concentrate. He found that he could not take off his watch except to shower or he would lose it. He had to use a notebook or a tape recorder so that he could keep track of where he was going and to record any changes which might be made in his schedule. On one occasion, he tried to carry a small message recorder but was unsuccessful because it had five buttons that had to be pressed in order to make it work. Even though these buttons were clearly marked he could not keep the sequence of the five numbers in his head to permit the instrument to function. The tape recorder, however, had only a start and stop button and he could handle that.

The decreased sexual function was creating a problem in his marriage and he diligently went to a sexual disorder clinic, as well as consulting a marriage counselor, but none of this had a favorable impact on this symptom. Combined with the distinct change in his personality as a result of his injury, these persistent symptoms led his wife to give up and finally to divorce him. For many months he had consulted a psychiatrist twice a week with no beneficial response. It was impossible for him to function in his business and he had to sell the two restaurants he owned and they eventually folded without his input.

The laboratory evaluations, consisting of an enhanced CT scan, a magnetic resonance imaging (MRI) scan of the head, EEGs, and an LP, were all within normal limits. Neurocognitive testing supported short-term memory impairment and slow cognitive responding and was otherwise normal.

Over time his headaches and other symptoms were treated with numerous medications including tricyclic antidepressants, beta-blockers, nonsteroidal anti-inflammatory drugs, methysergide, antiseizure medications, lithium, verapamil, and benzodiazepines. Many of these were used in combination and none added appreciably to the control of his headaches. The most effective control, although unusual for this problem, was the use of codeine to keep the intensity of the pain down so that he could live with his headaches. He used codeine two to three times per week. He was taken off it on more than one occasion for a month to be sure that he was not having a rebound effect and none could be demonstrated. He was allowed to continue this schedule as the lesser of the two evils.

He continues to the present time with these headaches but they are no longer interfering significantly with his quality of life. The most debilitating and persistent symptoms are the short-term memory loss and the impaired concentration. The memory loss is entirely limited to anything which has happened since the fall and he retains a perfect memory for those things that happened before his second fall. For example, if he is asked who the president of the United States is, or who our mayor or governor is, he has no idea. If he is asked who was president during World War II, he answers without the slightest hesitation—Roosevelt and Truman. If he is asked what a Lexus is, he has no idea but if he is asked what a Desoto is, he will respond promptly that it is an automobile. He cannot tell anyone how old he is but he can respond immediately with the month, day, and year in which he was born. He cannot recall a street name, a color, or a four-digit number (seven digits are usually used) within seconds of being asked to remember them. He has to write down where he parks his car otherwise he would have no idea where it is. This sort of scenario occurs constantly in his daily life.

Questions about This Case

- This patient had two essentially identical injuries to the head in a 5-year period. One left him with no sequelae and the other left him with permanent disabling symptoms. Do you have an explanation for that?
- Does he have an organic disease ?
- Is this a psychiatric disorder or a combination of both organic disease and a psychiatric disorder?
- Could he be a malingerer, looking for a lifetime of relative leisure by getting a bundle of money from an insurance company?
- What diagnostic studies would you have suggested when he was first referred by his primary care physician for help in the management of his headaches?
- Do headaches following trauma differ from those of primary origin?

- Are the headaches the primary reason for his incapacitation, or are there other issues involved?
- What would you consider doing in trying to bring his headaches under control?
- He developed many other symptoms in addition to his headaches. How would you handle these?

Case Discussion

This 47-year-old, married male was a highly motivated, happy workaholic who owned two very well-known and successful seafood restaurants in his home town. He had good employees and he went to these restaurants each day simply to oversee the operations, and to have something to do.

The first time he slipped on a wet spot in the kitchen of one of these restaurants and struck his head on the concrete floor, he received a blow sufficient to require a 1-week stay in hospital for observation. A brain scan (there were no CTs then), a skull radiograph, and an EEG were normal. He had a headache for 2 weeks and after that he became totally asymptomatic and remained so until his next head injury which was 5 years later and under very similar circumstances.

Let us address the first question as to whether there may be an explanation for that. There is no clear-cut scientific evidence to explain this series of events. However, there are many studies and reports in the literature which give us a basis for drawing reasonable conclusions about what might have happened. It is clear that there is room between the brain and the skull to allow for sufficient acceleration/deceleration motion of the brain, when subjected to closed injury, to permit stress (shear) injury to axons. Although impact on the skull may produce this, it also has been shown to occur as a result of flexion/extensional/rotational movements such as one might experience in a cervical "whiplash" situation without the skull impacting on anything. Many animal studies clearly show that damage does occur to axons and probably to neurons as well. There are autopsy data on patients with a prior history of closed head injuries, but dying later of other causes, that allow one to conclude that such axonal damage has occurred also in humans.

There are many reports in the literature analyzing the persistent symptoms resulting from closed head injuries. These reports indicate that about 70% of individuals who receive a closed head injury will be free of headache within 2 months—many in far shorter time than this. This leaves 30% who will continue with headache beyond 2 months and these are called chronic post-traumatic headaches (or syndrome if other symptoms are involved). Eighty percent of this group will be free of symptoms within 1 year with appropriate management and the remaining 20% are considered to be essentially permanently disabled.

Post-traumatic headache may occur as an isolated symptom but is also commonly associated with other symptoms such as impaired short-term memory, impaired concentration, easy fatigability, anger outbursts, depression and/or frustration, irritability, insomnia, loss of sexual desire, and lightheadedness and/or vertigo. It is quite interesting that these symptoms, including the headache are characteristic sequelae to a closed head injury. Physicians who see large numbers of closed head injury problems see the same symptoms over and over again regardless of the circumstances under which the injury occurred. It does not matter whether litigation is involved, or whether someone else was responsible for the injury, or whether the patient was responsible for the injury, the symptoms remain clearly stereotyped. Considering this fact, and the evidence for brain damage following a closed head injury, one may conclude that the force applied to the brain at the time of a closed head injury always follows a common pathway interfering with axons, and possibly neurons, that are involved in the generation of headache and the other symptoms just described. Most often this results in brain disturbances which may be relatively short lived, but not infrequently the disturbances may be permanent. The differences in the degree of traumatic force delivered to the brain under similar circumstances may not be great but this difference is likely to be sufficient to account for the fact that this patient had no long-term residua from his first fall but became permanently disabled from the second.

Does he have an organic basis for his long-term disability? It is almost certain that the answer to this is yes. There are no tests to prove this except perhaps for the confirmation of the clinical findings by the neuropsychologic testing. From what is known from both animal and human studies there is no doubt that the brain sustains significant injury in many cases of the closed head injury type.

Does he have a psychiatric disorder in addition to the organic problem or a combination of both? It is difficult to rule out completely some degree of pyschogenic component in someone whose quality of life has been so severely disrupted as has his. However, there is nothing to suggest that any of this is a primary issue and he consented to see a psychiatrist on a twice-weekly basis for many months with no resulting therapeutic benefit. Few of us would escape some psychogenic component under these circumstances, so one would suspect there is some degree of both with the organic injury side playing the major role.

Could he be a malingerer? There is no way that this is a possibility. He was a highly motivated workaholic running two successful restaurants who tried desperately to go back to work following his discharge from hospital. Not only were the headaches of sufficient intensity to keep him from working but so were the other symptoms described in his history. He had no one to sue except himself as the owner of the business and absolutely nothing to gain by not working. A true malingerer is someone who consciously simulates the symptoms of disease in order to deceive and often there is a financial motive for this. None of this was present in this patient.

When he was first referred for a headache evaluation 5 months after his second closed head injury, he had already had a skull radiography, a CT scan with contrast, an EEG, an LP, a complete blood count (CBC), chemistries, and urinalysis, all of which were normal. Would you consider requesting any other studies in this patient? Except for a neurocognitive assessment, none was needed. An MRI was obtained and was within normal limits. Some might argue that the contrast CT scan was adequate and that no further intracranial studies would be likely to throw any further light on his problem. Actually, the same thing might be said about ordering the neurocognitive testing. After all, one could find everything reported by the neuropsychologists

by doing an in-depth history of this patient. Sometimes these studies are more useful at a later date when they can be compared with follow-up neurocognitive studies to provide a more objective view of what progress, if any, is being made. This is a judgment call the physician has to make. Such studies are not always necessary either from the diagnostic or therapeutic viewpoint. They may be helpful when one is asked to testify in court, but one needs to weigh that against the possibility that such a study would be normal when the clinical evidence suggests otherwise. These tests still lack some degree of sensitivity.

It is essential to keep in mind that running tests in these individuals may be important, but this is far outweighed by the importance of an in-depth history and physical examination. Since many of these patients have memory problems, it may be useful to obtain information from a spouse or a close friend as well. Unfortunately, no one but the patient can tell you the details about the headaches, since this is a totally subjective symptom.

Let us look at the history the patient provided us with about his headaches. He recalls that he had a lifetime history of headaches, but it is difficult to say whether these were diagnostically significant or not. He remembers having them but could only tell us that they were two or three times a year, each lasting only 1 or 2 hours. He could neither tell us the location nor the intensity levels of these headaches. These could suggest that he has a migraine background, but the information is too meager to be conclusive. It is certainly not essential information, but it is known that individuals who have a history of migraine are likely to experience a significant exacerbation of their headaches as a result of a closed head injury. It is for this reason that many physicians interested in caring for headache patients will warn a known migraineur not to participate in activities such as football, boxing, wrestling, or soccer, as sufficient jarring of the head has the potential to aggravate the migraine mechanism.

The headaches experienced by those who have had a closed head injury do not differ from those seen in the noninjured headache population. Many of them have characteristics which are compatible with migraine and others are, perhaps, more like chronic tension-type headache. Fundamentally, it does not matter whether you want to call these simply post-traumatic headaches and let it go at that or whether you want to try to subdivide these into other categories. The treatment will be the same.

When the patient was first referred, he had chronic daily headaches occurring two to three times a day and lasting from 30 minutes to 4 hours each time. These were moderate to severe to incapacitating headaches and the intensity was always highest when he tried to work. The medications described in the case history were used over time in various combinations and dosages and none of these produced any significant improvement in his headaches. This poor response should be looked at in context. The majority of these patients will do well with the medications used in this case, but not all of those who are good responders will be on the same combination of medications. The statistics cited above show that there will be about 15 to 20% of the headache individuals who meet the chronic post-traumatic headache definition (i.e., having chronic headache persisting for more than 2 months after the closed head injury) and who will continue to be symptomatic regardless of the management program. Essentially, that is what happened to this patient.

This patient, nevertheless, was controlled to the degree that the headaches were no longer having an adverse impact on his quality of life. Remember, he was able to reduce the frequency of his headaches from daily to three to four times a week simply by reducing his activity level to staying at home. It was determined that codeine sulfate, 60 mg, given after the headaches started, would keep them from reaching a severe or incapacitating level. As long as he was allowed to do this, the headaches were not a problem to him. He used codeine no more than 2 to 3 days a week, and as stated in the case presentation he was taken off it completely for a month on several occasions to be sure that this was not creating a rebound factor in his headaches. This was never demonstrated and he was miserable without the codeine. This therapeutic method is not one that should be taken lightly in view of our knowledge regarding rebound headaches, but in this unusual instance it worked for him when more traditional approaches did not.

Although post-traumatic headache can occur without other symptomatology, it is more likely to occur in association with other symptoms. Therefore, it would not be complete to refer only to the headache manifestations of this patient's case history. As mentioned in the case presentation, this patient also had symptoms that had a severe impact on his quality of life, including loss of short-term memory, impaired concentration, depression without suicidal thoughts, anger outbursts, decreased sexual desire, insomnia, easy fatigability, and vertigo. Over the first 3 to 4 years following his injury, there was gradual improvement in the fatigue, anger outbursts, depression, insomnia, and vertigo, but no improvement has occurred in the short-term memory loss or the impaired concentration. The case history outlines the way in which this forces him to "self-help" methods that allow him to keep his life as close to normal as possible.

The combination of symptoms enforced a marked change in his way of life and in his ability to play the role of a normal husband. This eventually led to a divorce. He lost his restaurant business because others were not able to maintain it over time in the same way that he had been able to.

Are there proven methods of helping patients with post-traumatic symptoms other than headaches? None shows any benefit over another. If you do not feel that you have the experience or knowledge to give patients guidance in this area, then by all means send them to a reputable rehabilitation center. Here they may be taught self-help measures which will let them obtain the maximum possible degree of improvement of these disabling symptoms. Refer to the case history to review the measures this patient used to help with his poor memory and impaired concentration. Also note how very specific his memory impairment is. He can clearly recall all of those events that took place prior to the injury but cannot recall many events that have taken place since the injury. He is either incapable of laying down memory or if that is being done, then he is unable to use the process which can bring it back to a conscious level. Maybe both these processes are lost in many patients with symptoms resulting from a closed head injury.

Management Strategies

Always be sure that you have established the correct diagnosis. This requires you to do a thorough history for which there is no short cut. You will need to know at least the patient's headache history, if there was one prior to the injury, then a detailed history of the headache that has developed since the injury. This should include determining when the headache was first noticed in relation to the injury, whether it is similar to those present prior to the injury, where it is located, what kind of pain it is, whether it varies in intensity, how often it occurs, and how long it lasts. If you are not prepared to spend the time to do this and complete a full physical examination, then you should refer this patient to someone who will. Post-traumatic headache problems are usually complex and the primary care physician should be prepared to refer them to physicians who treat large numbers of headache patients in their practice. If you are not a specialist, you may wish to refer this patient early on.

A contrast CT scan or an MRI should be done if one has not been done prior to your seeing the patient.

Common treatment strategies for these headaches are essentially the same as they would be for migraine or tension-type headache not related to a traumatic event and would include a low-vasoactive-substance diet (Appendix 36–1). This diet eliminates known chemical triggers (phenylethylamine, monosodium glutamate (MSG), sodium nitrate, and tyramine) for migraine found in certain foods and is useful in about 60% of migraine patients, though pharmacotherapeutic measures are also usually needed. Unless contraindicated by asthma, hypotension, etc., use a beta-blocker you are familiar with, e.g., atenolol, nadolol, metoprolol, propranolol, or timolol, in combination with one of the tricyclic or related compounds, e.g., amitriptyline, nortriptyline, imipramine, or trazodone. The dosage may need to be pushed to accepted upper limits or individual patient tolerance. Then consider adding phenelzine a monoamine oxidase (MAO) inhibitor to this combination, but do not do this unless you are familiar with the precautions the patient must follow in order to avoid disastrous and dangerous side effects.

One can usually determine within a month to 6 weeks whether this combination of medications is appropriate for a given patient. If this should fail, then you still have available to you methysergide, and divalproex sodium, as well as hospitalization for the Raskin treatment (intravenous dihydroergotamine mesylate [DHE] and possibly a short course of prednisone).

There may be occasions in chronic headache problems when it is appropriate to use long-acting opiates such as oxycodone. This was not done in this patient because this method was not being used when his present management program was finalized, and the control of his headaches was satisfactory enough that this approach was not likely to improve the control he already had.

Keep in mind that patients who are suffering from post-traumatic headache often have other symptoms which are directly related to the trauma and these must be addressed along with the headache management.

Remember how important it is to involve the spouse or other close family members. This is a devastating disorder which can be very frightening to the patient. Not only should the patient be given a thorough explanation about what is wrong with him or her and why, but this same information should be given to close family members. The nonheadache symptoms may be subtle but, yet, prove very distressing to the patient. So always inquire about the related symptoms that have been outlined above.

Case Summary

- The patient does have a post-traumatic headache which is still present 15 years after onset but is no longer interfering with his quality of life.
- The use of short-acting analgesics is usually contraindicated in these patients because of the real potential for rebound. Nevertheless, this has worked for this particular patient and he has shown no evidence of the rebound phenomenon.
- There is no single management strategy which works well in all patients, and there is not one best therapy. Fortunately, there are a large number of therapeutic measures, usually in some combination form, that will greatly benefit the majority of these patients.
- In post-traumatic situations it is common to find, in addition to headache, other associated sympto-

matology which can be subtle and should be searched for so that your patient can be given the maximum support available to him/her.

Overview of Post-traumatic Headache and the Post-traumatic Syndrome

This overview is designed to give you brief background information concerning this important topic that should supply you with useful information and help to put this particular case in perspective.

The early assumption that post-traumatic headaches and related symptoms had a psychologic basis, and were motivated by greed, a desire not to work, the fulfillment of dependency needs, and the desire to seek sympathy from others, has finally given way to the understanding that the brain has suffered an injury and that these symptoms are a consequence of that injury. The onset of symptoms occurs immediately at the time of injury or within a few days thereafter, which would be quite unlikely as a psychologic response to an injury.

The clinical features of the headaches may mimic any of the headache disorders but are most likely to resemble migraine, tension-type headache, or a combination of both. Both migraine with aura and migraine without aura may be seen, but the majority are likely to be all over the head and neck, and may or may not include the face. Most often they are present constantly but may vary in intensity from time to time. Because they have a tendency to become aggravated by jarring of the head, bending over, lifting, straining, and exposure to lights and noises, the headaches may prevent the patient from participating in many forms of physical activity, including such innocuous things as riding in an automobile. This can have an adverse impact on the ability of someone to return to work. Even intense mental concentration may aggravate the level of headache intensity, making a job requiring only mental activity difficult to carry out. There are occasions when the neck may also receive an injury and may be responsible for headaches either located in the neck and occipital areas or the headache may be generalized and aggravated by neck movement. These are called cervicogenic headaches and apparently result from stimulation of the headache

generator thought in part to inhabit the upper cervical cord.

Injury to the brain can occur from flexion/extensional/rotational movement of the head without the head itself impacting on anything. There are experimental studies which show that this action sets up shear (tearing) forces along planes in the head that result in disruption of some axons. Some of these are anatomic disruptions and some may be physiologic ones. The association of these experimental findings and the clinical picture one sees in patients is speculative, but the probability is very high that there is such a relationship.

Only a brief summary can be given here of the experimental data that supports the above statements. You can find more details by referring to the Selected Readings at the end of this article. Evidence that closed head injury induced abnormalities in brain function, as well as structural abnormalities of the brain, began to develop in earnest in the 1940s. Denny-Brown and Russell used cats to demonstrate that less force was needed to produce concussion if the head was free to move than if it was fixed. Holbourne, using gelatin models and applying the theory of elasticity, showed that shear forces occur in relation to acceleration/deceleration. Others using guinea pigs showed loss of nerve cells and structural alteration of the brain after concussion and that these guinea pigs performed poorly in maze-running tests. Then Pudenz and Sheldon, using monkeys whose skulls were replaced by Lucite material, thus making the brain visible, confirmed that the brain moved within the skull on acceleration/deceleration as previously predicted by Holbourne using the gelatin model of the brain. Later, neuropathologists found in humans that in a few who subsequently died of a cause unrelated to their head injury, there were ruptures, tears, or other injuries to axons and that these were most prominent in the cerebral hemispheres, and brain stem—the areas likely to be involved in the production of headache. Finally, in the 1980s, Povlishock, using cats in precisely controlled experiments, confirmed that extensive axonal injury occurred after relatively minor head injury, usually axonal tears or ruptures, but also that interruption of the axonal transport system may occur without actual axonal tear or rupture.

This data gives us a scientific basis to understand that definite injury to the brain occurs with closed head injuries. We know the clinical manifestation presented by many patients after such an injury and we know that most often these symptoms begin immediately, or almost immediately, after injury. This is strong circumstantial evidence that the experimental findings and the clinical symptoms seen in patients are locked hand in hand. Strict scientific proof of this, however, must await further studies possibly by techniques that are not yet available.

Because, as a rule, there is little in the way of objective findings in these patients, they frequently find themselves in a position of frustration. They know there is something wrong with them, but others may suggest to them that they seem fine and wonder how could a minor injury cause all that trouble. Sometimes this may even come from a physician who either has a poor understanding of closed head injury and its consequences, or believes that all the symptoms are simply psychologic. This does not need to be said, as the patient is likely to be very good at reading tone of voice or body language, and when that happens, the physician has little chance of being helpful and should refer the patient to someone else. Neurocognitive testing may be useful as an objective finding if it is abnormal, but there are times when this is not the case, even in the face of a clinically stereotyped symptomatology. Always keep in mind that the diagnosis of this condition is largely a clinical one, and that negative "tests" do not exclude it at all.

Fortunately, there are excellent treatments for the headaches of the post-traumatic syndrome. This is the same treatment as for other headaches such as chronic migraine and chronic tension-type headache described in other chapters. As a guide, one approach to be considered is to do the following:

- If your patient is taking analgesics, ergots, or triptans on a frequent basis, then these will need to be discontinued to be certain you are not dealing with a rebound effect.
- Start all of these patients on a low vasoactive-substance diet. Clinical experience suggests that at least half of these patients will benefit from this, but it seldom will do enough good alone so it should be used along with the pharmacotherapeutic measures listed below.

- Prescribe a beta-blocker (e.g., metoprolol, timolol, nadolol, atenolol, or propranolol) in combination with one of the tricyclic or related compounds (e.g., amitriptyline, imipramine, nortriptyline, doxepin, desipramine, trazodone, or fluoxetine). Use those with which you are most familiar. The doses used need to be adjusted to response, tolerance, or maximum allowable recommendations. It may take 3 to 4 weeks before one can suspect that no improvement is going to occur at the dosage level being used.
- To a beta-blocker and tricyclic compound one may add a calcium channel blocker (long-acting only) such as verapamil SR, provided that there are no contraindications such as bradycardia or hypotension. Calcium channel blockers are slow to produce results but 4 to 6 weeks should be long enough to show whether they are effective or not.
- If this is ineffective, then one may stop the calcium channel blocker and add to the beta-blocker and the tricyclic compound an MAO inhibitor such as phenelzine or tranylcypromine. Although this combination is quite safe when used properly and with both verbal and written warnings given to the patient, it is potentially very dangerous to the point of causing death if the appropriate precautions are not taken. One should use this combination only if completely familiar with its food and drug interactions. This combination will show a response in 3 to 6 weeks if it is going to happen. Always remember, that if you use an MAO inhibitor, the restrictions you give the patient must be adhered to for 2 weeks after the MAO inhibitor has been discontinued.
- If none of the above is helpful after a reasonable trial period then consider divalproex sodium or gabapentin.
- Next, add methylergonovine. The patient should show improvement within a week.
- The role of long-acting opiates has not yet been clearly established, so one must be cautious about instituting them. However, for some patients who have failed with all other forms of treatment this may be appropriate.
- Inpatient management may play a definite role in the therapeutic management of these headaches. This becomes a judgment call on the part of the

physician as to when it is appropriate to consider this. At times it is necessary to contemplate this early on in the management of this problem and yet, at other times it may be correct to exhaust outpatient measures first. Inpatient management enhances the ability of the physician to maneuver medications more frequently than can be done outside a hospital since these patients are under 24-hour observation. The goal of inpatient management is to get patients off medication associated with rebound and to use intravenous DHE, following protocols established by Raskin and by Silberstein. Many of the medications described above may be used during this period as well.

- Finally, the symptoms associated with post-traumatic syndrome in addition to the headache should be addressed. There are no clearly established uniform management procedures which can be applied to the nonheadache post-traumatic syndrome symptomatology itself. A variety of techniques may be used such as memory and concentration practice. You can institute these yourself if you feel competent to do this, or you may refer them to rehabilitation centers where patients with closed head injury symptomatology are frequently treated.

There is nothing hard and fast about the order in which these suggestions have been presented. Individual circumstances in a given patient may dictate a different priority than that outlined here. That must be entirely a judgment call on the part of the physician.

Selected Readings

Goldstein J. Post-traumatic headache and post-traumatic syndrome. Med Clin North Am 1991;75: 641–51.

Povlishock JT, Becker DP, Cheng CL, Vaughan GW. Axonal change in minor head injury. J Neuropathol Exp Neurol 1983;42:225–42.

Raskin NH. Repetitive intravenous dihydroergotamine as therapy for intractable migraine. Neurology 1986;36:995.

Saper JR. Headaches that occur after trauma. In: Help for headaches (A guide to understanding their causes and finding the best methods of treatment). New York: Warner Books;1987. p. 129–40.

Saper JR, Silberstein SD, Gordon CD, Hamel RL. Post-traumatic headache and syndrome. In: Handbook of headache management (A practical guide to the diagnosis and treatment of head, neck, and facial pain). Baltimore: Williams & Wilkins; 1993. p. 138–45.

Silberstein SD, Schulman EA, Hopkins MM. Repetitive intravenous DHE in the treatment of refractory headache. Headache 1991;31:334–9.

Speed WG. Psychiatric aspects of post-traumatic headaches. In: Adler CA, Adler SM, Packard RC, editors. Psychiatric aspects of headaches. Baltimore: Williams & Wilkins; 1987. p. 201–6.

Speed WG. Closed head injury sequelae and changing concepts. Headache 1989;29:643–7.

Speed WG. Post-traumatic headache. In: Samuels MA, Feske S, editors. Office practice of neurology. New York: Churchill Livingston; 1996. p. 1137–41

Editorial Comments

Understanding and managing patients with headache following a closed head injury requires a very special knowledge of the disorder, and its putative pathophysiology, and experience in headache management in general. It truly is an art as well as a science and the clinician who remains honest with himself or herself and his or her patient will be the most successful. Dr. Speed's case and discussion as well as the case management are a model of such effective strategies for the management of these complex patients. Not everyone will agree with everything found in this chapter, or with some of the medications used, but one suspects that Dr. Speed would prefer it that way. He advocates a positive role for the physician in such cases, and reveals numerous clinical pearls throughout his excellent chapter.

Appendix 36–1

A low vasoactive-substance diet avoids the following foods that contain chemical substances that may trigger headaches in susceptible people:

Chocolate	Bananas
Tea	Pickled herring
Coffee, including decaffeinated coffee	Foods containing MSG
Alcohol	Canned figs
Aged cheese	Avocado
Nuts	Fermented sausages (bologna, salami, pepperoni, summer sausage)
Onions	
Citrus fruits (orange, lemon, lime, grapefruit, and their juices)	Hot dogs
	Chicken livers

CHAPTER 37

TWO HEADACHE PATIENTS WITH THE SAME INFECTION

JEROME GOLDSTEIN, MD

RAGUI H. MICHAEL

Case 1 History

The first case is that of a 50-year-old male who was diagnosed as having human immunodeficiency virus (HIV) infection in 1985 when HIV testing became available. He believes that he was infected as early as 1977. His headache history started in 1979 with a unilateral headache, primarily on the right side, that occurred about twice a week. He was prescribed propranolol, and the headaches completely disappeared within 6 months. In 1985, his headaches returned. He was re-evaluated at that time, and no obvious reason for the recurrence of his headaches was found. A magnetic resonance imaging (MRI) scan did not reveal the cause of the headaches. Since 1985, the headaches have been intermittent and without a definite pattern. A cytomegalovirus (CMV) infection was discovered in 1994 but there was no change in the headache pattern.

In November of 1997 he complained of motor incoordination manifested by his inability to use a typewriter, lethargy, and some confusion. He characterized the symptoms as "My motor control was turned off." A repeat MRI revealed an increase in brain atrophy. Extensive psychometric testing was done that did not confirm a new-onset dementia. With a change in antiretroviral medication, the neurologic symptoms did improve but there was a perceptible increase in the frequency of headache. He noticed that didanosine precipitated his headaches.

The headaches became more left sided and the use of a butalbital, acetaminophen, and caffeine preparation with codeine and opioids increased. In an effort to treat the headaches more effectively, the patient was prescribed meprobamate, 400 mg, three times a day, and there was a significant reduction in the codeine and opioid use. He also stopped taking didanosine. His headache episodes decreased significantly since then.

Questions about Case 1

- Are all HIV-related headaches due to secondary infection or could they be due to to the HIV infection itself?
- Can reccurent headaches in patients with HIV be controlled effectively with analgesic medications?
- Is there an association between HIV-associated headache and the medications used to treat HIV?
- Does dementia play a role in the onset of headache in patients with HIV?

Case 2 History

The second case is that of a 38-year-old male who was diagnosed with HIV infection in 1984, when he was 24 years old. His past medical history is significant for multiple head injuries, throughout his life, resulting in chronic headaches. His first head injury occurred at age 7 years when he was hit by a piece of concrete. Later, he suffered seven more head injuries, all from motor vehicle accidents. Other symptoms include tinnitus at the age of 19, and right-sided Bell's palsy for 6 months followed by left-sided palsy with a residual effect on the left side at the age of 21. The patient was noted also to have scintillations that were greater on the left side.

In 1994, his chronic headache changed. He noted that his headaches were increasing in frequency and duration; they usually started in the afternoon and were triggered by stress. The headache was located over the bifrontal, temporal, and occipital regions of the head. The pain was throbbing and stabbing in nature. The patient also noted that photophobia and phonophobia accompanied the headache. When seen at our office, he was using an ASA and oxycodone preparation and a combination of ASA, butalbital, and caffeine with codeine to treat his headache, without any success. He was also on atenolol, 50 mg every night at bedtime and was also using sertraline and clonazepam for depression. The patient was advised to increase his dose of atenolol to 100 mg every night at bedtime, and amitriptyline was added in a dosage of 25 to 50 mg daily, which resulted in significant improvement in the headache problem.

Recently, he was assaulted while walking on the street. The assault resulted in a right frontal head laceration and daily headache. The computed tomography (CT) scan done to rule out a subdural hematoma was normal.

Questions about Case 2

• Can HIV infection affect the pattern of a pre-existing headache?
• Is there any interaction between the medications used to treat HIV infection and those used to treat headache?
• What is the role of head trauma in the evolution of HIV-associated headache?
• What is the relationship between Bell's palsy, HIV infection, and HIV-associated headache?

Case Discussion

Neurologists will be evaluating a large number of the currently asymptomatic HIV-1 infected patients with a new complaint of headache. In the past, HIV-associated headache was thought to be mainly secondary or organic. As the disease continues to change in its evolution and pattern, more primary HIV-associated headaches are being reported. The first case is a clear-cut example of this type of headache. It is also evident that the medication regimen of this patient played a significant role in the headache condition. Later in the evolution of his illness, there was also concern that dementia and/or cerebral atrophy might be contributing to the headache problem by virtue of a secondary process. This was not found to be the case. The introduction of an anxiolytic agent, meprobamate, resulted in significant reduction in the use of opioids and other analgesics.

The second case is that of a pre-existing muscle-contraction and migraine headache condition which changed significantly over the course of the HIV infection. Modifications in the therapy for both the muscle-contraction-type headache and the migraine-type headache resulted in improvement in both conditions.

Neither of the cases reported here revealed any type of opportunistic infection or tumor, confirming more recent reports of a changing distribution of the headache associated with HIV infection.

Overview of Headache Associated with HIV Infection

An estimated 1 to 2 million people in the United States are currently infected with HIV-1. In 1995, HIV-1 infection was still the leading cause of death in males aged from 25 to 44 despite the substantial decrease in death rate among people with acquired immunodeficiency syndrome (AIDS).

HIV-1 is a neurotropic virus that can readily invade the central nervous system causing a variety of neurologic disorders. These disorders (Table 37–1) may present as an early finding of the disease or more commonly as a late finding. They are associated with a wide spectrum of symptoms.

One of the most common of these symptoms is headache. Goldstein was the first to report on the importance of HIV-associated headache in the early 1990s. The exact prevalence rate of headache in HIV-1 infection is still unknown. However, there is a predictable increase in the prevalence of headache in the HIV-infected population versus the general population. Recent studies indicate that about 50% of all patients with HIV infection will present with headache at some time during the course of the disease.

HIV-related headaches can be due to HIV-1 infection itself or more commonly to the HIV-associated neurologic disorders. Increased rates of anxiety and depression also act as comorbid factors that increase the prevalence of headache in HIV-infected patients. In addition, the higher prevalence of substance abuse in the HIV-infected population can result in headache associated with the substances or their withdrawal. Late in the disease, medications used to treat HIV infection or its complications can cause headache. Diagnostic procedures may also increase the prevalence of headache in the HIV-infected population.

During HIV-1 infection, pre-existing migraine headache tends to decrease in frequency. Evers et al. reported in 1998 that HIV infection causes a reduction in the migraine-specific neurogenic inflammation of the cerebral vessels. In contrast, pre-existing tension-type headache tends to increase in frequency, partially due to a significant incidence of aseptic meningitis.

Primary HIV-Associated Headache

In recent years, a primary type of headache that is associated with HIV-1 infection is being recognized as a distinct clinical entity. Brew and Miller reported in a retrospective study that acute aseptic meningitis was associated with primary HIV-1 infection. It has been estimated to occur in about 2% of all HIV-1 infections. Acute aseptic meningitis can occur as early as at seroconversion and is usually self-limited but can recur later at any time during the disease. Other causes of primary headache in HIV-1 infection include late-stage HIV-related headache without pleocytosis and chronic headache with a persistent pleocytosis. This kind of headache is usually generalized or unilateral and is not accompanied by nausea, thus resembling tension-type headache.

Primary HIV-associated headache is thought to occur through several mechanisms. One possible mechanism is the alteration of the central pain mechanisms at the level of neurotransmission. This mechanism has been suggested along with the discovery of a definite alteration in serotonin and tryptophan metabolism in HIV infection. Another mechanism proposed is the neurotoxic effect of substances released by HIV-infected macrophages. This mechanism was postulated originally to explain the dementia and neuropathy associated with HIV infection. The precise mechanism of primary HIV-associated headaches, however, remains obscure.

Analgesics can be used to treat the primary headache of HIV infection. Antidepressants in moderate doses are also effective in treating primary HIV-associated headache. It is known that certain analgesics interact with drugs used to treat HIV infection. Acetaminophen and indomethacin decrease the blood levels of zidovudine. On the other hand, valproic acid increases zidovudine blood levels.

TABLE 37–1. HIV-1-Infection-Associated Neurologic Disorders

Etiology	Disorder
Infection	Aseptic meningitis
	Cryptococcal meningitis
	Cerebral toxoplasmosis
	Progressive multifocal leukoencephalopathy
	Cytomegalovirus encephalitis
	Cytomegalovirus polyradiculopathy
	Cytomegalovirus mononeuritis multiplex
Neoplasm	Primary central nervous system lymphoma
	Metastatic lymphoma
Systemic	Hypoxic encephalopathy
	Sepsis
	Stroke
Functional	Anxiety disorder
	Psychotic depression
Primary aids	AIDS dementia complex
	Distal sensory polyneuropathy
Autoimmune	Guillain-Barré syndrome
	Chronic inflammatory demyelinating polyneuropathy

Secondary HIV-Related Headache

This kind of headache tends to occur later in the disease. Opportunistic infections and tumors are the most likely causes. The most important opportunistic infections are cryptococcal meningitis and toxoplasmosis. The most important tumor associated with HIV infection is primary central nervous system lymphoma. HIV-related headache secondary to opportunistic infection is usually constant and gradual in onset. It is also associated with fever, nausea, and vomiting. HIV-related headache secondary to a space-occupying lesion is usually variable in onset and associated with focal neurologic deficits.

Headache can also be secondary to systemic illness. Patients with *Pneumocystis carinii* pneumonia (PCP) may complain of headache initially before other symptoms such as dyspnea or cough occur. Syphilitic meningitis can present at any time during the course of HIV infection and may be associated with headache. Increased sinusitis is common with HIV infection and is another cause of secondary headache, occurring in 33 to 50% of patients.

Medications used in the treatment of HIV-1 infection or its complications can cause headache. Headache is one of the side effects of antiretroviral medications used to treat HIV-1 infection. Zidovudine was shown to induce headache in up to 50% of patients using the medication. This can result in decreased compliance. The high prevalence of painful conditions associated with the HIV-infected population, including peripheral neuropathy, predisposes that group to analgesic abuse, which, when present and untreated, can induce headache.

New-onset headache in the late stages of HIV infection should always raise the possibility of an opportunistic infection or tumor. An MRI and a CT scan should be done for HIV-associated headache occurring late in the disease. A lumbar puncture is also indicated for cerebrospinal fluid analysis and measuring pressure. The incidence of lumbar puncture headache is lower in HIV-infected patients due to the pathophysiologic changes in the brain caused by the HIV infection.

Selected Readings

Brew BJ, Miller J. Human immunodeficiency virus-related headache. Neurology 1993;43:1098–100.

Centers for Disease Control. Update: mortality attributable to HIV infection among persons aged 25–44 years—United States, 1991 and 1992. MMWR Morb Mortal Wkly Rep 1993;42:869–72.

Centers for Disease Control. Update: trends in AIDS incidence, deaths, and prevalence—United States, 1996. MMWR Morb Mortal Wkly Rep 1997;46:165–73.

Epstein LG, Gendelman HE. Human immunodeficiency virus type 1 infection of the nervous system: pathogenetic mechanisms. Ann Neurol 1993;33:429–36.

Evers S, Brilla R, Husstedt I. Headache and human immunodeficiency virus infection—a systemic review. Headache Q 1998;9;129–33.

Fuchs D, Möller AA, Reibnegger G, et al. Decreased serum tryptophan in patients with HIV-1 infection correlates with increased serum neopterin and with neurologic/psychiatric symptoms. J Acquir Immune Defic Syndr 1990;3:873–6.

Goldstein J. Headache and acquired immunodeficiency syndrome. Neurol Clin 1990;8:947–60.

Holloway RG, Kieburtz KD. Headache and the human immunodeficiency virus type 1 infection. Headache 1995;35:245–55.

Katz DA, Berger JR, Duncan RC. Neurosyphilis. A comparative study of the effects of infection with human immunodeficiency virus. Arch Neurol 1993;50:243–9.

Levy RM, Bredesen DE, Rosenblum ML. Neurological manifestations of the acquired immunodeficiency syndrome (AIDS). J Neurosurg 1985;62:457–95.

Lipton RB, Feraru ER, Weiss G, et al. Headache in HIV-1-related disorders. Headache 1991;31:518–22.

Markowitz JC, Rabkin JG, Perry SW. Treating depression in HIV-positive patients. AIDS 1994;8:403–12.

McArthur JC. Neurological diseases associated with human immunodeficiency virus type 1 infection. In: Johnson RT, Griffin JW, editors. Current therapy in neurological disease. 4th ed. St. Louis (MO): Mosby-Year Book, Inc.; 1993. p. 146–52.

O'Neil WM, Sherrard JS. Pain in human immunodeficiency virus disease: a review. Pain 1993;54:3–14.

Price RW. Management of the neurologic complications of HIV-1 infection and AIDS. In: Sande MA, Volbberding PA, editors. The medical management of AIDS. 5th ed. Philadelphia: WB Saunders; 1997. p. 197–216.

Richmond DD, Fischl MA, Greico MH, et al. The toxicity of azidothymidine (AZT) in the treatment of patients with AIDS and AIDS-related complex. N Engl J Med 1987;317:192–7.

Sanford JP, Sande MA, Gilbert DN, Gerberding JL. Guide to HIV/AIDS therapy. Dallas (TX): Antimicrobial Therapy, Inc.; 1993. p. 95–9.

Singer ES, Kim J, Fahy-Chandon B, et al. Headache in ambulatory HIV-1-infected men enrolled in a longitudinal study. Neurology 1996;46:487–94.

Small CB, Kaufman A, Armenaka M, Rosenstreich DL. Sinusitis and atopy in human immunodeficiency virus infection. J Infect Dis 1993;167:283–90.

Editorial Comments

The challenge to neurologists in evaluating patients with HIV infection is to diagnose and exclude serious secondary causes of headache and to help with their management. Exacerbation of common primary headache disorders is emphasized in Dr. Goldstein's second case. However, the first case represents an increasingly more common headache seen in HIV patients, that of primary HIV-associated headache. This entity requires special attention and must be differentiated from all other types of headache in HIV patients. Once recognized, it usually can be managed successfully, as in the case presented.

The Patient with Bruxism and Headache

Sheldon G. Gross, DDS

Case History

Since the age of 12, this 18-year-old woman has periodically ground her teeth. She generally knows when she bruxes, because she awakens with a headache that is usually confined to her temples, face, and neck. If the headache is mild, it subsides following a hot shower. Occasionally, the headache is more intense, lasting 1 or 2 days. During these times, chewing aggravates her symptoms, also causing her jaw to ache.

Three years ago, the patient awakened with a more intense headache. Even though her jaw was sore, she joined her family for a barbecue. Her mouth opening was somewhat restricted and chewing was painful. Not being a complainer, she suffered through the meal. The increased pain lasted all evening. Although the intensity decreased, her jaw ache never fully subsided. The dull ache was present on awakening and progressively worsened throughout the day. She stopped chewing gum and avoided eating large sandwiches. She consulted with her physician and an otolaryngologist because she was concerned about frequent sinus and earaches. Sometimes, her teeth even hurt but all her medical and dental evaluations were negative. When she experienced additional symptoms of tinnitus and blurred vision, a more thorough medical work-up included a brain magnetic resonance imaging (MRI) scan and a Lyme test; both were normal. Her complaints were now daily and extended into her neck, often worsening with reading or working at her computer.

During her college interviews, at the start of her senior year, she awakened sensing that her jaw was "stuck." She experienced no pain, but her mouth opening was notably limited until she provoked a right temporomandibular joint (TMJ) noise. Full range was immediately restored, and no additional joint noises occurred for the remainder of the day. She began to experience this same problem most mornings, until it eventually became a daily occurrence. As the problem progressed, opening her mouth on awakening became more difficult. Some mornings, the resistance to opening was so great, that she needed to first "pop" her jaw, a painful maneuver that sometimes provoked a headache similar to the ones which accompany her menstrual cycle. This 1-day pounding pain was accompanied by photophobia, sonophobia, nausea, and vomiting. A codeine/ASA/butalbital compound, prescribed by her family doctor, or sleep were her only means of relief.

The patient's joint noise now occurs daily, and no longer just on awakening. For the past 6 months, all jaw openings have been accompanied by a subtle, right TMJ clicking noise, followed by a second quieter noise when she closes her mouth. Her headaches have worsened on the right side. At times, chewing provokes a louder noise, that others can hear. Her TMJ may even "catch" forcing her to wiggle it or push on the right side of her jaw in order to fully open her mouth. She has now confined her diet to softer foods. Foods that are difficult to chew now trigger sharp, stabbing ear pains, which are often a precursor to a more intense, throbbing headache.

With the increased frequency of clicking, she experiences more right ear and periorbital aches. Her headaches are more global, and she now takes over-the-counter medications for partial relief.

Questions about This Case

- What is the probable cause of this patient's bitemporal and frontal morning headaches?
- What are the different diagnostic considerations?
- Why are her migraines becoming more frequent?
- What is the relationship between her headaches and jaw dysfunction?
- How would you have managed this case at the beginning?
- How would you manage it now?
- What long-term strategies would apply to this patient?

Case Discussion

The patient's history may appear as a group of unrelated problems but, actually, it portrays several of the more common temporomandibular joint dysfunction (TMD) symptoms. She initially suffered from a myalgia that became compounded by a true joint arthropathy. Her first symptom was that of a dull headache that subsided with a hot shower. Infrequently, her headache lasted all day.

The first major change occurred when she awakened with a sore jaw and nevertheless decided to attend the family barbecue. Her pain became daily and intensified as the day progressed. Next, she awakened with a joint noise that became a forerunner of a temporomandibular disk derangement. As her symptoms increased in frequency, she also experienced an increase in her tension-type and migraine headaches. The finding that her symptoms occurred on awakening and, initially, were not present during the day, points to an association with nocturnal events. It seems logical to pursue the relationship between her sleep disturbance and jaw dysfunction influencing both types of headaches. Her case is much easier to understand if her symptoms are divided into separate myalgia and temporomandibular joint discussions.

Myalgia

She initially awakened with a dull morning headache that responded to a hot shower, which is characteristic of muscular soreness. Her symptoms were infrequent and indicative of nocturnal clenching causing muscle fatigue, a condition which decreases rapidly when the provoking exercise is stopped. Although, in the past, morning complaints like hers were usually attributed to muscle spasm, current studies show that increased electromyogram (EMG) activity is not present when the involved muscles are at rest, thus ruling out a true myospasm. The hypothesis of TMD being perpetuated by a pain/muscle hyperactivity cycle has never been proved, and, in fact, research tends to show that pain is inhibiting, rather than stimulating, to muscle.

Her form of myalgia has been referred to as delayed-onset muscle soreness or postexercise muscle pain. Even though algesiogenic substances such as bradykinins and substance P are released, local cellular changes characteristic of an inflammatory process are not evident and no change in EMG activity of the sore muscles has been observed. Presenting symptoms of muscle stiffness, palpable tenderness, and pain with active muscular contractions are seen in episodic bruxers and are believed to occur because a poorly exercised muscle is overexerted. Those individuals who grind their teeth on a daily or almost daily basis, like anyone who exercises every day, develop muscles that are capable of adapting to larger demands, without pain. Although inflammation in post-exercise muscle soreness is not evident at the clinical level, changes of the Z-bands have been observed at the ultrastructural level; this is believed to be due to overloading muscles unaccustomed to heavy exercise. During treatment, emphasis must be placed on decreasing muscle soreness and its cause. Medications that influence sleep and nocturnal bruxism may be necessary to facilitate recovery in a refractory patient.

Nocturnal bruxism (NB) is the nocturnal clenching, grinding, or gnashing of the teeth during nonfunctional movements of the mandible. Nocturnal bruxism is an orofacial motor disorder and should not be confused with other facial movement activities such as sleeptalking, grunting, or alternating jaw opening and closing. Lavigne and Montplaisir (1995) recommend that "phasic jaw muscle activity, in the absence of obvious tooth grinding or contact, be named rhythmic masticatory muscle activity." Nocturnal bruxism usually occurs in sleep stages I and II as well as in rapid eye movement (REM) sleep, often when a person is transitioning from a deeper to lighter sleep. It is believed to function as part of an arousal mechanism and is rare in sleep stages III and IV. The American Sleep Disorders Association refers to bruxing as a "parasomnia" rather than a sleep disorder. Parasomnias are considered an episodic disorder of sleep that occurs during arousal, partial arousal, or sleep-stage transition.

During NB, masseter muscle contractions occur equally in both muscles as opposed to the greater unilateral muscle loading seen when grinding occurs in the awakened state. This important finding offers additional support that NB is a central mechanism and is different from diurnal bruxism. Nocturnal bruxism decreases with age and may be influenced by other factors such as drugs, disease, and personality. For example, alcohol has been shown to interfere with sleep and increase bruxism. Therefore, the recommendation of a glass of wine at bedtime to enhance sleep is incorrect and actually contraindicated.

The tricycic antidepressant medications, such as amitriptyline, doxepin, and nortriptyline, have been shown to decrease REM and enhance delta sleep making this family of medications effective in reducing symptoms of NB. Cyclobenzaprine is related to the tricyclic antidepressants, which may explain why this medication has also been found effective. Benzodiazepines exhibit good muscle-relaxant properties but are not analgesics. They influence sleep onset by causing sedation, but they prolong REM latency, increase stage II sleep, and decrease stage IV sleep. Some benzodiazepine studies imply a decrease in central serotonin levels, possibly predisposing the patient to a future sleep disturbance or other decreased serotonin problems. These effects occur in concert with the typical adverse reactions associated with benzodiazepines.

No single panacea exists for treating NB. Medications may be used to modify sleep habits, allowing for an immediate approach to symptom reduction. When effective, a nocturnal appliance offers a nonpharmacologic approach to reducing morning TMD complaints. Night bruxing appliances have been popularized by dentists as an effective treatment modality used to minimize morning TMD symptoms. The success of these appliances has been attributed to both psychologic and to mechanical benefits. The results have been shown to be as or more effective than other treatments, and appliances may offer a rapid nonmedicinal approach to symptomatic relief. Behavioral approaches, which usually do not produce immediate results, may influence sleep onset by altering the patient's responses to daytime stress or by modifying habits that interfere with sleep. Although stress is not considered a cause of bruxism, some studies that monitor bruxing activity portray a strong temporal pattern concomitant with stressful events.

A close association between NB and TMD symptoms has been shown in many studies, and the consistency of these reports imply causality. Nevertheless, the true relationship between the two conditions may not be fully established and the association may not be as simplistic as that presented above. Temporomandibular joint dysfunction has been shown to be a complex condition resulting from numerous predisposing and initiating factors, one of which may be NB.

After this patient's barbecue experience, her complaints transformed from being a morning problem to a dull ache that lasted all day. Her symptoms now worsened as the day progressed. She developed additional complaints ranging from blurred vision to earaches. The various complaints may seem unrelated but are typical for TMD patients and are characteristic of masticatory myofascial pain. Myofascial pain occurs in any skeletal muscle, but is often improperly referred to as myofacial pain when it is present in the head region.

Myofascial pain (MFP) is a regional muscle disorder, typified by a dull aching pain and tender sites capable of producing pain reference to nondermatomic areas. Myofascial pain usually begins with a definable onset and often a recognizable cause. The onset of this patient's progressive pains began after the barbecue. She also developed other related symptoms, such as blurred vision, tinnitus, and ear pains. These new complaints can be explained by current concepts that pertain to "convergence." Convergence may occur via afferent, efferent, and/or autonomic routes. This is how symptoms can spread or be referred to a region remote from the original source. Studies have already shown that multiple neuronal inputs may converge upon one dorsal horn neuron. In MFP, symptoms are experienced in other areas because the converging transmissions not only originate from nociceptors in the painful muscle, but also from other locations such as the skin, viscera, and joints. Under normal conditions, it is believed that some converging connections cannot be activated except during certain pathologic states, helping to explain why not every muscle pain is referred. Mense (1995) has offered other possible explanations to further clarify convergence. For example, ineffective or "somatotopically inappropriate" connections occur between certain neighboring neurons carrying input from different muscles. Under routine function, weak or normal stimuli from one neuron do not excite the neighboring nerve cells. On the other hand, strong or long-lasting stimuli may excite or lead to subthreshold depolarization of these adjacent neurons making them more excitable.

Symptoms from MFP sensory convergence include ear and head pains referred from some masticatory and cervical muscles. Motor symptoms are usually exemplified by muscle twitching or tightness. Autonomic complaints are varied and have been shown by Travell and Simons (1983) to present in the facial region as tearing, ear fullness or blockage, dizziness, tinnitus, and/or sinus congestion. It is generally believed that the myofascial trigger point must be treated before total resolution of the symptoms can occur. Frequently, when improperly treated, the myofascial trigger point may change from an active to a latent state where it remains asymptomatic until an event such as stress or trauma initiates a recurrence.

Myofascial pain improves with local therapies as long as the source of pain has been removed. The patient's initial complaints of bilateral, dull, temporal, and frontal headaches, as well as episodic ear-

aches, are characteristic of referred symptoms from masticatory muscles. As her symptoms expand, she complains of dizziness and facial fullness, described as sinus discomfort. Sinus congestion may even occur. Her symptoms worsen as the day progresses, and increase with provocation so that simple activities are now capable of increasing her pain. This response contrasts with her initial symptoms of postexercise muscle soreness which decreased as the day progressed.

According to Travell and Simons, the following muscles are each capable of causing pain reference with symptoms characteristic of a tension-type headache: masseter, temporal, trapezius, occipital, suboccipital, sternocleidomastoid, occipitofrontal, and the semispinal muscles of the neck and head. Any of these muscles may be involved as a primary source of myofascial pain. The finding that so many muscles can produce similar symptoms makes it easy to appreciate the confusion in establishing the role of TMD as a cause of tension-type headache. This confusion becomes more apparent when we realize that studies show that 75% of TMD patients complain of recurrent headaches as opposed to 20% of the general population.

As with tension-type headaches, stress may inappropriately be defined as a cause of TMD. A small population of TMD patients may demonstrate a specific, reproducible, muscular response to stress (response specificity), in much the same way as certain patients with lower back problems experience increasing back pain, but efforts to use EMG recordings during stress to distinguish headache from nonheadache patients have been unsuccessful. Supporting this concept is the finding that muscle hyperactivity does not seem to be a predisposing factor for TMD symptoms. In any case, as with all musculoskeletal complaints, stress may generate an exaggerated response or worsen symptoms.

Treatment of myofascial pain involves eliminating the cause, modifying behaviors that perpetuate symptoms, restoring muscle length, and minimizing discomfort. The patient's sleep habits, daytime activities, and stresses must be reviewed. Factors that have a negative impact on sleep, such as caffeine intake and other dietary habits, may need to be quantified. Physical therapy and exercise may be necessary to restore muscle length. Symptoms that do not respond initially may need to be treated more aggressively. The judicious use of trigger-point injections has been shown to facilitate recovery.

Temporomandibular Joint

The first indication that the patient may be developing a true joint derangement occurs when she begins awakening with a subtle joint "catching." Initially, the noise is only present on awakening, and the description of the noise implies that the articular disk in the right joint is adhering slightly to the articular eminence (sometimes referred to as a "suction-cup effect"). Disk "sticking," in this situation, is believed to occur from alterations in the synovial fluid and/or pressure as a result of sustained nocturnal clenching. Opening her mouth dislodges the disk, allowing joint lubrication to occur, so that the joint function remains symptom free for the remainder of the day. The wear and tear of persistent disk sticking slowly results in the development of minor surface irregularities within the joint.

Treatment for articular disk sticking depends upon the cause, frequency, and severity of the condition. Infrequent morning catching may only require monitoring. When a patient is symptomatic, as portrayed when the patient needed to painfully "pop" her jaw, treatment approaches may include medications to decrease nocturnal bruxing and clenching, behavioral modification, and/or the fabrication of a nocturnal appliance.

A further review of the patient's history reveals progressive worsening of her TMJ symptoms. Over time, she has found it consistently more difficult to dislodge the articular disk in the morning. Her maneuvers have caused repeated minor strains and trauma to the disk ligaments, resulting in ligamentous tears and elongation. Eventually, she developed a clicking noise occurring throughout the day, indicative of an articular disk displacement.

The TMJ is comprised of two separate joints: a lower hinge joint between the head of the condyle and the inferior surface of the articular disk and a sliding upper joint between the superior surface of the articular disk and the articular eminence. It may be easier to visualize the TMJ as a hinge joint within

a sliding socket. Disk displacement implies that irreversible changes have occurred in the ligaments attaching the disk to the condyle which allow the disk to be displaced usually anterior or anteromedial to the condyle. The noise the patient experiences occurs during mouth opening as the disk reduces to a more proper position when the condyle translates forward. A second, often very quiet, closing noise occurs when the teeth are near contact and the disk again dislocates. Since this problem is the result of irreversible alteration in the ligaments and possibly the disk shape, the noises continue to occur throughout the day.

Most patients are able to adapt to a reducing disk displacement. However, in some patients, disk displacement may progress allowing the disk to gradually assume a position further off the condyle, thus interfering with joint function. Pain usually occurs from strain to the collateral disk ligaments and tears within the highly vascular, innervated posterior disk attachment. Often, this condition is self-limiting, and the disk eventually becomes dislocated and afunctional. Sometimes the repetitive trauma to the posterior attachment tissues may result in tissue alteration and the formation of a "pseudo" disk. Many patients suffer from joint noises that have been shown not to require treatment but other patients experience severe pain, joint inflammation, and adhesions. Random MRI studies have shown that as many as 34% of asymptomatic patients may have a disk displacement but the percentage increases to 86% in symptomatic patients.

The loss of the cushioning effect of the fibrous articular disk is often accompanied by degenerative joint changes, believed to be due to the change of biomechanics. If the changes have accompanying inflammation causing pain, treatment is indicated. Patients present with point tenderness over the joint, pain with function, and a limited range of motion. Treatment of these symptoms should also include ruling out the systemic arthritides and other causes of joint inflammation such as Lyme disease. Patients with symptoms of osteoarthritis should be placed on a soft diet and encouraged to function within a pain-free range of motion. NSAIDs may help the inflammation. When refractory, a steroid injection into the joint may be beneficial.

The term osteoarthrosis is often used to describe the noninflammatory, degenerative changes within a joint. Osteoarthrosis may follow osteoarthritis, or occur as a result of mechanical overloading of the TMJ. The patient may present with joint crepitus and a painless limitation of range of jaw motion. Treatment is only necessary when structural changes or limitations in function are necessary for proper function.

The patient first develops joint pain when she must "pop" her jaw in the morning. Her pain results from strained collateral disk ligaments that trigger an intense headache with the characteristics of a migraine. Peripheral trigeminal pains have been shown to influence the frequency of migraine headaches. Temporomandibular joint and muscle pains are sources of deep somatic pain and, along with other facial pains such as an otitis or sinusitis, are peripheral trigeminal sources capable of triggering a migraine in a migraineur. Her menstrual migraines have laid the foundation for her propensity toward this increase in headaches.

As the patient's right joint condition progresses, the articular disk ligaments elongate, allowing for greater disk displacement with mouth closure. During chewing, rapid changes in the intra-articular pressure may result in the articular disk being forcibly displaced or reduced, causing louder clicking noises. Most patients can sense a disk displacement as it produces pressure and discomfort as well as the urge to correct the altered disk position. Often the disk is displaced medially as well as anteriorly and patients find that pressing on the lateral surface of the jaw helps them to reduce the disk or relieve the pressure within the joint. This patient feels the need to wiggle her jaw or push on her face. Now she avoids chewing hard foods for fear of producing joint pain and provoking a migraine headache. She experiences sharp ear pains on chewing that, most probably, result from strained disk ligaments and pressure against the highly vascular and innervated posterior disk attachment. As her joint symptoms become constant, the pain continuity of the arthralgia becomes a source of trigeminal nerve input and a significant contributing factor for increasing both migraine and tension type-headache symptoms.

Overview of Temporomandibular Joint Dysfunction

Temporomandibular joint dysfunction (TMD) is a broad term used to identify a group of medical and dental conditions with overlapping signs and symptoms. The term includes the primary and secondary causes of jaw dysfunction problems that range from developmental anomalies to the arthritides and myalgias. The tissues that may be affected include the TMJ, muscles of mastication, and adjacent structures. The main signs and symptoms are pain and tenderness in the face, head, neck, and shoulders as well as in the temporomandibular joints. The severity may range from barely noticeable to debilitating. The estimated prevalence in the general population has been reported to be 6% with a minimum ratio of 3:1 of women seeking treatment over men.

Temporomandibular joint dysfunction may occur independently of headache symptoms or as a comorbid condition. Confusion often exists regarding the primary diagnosis, as any source of deep somatic pain may be accompanied by a secondary myalgia. Therefore, it is not uncommon for such diverse conditions as migraine headache, otalgia, pharyngitis, sinusitis, and toothache to present with symptoms characteristic of TMD. Conversely, peripheral trigeminal pains, including TMD, may trigger or increase the frequency of migraine or tension-type headaches as well as mimic other medical illnesses. Temporomandibular joint dysfunction therefore, has garnered the reputation of being yet another condition labeled as "a great impostor" with myriad presenting complaints, such as headaches, earaches, neck aches, eye pains, lightheadedness, or sinus congestion with or without the symptoms of jaw noise, pain, or limitation.

This dysfunction may also have a close relationship with cervical symptoms. Both conditions may occur separately or concomitantly as two independent illnesses responsible for causing pains in the jaw, head, and/or neck regions. For example, cervical myofascial trigger points, as mentioned earlier, frequently refer pains into the head and facial region. Furthermore, anesthesia of a trapezius myofascial trigger point has been shown to effect a decrease in ipsilateral masseter muscle EMG activity. Studies with animals show that deep posterior cervical muscle inflammation is accompanied by increased masseter muscle tension. Pharyngeal pain or ninth nerve irritations are both capable of causing ear and face complaints. The dermatomes of C2 and C3 may encompass the ears, the angle of the mandible and the mandibular border, and the cervical nerves that innervate the infrahyoid and geniohyoid muscles. Cervical flexion/extension injuries show a higher incidence of limited jaw mobility and facial pain. Conversely, studies show an increased prevalence of cervical symptoms in patients diagnosed with TMD as compared to controls. Other studies show a decrease in cervical complaints with TMD treatment. Thermography studies of patients with unilateral TMD symptoms reveal increased bilateral trapezius muscle temperatures. The first synapse of trigeminal afferent fibers occurs in the trigeminal spinal tract nucleus which extends caudally to the region of the upper cervical nerves and is structurally similar to the dorsal horn of the spinal cord. Communication between cervical and trigeminal neurons has been shown to occur. Therefore, the practitioner must take a careful history in order to differentiate between head, neck, and face pains that result from primary TMD, primary cervicogenic, or unrelated causes of facial pain. The American Academy of Orofacial Pain has published its recommended guidelines for obtaining a basic history and clinical examination information, which can be found in Appendix 38–1.

Management Strategies

Management always begins with a thorough history and clinical evaluation. The goals should be similar to those for other orthopedic disorders. Predisposing, initiating, and perpetuating causes of TMD must be assessed. Developmental or biomechanical abnormalities, genetic predisposition, medical illnesses, nutritional deficiencies, and psychologic factors illustrate predisposing conditions of concern. Macrotrauma or microtrauma are the most common initiating events. Macrotrauma usually occurs as a single event, ranging from external trauma to the face to intubation during general anesthesia. Microtrauma is really a situation of

repetitive loading, and, as such, is frequently overlooked as an initiating factor. Gum chewing, bruxing, and nail biting have all been discussed as initiating factors.

Perpetuating conditions interfere with or complicate treatment. Included are various conditions such as illness, sleep disturbances, oral habits, and attitude. In many instances, the same condition may serve as a predisposing, initiating, or perpetuating cause depending upon the circumstances.

The majority of patients suffering from TMD achieve good relief with reversible, conservative measures such as a soft diet, moist heat, and avoiding trigger factors such as gum chewing. Occasionally, TMD symptoms may be cyclical, thereby confusing patient management, as symptoms may regress spontaneously and not as a result of therapy. Some TMD conditions, like osteoarthritis, usually require a limited period of management. Other conditions, such as rheumatoid arthritis, are recurrent problems, requiring intermittent palliative therapy. Irreversible procedures, such as surgery or changes in occlusion, should never be considered as an alternative to a poor response to treatment. When a patient with a musculoskeletal problem fails to respond in a predictable manner, the diagnosis and treatment must be reassessed. A poor response may often stem from comorbid conditions such as fibromyalgia and migraine headaches, or may reflect contributing factors such as occupational or oral habits. For example, treatment of jaw muscle pain and tension with physical therapy or muscle-relaxant medication will be ineffective or only palliative when rebound headache symptoms are also present and are not addressed.

When TMJ derangements do not respond to conservative measures and contributing factors have been ruled out, more aggressive treatment approaches may be necessary. Invasive treatments include steroid injections, arthrocentesis, arthroscopy, and open joint procedures. The choice of an irreversible procedure, such as surgery or changes in occlusion, should not be based on a poor response to nonsurgical therapies but should be made after arriving at a specific diagnosis requiring such an intervention. Approximately 5% of TMD cases present with indications for surgical intervention that fulfill the criteria of moderate to severe refractory pain, disabling dysfunction, and/or evidence of pathologic conditions.

Because TMD is multifactorial, it requires a multidisciplinary approach. Treatment must take into consideration predisposing, initiating, and perpetuating factors, and may include any or all of the following strategies.

Education is a primary tool in the treatment of TMD. Patients must be reassured that TMD is a treatable condition. Many patients seeking treatment fear that as their pain is so terrible, it must stem from a brain tumor or other form of cancer. Patients need to be taught to recognize their habits, personal stresses, and trigger factors and to map out appropriate coping strategies. Patients with chronic conditions must recognize that their symptoms may recur because treatment goals may be palliative, not curative.

Pharmacotherapy often facilitates recovery by decreasing pain and inflammation, and by improving sleep. When a sleep disturbance is present, judicious use of tricyclic antidepressants or cyclobenzaprine at bedtime is often very effective. In certain circumstances, benzodiazepines such as clonazepam, have proved effective in decreasing nocturnal bruxism. Occasionally, other medications may actually contribute to or complicate treatment. For example, within the past few years, some selective serotonin reuptake inhibitors (SSRIs) have been implicated as actually being responsible for triggering the onset of NB in certain patients.

Physical therapy has been an effective adjunct to the treatment of TMD. However, care must be taken not to overtreat the patient, a situation which may arise when comorbid conditions prevent the patient from responding as expected. Ice, heat, exercise, and massage are a few effective home treatments. Physical therapy is most beneficial in reducing acute myofascial pain, providing palliation in chronic conditions through exercise, correcting general posture and work positions, and facilitating recovery by restoring the patient's range of motion after surgery.

The myofascial trigger point must be recognized as a source of localized, deep tenderness in a taut band of skeletal muscle or tendon that has the ability to refer pain in a nondermatomic distribution. The pattern of pain referral is reproducible, consistent, and serves as a guide to the knowledgeable clinician. Palpation of the trigger point yields the characteristic "jump sign" typified by flinching or a response of "That's it." Myofascial trigger points generally respond to stretching techniques when contributing or causative factors are eliminated. Prolonged pain may result in maladaptive behaviors that may need to be addressed before improvement occurs. When the trigger point is refractory to medical treatment, injecting steroids directly into it often yields good results.

Behavior therapy and psychotherapy have an impact on TMD treatment through several different channels. These approaches vary from addressing orofacial and parafunctional habits, such as pencil chewing and nail biting, to coping skills when a chronic problem interferes with home, work, and social activities. A poor response to treatment may be influenced by factors such as dysfunctional family situations, poor compliance, accompanying anxiety and/or depression, poor eating habits, and abuse or improper use of medications.

Although many studies have shown that dental appliances are effective in decreasing muscle hyperactivity, the explanations behind the success remain controversial. The following are some explanations that have been offered. (1) In cases of internal derangements, changing temporomandibular joint condylar position to accommodate swelling or to temporarily improve joint function and decrease noise yields good symptomatic relief which is, often sufficient to resolve the symptoms. (2) Studies have shown that a temporary increase in vertical dimension of the jaws (as happens with appliances) results in a temporary decrease in muscle hyperactivity. (3) Although occlusion is not considered to be a primary cause of TMD, excessive force during heavy clenching may play a secondary role, and appliances may improve occlusal stability. (4) The presence of an intraoral appliance creates a behavioral change or cognitive awareness by reminding the patient of functional and parafunctional habits. (5) Proprioception and delicate sensitivity of tooth to opposing tooth is altered by the appliance to that of a tooth against an opposing plastic surface. (6) Placebo effects occur with all treatment modalities, especially if an early doctor-patient rapport is established. (7) Appliances change peripheral sensory input and may, therefore, alter the influence of the central nervous system (CNS) on muscles, resulting in a central inhibitory effect.

Two basic types of TMD appliances are currently advocated by dentists. Although modifications occur, most appliances can be categorized as a stabilization or repositioning appliance.

A stabilization or muscle-relaxation appliance may fit over the mandibular or maxillary teeth, although maxillary appliances are more popular. Its treatment objective is to decrease muscle complaints or symptoms of minor joint pains. The design usually allows for one point of even contact with each posterior tooth of the opposing dental arch. Parafunctional activity and muscle hyperactivity have been shown to decrease with this mode of treatment. Although some patients may experience a reduction in symptoms with a soft appliance, evidence favors the use of hard appliances for the reduction of symptoms from parafunctional activity. Intraoral appliances, used for nocturnal bruxism, are similar in design to the stabilization appliance and have been effective in either reducing bruxism and/or relieving masticatory muscle pain.

The joint repositioning or anterior repositioning appliance has a built-in ramp that repositions the mandible in an anterior direction with the intention of correcting an anterior displaced articular disk. It can also reduce refractory joint pain and clicking secondary to an internal derangement or inflammation. Clicking is usually the most difficult symptom to treat. The primary intention of the repositioning appliance may not be to permanently alter the mandibular relationship, but to allow for healing or for a reduction of symptoms before permitting the lower jaw to again function in its prior occlusal relationship. Repositioning appliances have the potential for creating irreversible changes in occlusion that may initiate additional problems. Sometimes patients function extremely well in the new relationship and experience acute recurrences of pain when the new relationship is modified. In this situation, it may be more advantageous to maintain the new relationship by altering the patient's occlusion via orthodontic therapy or prosthetic restorations.

Case Summary

The patient's symptoms began as a morning problem that seemed to be associated with her sleep disturbance. Many of her complaints may have been minimized if early treatment had been provided. Medication could have offered early symptomatic relief but it is very likely that her symptoms would have recurred as soon as the medication was stopped. Recurring symptoms warrant a better long-term management approach for this young individual. When effective, an intraoral appliance minimizes future problems without medication. When these approaches prove inadequate, long-term considerations may include an evaluation at a sleep clinic or a more comprehensive cognitive-behavioral therapy. Not addressing her immediate complaints only led to additional problems that continued to escalate.

As this patient's symptoms have progressively worsened, she has experienced a gradual increase in both types of headache, which eventually resulted in her taking over-the-counter medications. Inevitably, she can be expected to receive a diagnosis of rebound headaches and/or transformed migraine headaches. Her treatment will, most probably, involve medications that may have an impact upon her sleep disturbance, also resulting in a reduction of complaints. A complicating factor that may interfere with recovery will be the degree of myofascial pain and temporomandibular joint disease.

Selected Readings

Fricton JR, Dubner, R, editors. Advances in pain research and therapy: orofacial pain and temporomandibular disorders. New York: Raven Press; 1994.

Lavigne GJ, Montplaisir JV. Bruxism: epidemiology, diagnosis, pathophysiology, and pharmacology. In: Fricton JR, Dubner R, editors. Orofacial pain and temporomandibular disorders. New York: Raven Press; 1995. p. 391.

Mense S. Mechanisms of pain in hindlimb muscles: experimental findings and open questions. In: Sessle BJ, Bryant PS, Dionne RA, editors. Temporomandibular disorders and related pain conditions. Seattle: IASP Press; 1995. p. 63.

National Institute of Health. Technology Assessment Conference Statement, Management of Temporomandibular Disorders, 4/29–5/1/96. Bethesda (MD): U.S. Department of Health and Human Services.

Okeson JP, editor. Management of temporomandibular disorders and occlusion. 3rd ed. Boston: Mosby; 1993.

Okeson JP, editor. Orofacial pain: guidelines for assessment, diagnosis and management. Chicago: Quintessence; 1996.

Pertes R, Gross S, editors. Clinical management of temporomandibular disorders and orofacial pain. Chicago: Quintessence; 1995.

Sessle BJ, Bryant PS, Dionne RA, editors. Progress in pain research and management: temporomandibular disorders and related pain conditions. Seattle: IASP Press; 1995.

Travell JG, Simons DG. Myofacial pain and dysfunction: the trigger point manual. Baltimore: Williams & Wilkins; 1983. p. 166.

Editorial Comments

For neurologists and most physicians who deal with headache patients, it can be exceedingly difficult to properly assess, diagnose, and treat patients who have predominant dental disorders and, in particular, temporomandibular joint dysfunction. In a very thorough and clear fashion, Dr. Gross overviews the latter condition in the context of the specific case he presents. Some will be entirely comfortable employing the management strategies outlined; most will benefit from the discussion and conservative opinions given; and all would be better off if they had the guidance and advice of an experienced colleague like the author in close proximity to their practice.

Appendix 38–1

Recommended Screening Questionnaire for TMD

1. Do you have difficulty, pain, or both when opening your mouth, for instance when yawning?
2. Do your jaws "get stuck" or "go out?"
3. Do you have difficulty, pain, or both when chewing, talking, or using your jaws?
4. Are you aware of noises in the jaw joints?
5. Do your jaws regularly feel stiff, tight, or tired?
6. Do you have pain in or about the ears, temples, or cheeks?
7. Do you have frequent headaches, neck aches, or toothaches?
8. Have you had a recent injury to your head, neck, or jaw?
9. Have you been aware of any recent changes in your bite?
10. Have you been treated previously for unexplained facial pain or a jaw joint problem?

Recommended Screening Examination Procedures for TMD

1. Measure range of motion and note any incoordination in movement of the mandible on opening and right and left lateral movement..
2. Palpate for preauricular tenderness.
3. Auscultate and/or palpate for sounds (e. g., clicking).
4. Palpate for tenderness in the masseter and temporalis muscles.
5. Inspect symmetry and alignment of the face and jaws.

International Headache Society Classification for Headache Disorders, Cranial Neuralgias, and Facial Pain

1. Migraine headache
2. Tension-type headache
3. Cluster headache and chronic paroxysmal hemicrania
4. Miscellaneous headaches, unassociated with structural lesion
5. Headache associated with head trauma
6. Headache associated with vascular disorders
7. Headache associated with nonvascular intracranial disorders
8. Headache associated with substances or their withdrawal
9. Headache associated with noncephalic infection
10. Headache associated with metabolic disorder
11. Headache or facial pain associated with disorder of cranium, neck, eyes, ears, nose, sinuses, teeth, mouth, or other facial or cranial structures
12. Cranial neuralgias, nerve trunk pain, and deafferentation pain
13. Headache not classified

Diagnostic Classification Recommended for the International Headache Society[*]

11.0 Headache or facial pain associated with disorder of cranium, neck, eyes, nose, sinuses, teeth, mouth, or other facial or cranial structures

11.1 Cranial bones including the mandible

11.2 Neck

11.3 Eyes

11.4 Ears

11.5 Nose and sinuses

11.6 Teeth and related oral structures

11.7 Temporomandibular joint

11.8 Masticatory muscle

Recommended diagnostic classification for:

11.1 Cranial bones including the mandible
- 11.1.1 Congenital and developmental disorders
  - 11.1.1.1. Aplasia
  - 11.1.1.2. Hypoplasia
  - 11.1.1.3. Hyperplasia
  - 11.1.1.4. Dysplasia
- 11.1.2 Acquired disorders
  - 11.1.2.1. Neoplasia
  - 11.1.2.2. Fracture

Recommended diagnostic classification for:

11.7 Temporomandibular joint articular disorders
- 11.7.1 Congenital or developmental disorders
  - 11.7.1.1 Aplasia
  - 11.7.1.2 Hypoplasia
  - 11.7.1.3 Hyperplasia
  - 11.7.1.4 Neoplasia
- 11.7.2 Disk derangement disorders
  - 11.7.2.1 Disk displacement with reduction
  - 11.7.2.2 Disk displacement without reduction
- 11.7.3 Temporomandibular joint dislocation
- 11.7.4 Inflammatory disorders
  - 11.7.4.1 Capsulitis/synovitis
  - 11.7.4.2 Polyarthritides
- 11.7.5 Osteoarthritis (noninflammatory disorders)
  - 11.7.5.1 Osteoarthritis: primary
  - 11.7.5.2 Osteoarthritis : secondary
- 11.7.6 Ankylosis
- 11.7.7 Fracture (condylar process)

11.8 Masticatory muscle disorders
- 11.8.1 Myofascial pain
- 11.8.2 Myositis
- 11.8.3 Myospasm
- 11.8.4 Local myalgia—unclassified
- 11.8.5 Myofibrotic contracture
- 11.8.6 Neoplasia

[*]From Okeson JP, editor. Orofacial pain: guidelines for assessment, diagnosis and management. Chicago: Quintessence; 1996. p.46–7.

CHAPTER 39

Two Patients with Headache and Systemic Symptoms

Oscar Bernal, MD

Patricia K. Coyle, MD

Case 1 History

This patient was a 35-year-old woman who had had headache for the last 3 months. It started 2 weeks after returning from a July vacation trip to Montauk, Long Island, when she spent a lot of time outdoors hiking and biking. Her headache began as part of an acute febrile illness (characterized by myalgias, chills, and a generalized malaise) that lasted for several days. She denied having had a recent insect bite or an unusual rash. Initially, the headache was sporadic occurring once or twice a week but for the last 2 months it had been present 24 hours a day. There were no associated visual symptoms. The pain had a pressure-like quality. It was mainly frontal but occasionally generalized. It was made worse by physical activity.

Although the headache was persistent, it did not interfere with the patient's job or prevent her from falling asleep. She rated the severity of her pain as mild, and she had been using over-the-counter medication with moderate relief. Her examination was normal, as was a noncontrast computed tomography (CT) scan of the brain. She was prescribed amitriptyline, 50 mg at bedtime, and given a follow-up appointment in 1 month.

On her return visit she reported some improvement in the headache intensity, although it was still present. She also reported new problems such as extreme fatigue and malaise, myalgias, and migratory joint pains, which involve the elbows, knees, and shoulder. Physical and neurologic examinations showed mild posterior cervical muscle tenderness. There was no joint swelling.

Questions about Case 1

- What is the differential diagnosis of this patient's headache problem?
- Would you ask any other questions?
- Are there any helpful clues in the history and examination?
- What further diagnostic procedures would you do?

Case 1 Discussion

This young woman had a chronic headache problem. The differential diagnosis involved both primary and secondary headache disorders. Primary disorders included a transformed-migraine problem (either drug induced or not drug related), chronic daily headache with pericranial muscle tenderness, and new daily persistent headache. Secondary disorders included post-traumatic, structural, metabolic, and infectious/inflammatory conditions.

A further history would be helpful. The physician would want to know whether there was a prior history of headaches or paroxysmal attacks as a child, and whether there was any family history of headaches. It was unlikely to be a vascular headache problem, as the patient's pain was mild, nonthrobbing, nonradiating or lateralizing, and was not associated with visual or gastrointestinal symptoms. Rebound headache was also improbable, since she was not using large quantities of analgesics. Her headache was not described as band-like, nor was it associated with a stiff neck, which pointed against a muscle-contraction problem. Primary chronic daily headache does not usually start abruptly. It generally results from analgesic abuse or psychiatric comorbidity in patients with chronic intermittent headache or migraines. None of these factors were present in this patient. Finally, the fact that her headache worsened with physical activity excluded a diagnosis of primary headache.

With regard to secondary headache, there was no history of prior physical trauma or head injury to suggest a post-traumatic disorder. Her normal examination and brain CT scan excluded structural problems such as brain tumor, foramen magnum lesion, or subdural hematoma. Metabolic causes also did not seem likely. Although formal blood work had not been done, there were no obvious indications of organ disease or a toxic condition from her history or her examination.

What was left was an infectious or inflammatory cause for her chronic headache. The fact that the problem began with a flu-like syndrome was highly suspicious for infection. Viruses are statistically the most common cause of such symptoms but they typically produce an acute monophasic syndrome, which spontaneously clears. In rare instances, prior viral infection can lead to a chronic vascular or muscle-contraction headache problem. This has been reported, for example, in some patients after Epstein-Barr virus infection; however, this patient did not seem to have a vascular or muscular-contraction problem.

The major red flag in this case was an epidemiologic clue. Her headache and flu-like illness began shortly after a summer vacation in an area where Lyme disease is highly endemic. A flu-like illness with sero-conversion is a recognized early infection syndrome (Table 39–1). The patient engaged in outdoor activities within this particular area, which is recognized as a major risk factor for Lyme-disease. It is not suprising that she did not recall a tick bite since only a minority of patients recall a bite. The disease vector, an Ixodes hard-body tick, is very small (poppy-seed size), has a painless bite, and is easy to miss.

The patient's later development of a multisymptom complex (profound fatigue, large joint arthralgias, myalgias) was nonspecific but certainly occurs in Lyme disease. Although she never noted the pathognomonic rash of erythema migrans (EM), 20 to 40% of patients either never develop or never see this rash.

Among the characteristic neurologic syndromes of Lyme disease is meningitis. Although typically acute, it can be chronic (defined as meningitis lasting a month or more). It is often mild, with minimal headache and stiff neck, and mimics a viral/aseptic process. Highly suggestive features of Lyme meningitis are associated unilateral or bilateral facial nerve palsy and associated painful radiculitis.

This patient showed none of these helpful signs. On her most recent examination, however, she had new neck pain. Although this could relate to muscular spasm, it could also suggest meningitis. The frontal and diffuse nature of her headache was certainly consistent with the headache seen in Lyme disease.

Other infections do need to be considered. The same tick vector that carries the Lyme disease spirochete *Borrelia burgdorferi* can also carry a parasite called *Babesia microti*, and a rickettsia-like agent which causes human granulocytic ehrlichiosis (HGE). The co-infection rate for *B. burgdorferi* and one of these other two pathogens ranges from 4 to 30%. Dual infections are significant because they lead to a more severe Lyme disease syndrome, one which is protracted and harder to treat.

Appropriate antibiotic therapy varies depending on the specific pathogen. *B. burgdorferi* infection is treated with oral agents such as amoxicillin, doxycycline, cefuroxime axetil, and intravenous third-generation cephalosporins such as ceftriaxone. Babesia infection is treated with a combination of clindamycin and quinine while Ehrlichia infection is treated with tetracycline agents such as doxycycline.

This patient had a very limited work-up. The brain CT scan ruled out any structural causes of headache. In retrospect, there was enough suspicion based on the initial history and examination to have considered neurologic Lyme disease as the explanation for her headache. A further work-up should include screening blood tests. In early Lyme disease, there may be mild elevations in sedimentation rate, liver enzymes, and quantitative IgM levels, and neurologic patients may have anticardiolipin IgM antibodies. Serology should be performed to look for *B. burgdorferi* antibodies. Since there is a high index of suspicion of Lyme disease, both a screening enzyme-linked immunosorbent assay (ELISA) and a confirmatory Western immunoblot should be done. At the same time, potential exposure to Babesia and Ehrlichia can be screened by checking serum antibodies to these agents.

Most importantly, a lumbar puncture is necessary to rule out Lyme meningitis. Cerebrospinal fluid (CSF) is sent for routine studies such as a cell count, and protein, glucose, and venereal disease research laboratory (VDRL). Other useful CSF studies can include an IgG index, oligoclonal bands, cytology, a Gram's stain, an acid-fast stain, and bacterial, mycobacterial, and fungal cultures. Specific CSF studies involve paired (CSF and serum) *B. burgdorferi* antibodies to look for intrathecal antibody production. Polymerase chain reaction (PCR) detects organism deoxyribonucleic acid (DNA), and this can also be done on CSF. Unfortunately, PCR has a low sensitivity (less than 40%) in neurologic Lyme disease.

This patient had serum antibodies to *B. burgdorferi*. Her positive ELISA was confirmed by Western immunoblot. The cerebrospinal fluid showed a white blood cell count (WBC) of 22 per cubic millimeter (all lymphocytes), consistent with meningitis. The level of protein in CSF was mildly elevated at 52 mg per deciliter, and glucose was normal at 65 mg per deciliter. All other CSF studies (including cultures) were negative. Intrathecal synthesis of *B. burgdorferi* antibodies was confirmed when a paired serology showed a higher ELISA titer in CSF than in serum. A diagnosis of Lyme meningitis was made, and the patient was treated with intravenous ceftriaxone (2 g once a day) for 4 weeks. Transient fever and worsening of flu-like symptoms developed

TABLE 39–1. Clinical Lyme Disease Syndromes

I. Early local infection (within 1 month)
- EM with or without constitutional symptoms

II. Early disseminated infection (within 3 months)
- Flu-like syndrome with seroconversion
- Skin: multifocal EM, lymphocytoma cutis in Europe
- Musculoskeletal: myalgias, brief arthritis
- Cardiac: AV block, pericarditis, myocarditis, arrythmias
- Ocular: conjunctivitis
- Neurologic: (Table 39–3)

III. Late-stage infection (after 3 months)
- Skin: acrodermatitis chronica atrophicans in Europe
- Musculoskeletal: episodic arthritis, chronic arthritis
- Ocular: episcleritis, keratitis, iridocyclitis, vitreitis, choroiditis, panuveitis
- Neurologic: (Table 39–3)

shortly after the first dose. These symptoms were felt to be a Jarisch-Herxheimer reaction, and were treated with acetaminophen. After the patient finished the course of antibiotics, her headache gradually cleared, and she was headache free by 3 months after therapy.

Case 2 History

This patient was a 23-year-old landscaper who presented 6 months ago with multifocal EM skin lesions and flu-like symptoms, including headache and a stiff neck. At that time IgM and IgG antibodies to *B. burgdorferi* were found through ELISA and a Western immunoblot. Antibodies to Babesia and Ehrlichia agents were negative. A lumbar puncture was entirely normal. A diagnosis of early disseminated Lyme disease was made, and the patient was treated with 3 weeks of oral doxycycline (100 mg twice a day).

All the symptoms resolved except for the headache. It continued to be present most of the day, and had a throbbing component superimposed on a mild dull ache. There were no other significant complaints. The patient's past medical history was otherwise unremarkable. His family history was positive for migraine headaches in several family members, including his mother and sister. The patient felt his headache was getting worse. He was worried about chronic Lyme disease, and was asking for intravenous antibiotics. His examination was entirely normal.

Questions about Case 2

- What would you tell this patient?
- Would you do any further testing?
- How would you treat this patient?

Case 2 Discussion

The patient had clear-cut early disseminated Lyme disease. Cerebrospinal fluid studies were negative, indicating that the central nervous system (CNS) was not infected. All the patient's complaints cleared with antibiotic therapy except for the headaches. The differential diagnosis included chronic tension-type headache and migraine headache, but it also included a poorly defined postinfectious entity referred to as chronic Lyme disease syndrome/post-Lyme-disease syndrome. In this case, migraine was the major consideration, in light of the strong family history as well as the intermittent throbbing nature of the headache. Nevertheless, since the headache began as part of a well-documented Lyme disease syndrome, it was reasonable to exclude active infection.

Chronic Lyme disease syndrome is a term applied to patients who are treated for Lyme disease, yet continue to complain of persistent problems which date back to their original infection. The persistent problems often involve varying combinations of a variety of symptoms, without much in the way of objective signs. Patients experience fatigue and malaise, arthralgias, myalgias, diffuse pain with muscle tender points (fibromyalgia syndrome), cognitive difficulties, mood disturbances, dizziness, sleep problems, and hearing abnormalities. These patients are often believed to have a chronic infection and are treated with repeated or long-term antibiotics. In fact, there are a number of possibilities that might explain persistent problems following treated Lyme disease (Table 39–2).

This patient was unlikely to have an active *B. burgdorferi* infection. His original Lyme disease syndrome did not involve the nervous system, and all his symptoms resolved after treatment except for the headache. The family history was strongly positive for vascular headache, and the headache features suggested that it was vascular. The most likely explanation in this case would be a migraine prob-lem brought on by the prior infection syndrome.

As part of a thorough work-up, a lumbar puncture was carried out to rule out an occult CNS infection. All CSF studies were normal. The patient insisted on treatment with intravenous ceftriaxone for 4 weeks. The headache was unaffected. Propanolol in escalating doses was then prescribed, with clearing of the headaches. The final diagnosis was migraine without aura.

Management Strategies

- Be sufficiently familiar with Lyme disease to suspect the diagnosis in patients with consistent syndromes and exposure to an area where the disease is endemic. As in Case 1, summer flu in such an area followed by multisystem complaints should raise the possibility of Lyme disease.
- To help establish the diagnosis, order a screening ELISA to look for *B. burgdorferi* antibodies. Proceed to a Western immunoblot if the ELISA is borderline or positive.
- If there are neurologic complaints, CSF should be examined to document neurologic Lyme disease.
- In patients with *B. burgdorferi* infection, exposure to other tick-borne pathogens (Babesia, Ehrlichia) should be assessed.
- Once the diagnosis is established, patients must be treated with antibiotics. In most cases with neurologic involvement, this means intravenous ceftriaxone, 2 g once a day.
- When patients require several weeks of therapy, insertion of a PICC line allows easy access. Antibiotic treatment is usually done at home although the first dose can be given under medical observation.
- It is important to warn the patient that problems often improve slowly after antibiotic treatment, and it may take months to get better. This does not indicate treatment failure.
- In complicated cases, evaluation by a Lyme disease specialist may be advisable.

Case Summaries

- The first patient had chronic Lyme meningitis with very subtle meningeal features. The diagnosis was established by CSF analysis. Appropriate ther-

TABLE 39–2. Possible Explanations for Chronic Lyme Disease/Post-Lyme-Disease Syndrome (Persistent Post-treatment Complaints)

Etiology	Clues
Persistent infection	• Worsening problems • Objective deficits • Abnormal spinal fluid • Sustained antibiotic response
Postinfectious immune/inflammatory condition	• Classic chronic fatigue/fibromyalgia syndrome • Deficit waxes and wanes, no consistent worsening • No evidence of current infection • No/transient antibiotic response • Consistent immune disturbances
Second diagnosis	• Problems consistent with alternative condition • Therapeutic response with treatment for alternative condition
Residual damage	• Deficit occurred with original Lyme disease syndrome • Deficits are fixed • No/transient antibiotic response
Prolonged recovery after treatment	• Within 6 months of treatment • An ongoing slow improvement
Re-infection	• Exposure to endemic area • New seroconversion or rising antibody titer • Consistent new syndrome
Co-infection	• Positive Ehrlichia or Babesia serology • Prominent anemia, leukopenia, liver enzyme elevation with original Lyme disease syndrome

apy involved intravenous antibiotics to eradicate this bacterial CNS infection.

• The second case represented a primary headache precipitated by Lyme disease. With a strongly supportive clinical history and no evidence of active infection, it would have been more sensible to treat with a prophylactic vascular headache agent first, rather than proceeding to costly and unjustified parenteral antibiotics.

Overview of Lyme Disease

Lyme disease is due to infection with a tick-borne spirochete named *Borrelia burgdorferi*. This systemic bacterial infection has specific target-organ involvement (skin, central (CNS) and peripheral (PNS) nervous systems, the musculoskeletal system, heart, and eyes). *B. burgdorferi* shares the properties of other human spirochetal infections such as syphilis, leptospirosis, and relapsing fever. It causes chronic infection with periodic clinical reactivations. The spirochete is quite heterogeneous, and there are a number of genospecies and strains. At least three distinct genospecies cause Lyme disease. Different *B. burgdorferi* strains can vary in their DNA, plasmids (extrachromosomal DNA), and protein composition. This heterogeneity probably has clinical significance. Some strains appear to be neurotropic while others cause skin or joint disease.

The tick vector for Lyme disease is the hard-body Ixodes tick. These ticks have a 2-year life cycle and go through three stages (larva, nymph, and adult). Each stage involves a single blood meal. Ticks feed on over a hundred different mammals and birds but wild mice (for nymphal ticks) and deer (for adult ticks) are the preferred hosts. Humans are accidental hosts. Virtually all Lyme disease cases are due to tick bite. Spirochetes are transmitted through tick saliva into the open bite. Successful transmission seems to require a prolonged blood meal, and experimental as well as clinical studies suggest that infected ticks must feed for 24 hours or longer to cause infection. Most human bites are due to questing nymphs which feed in late spring and early summer.

Lyme disease accounts for more than 90% of vector-borne infections in the United States. Although it was originally felt that the agent must have originated in Europe since skin (EM) and neurologic (painful lymphocytic radiculoneuritis or Bannwarth's syndrome) manifestations were described many years before the first American cases, recent data indicate that endemic foci of *B. burgdorferi* have existed in North America for a very long time.

A major feature of Lyme disease is its geographic restriction to areas with the tick vector. The United States has three regions where the disease is endemic: the coastal Northeast, the upper Midwest (Minnesota and Wisconsin), and the upper Pacific coast. The majority of infections are reported from five states (New York, New Jersey, Connecticut, Pennsylvania, and Rhode Island). Although Lyme disease occurs year round, there is seasonality in temperate climates because the ticks are not active during cold winters. Most cases occur from May through October, and particularly in June and July. The major risk factor for infection is time spent out of doors.

B. burgdorferi causes asymptomatic infections in at least 20 to 30% of cases. Asymptomatic infection may reflect nonpathogenic strains, a small inoculum, or else effective early responses. This is important to keep in mind since these individuals will be seropositive but will not have Lyme disease. There are no data on how to handle asymptomatic *B. burgdorferi* infection. Many individuals who practice where Lyme disease is endemic will give such patients several weeks of oral antibiotics, similar to the approach to individuals with an unexpected positive syphilis serology.

Symptomatic infections can be classified temporally and by stage of disease into early local, early disseminated, and late-stage disseminated syndromes (see Table 39–1). Patients may present at any point but the most common Lyme disease manifestation is the local-infection stage EM. This is an expanding red skin lesion at the site of the tick bite and is considered the only clinical pathognomonic marker for Lyme disease. It occurs or is noted in approximately 60 to 80% of infected individuals. In more than one half of patients, the EM is accompanied by various constitutional symptoms, which can include headache. Spirochetes are actually present within the EM skin lesion. Once they are inoculated into the skin at the site of the tick bite, they move outwards in a centrifugal fashion. Erythema migrans develops 1 to 30 (typically 7 to 9) days after the tick bite. A rash within 24 hours of the bite is not EM but an allergic reaction. Erythema migrans is usually painless. Its most characteristic feature is that it gets bigger over time and can get quite large; however, there are atypical forms of the skin lesion. It can be small, raised, itchy, or have a peculiar shape. It can be misdiagnosed as a spider bite, an insect bite, or contact dermatitis. The index of suspicion of Lyme disease needs to be high for anyone exposed to an area where the disease is endemic and who develops an unexplained skin lesion. Untreated EM clears spontaneously within days to weeks and clears faster with treatment. In addition to EM, early infection can also manifest as a summertime flu-like syndrome without rash. Headache is a prominent feature of this syndrome.

After a period of time (days to weeks), spirochetes disseminate from the skin inoculation site into the blood to spread widely throughout the body. A number of target-organ syndromes are associated with this early dissemination. Typically, they occur within 3 months of infection. Some patients develop multiple EM skin lesions. Other patients develop musculoskeletal complaints (arthralgias, myalgias, periarticular pain, and cervical or back pain), which are typically fluctuating and migratory. Dissemination may also be associated with cardiac (high degree heart block) and ocular (conjunctivitis) disease.

Late-stage disease (more than 3 months after infection) includes Lyme arthritis, a monoarticular, oligoarticular, or less frequently polyarticular joint involvement with effusion. Swelling of the joint is a helpful objective sign, and increases the likelihood of Lyme disease as the cause of joint pain. The most frequently affected joints are the knee, shoulder, and ankle. The inflammation and effusion subside spontaneously but can recur. In 10% of patients chronic arthritis develops, which appears to be an immune-mediated and nonantibiotic-responsive syndrome in people who have a genetic predisposition. Lyme arthritis can include temporomandibular joint (TMJ) involvement, which is unusual in most other systemic arthritides. This localized arthritis can give rise to focal pain and tenderness, including facial or periauricular pain associated with jaw claudication and unilateral headache. Late ocular disease is rare but can involve uveitis and keratitis.

Neurologic Lyme disease includes both CNS and PNS syndromes. Distinct syndromes are associated with early and late stage dissemination (Table 39–3). The most frequent early neurologic syndrome is Lyme meningitis (see below). Cranial nerve palsy is also a recognized feature of early dissemination. Approximately 80% of cranial nerve lesions involve the facial nerve. Within endemic areas, Lyme disease accounts for up to 25% of facial nerve palsies, particularly those that develop during summertime. Clinical clues to Lyme-disease-related facial nerve palsy include bilateral involvement (which occurs in up to a third of patients) and accompanying constitutional symptoms (headache, arthralgias, myalgias, fatigue, and cognitive difficulties). Although some cases of facial nerve palsy may reflect pure PNS involvement, there is increasing evidence that most reflect CNS infection. Cerebrospinal fluid is frequently abnormal, and even patients with otherwise normal CSF have been PCR positive for *B. burgdorferi* DNA. Other cranial nerves can also be affected, and in rare cases, there may be multiple cranial neuropathies. The third early dissemination syndrome is an acute painful radiculitis. This is the classic presentation of neurologic Lyme disease in Europe, where it is referred as to Bannwarth's syndrome. Acute radiculoneuritis is much less common in North America. Patients present with radicular pain in various areas, particularly between the scapulae, followed by development of asymmetric dermatomic and myotomic abnormalities. Pain is invariably a significant component, and headache and stiff neck are frequently accompanying features. Inflammatory CSF changes in acute radiculoneuritis are typically more marked than in the routine Lyme meningitis case. Variations in this early disseminated PNS syndrome include painful mononeuritis, mononeuritis multiplex, plexopathy, and painless symmetrical polyradiculoneuropathy resembling Guillain-Barré syndrome. Cerebrospinal fluid pleocytosis is an important clue to Lyme disease in patients with otherwise typical Guillain-Barré syndrome.

Unusual neurologic syndromes that can occur during the early dissemination stage include confusional states with behavioral abnormalities, transient ischemic attack-like episodes, and cerebellar ataxia syndromes.

The most common neurologic syndrome associated with late-disseminated infection is encephalopathy. This can develop months to years after the original infection. Deficits are subtle and affect memory, attention, processing speed, problem solving, and can include slowed reaction time. Cerebrospinal fluid shows very mild disturbances and can even be normal. Neuroimaging studies, single photon emission computed tomography (SPECT) of the brain, may show nonspecific abnormalities in cerebral blood flow. Late Lyme encephalopathy probably reflects CNS infection. This is supported by the fact that the organism DNA and its antigen as well as a low-grade pleocytosis have been detected in the CSF of these patients. Antibiotic treatment is associated with improvement in clinical symptoms, neurocognitive measures, and neuroimaging parameters. A second characteristic syndrome of late disseminated infection is a subtle axonal poly-radiculoneuropathy, with intermittent limb paresthesias or radicular pain. Neurophysiologic testing is generally needed to document the neuropathy. This PNS syndrome may occur along with CNS encephalopathy. The neuropathy also improves clinically and by neurophysiologic parameters with antibiotic therapy, supporting the fact that it reflects ongoing *B. burgdorferi* infection.

The most striking late syndrome is an encephalomyelitis referred to as progressive Borrelia encephalomyelitis. This is the least common of the six characteristic neurologic syndromes of Lyme disease. Most case series described come from Europe. Patients have parenchymal involvement, with progressive multifocal abnormalities that can affect the hemispheres, brain stem, spinal cord, or cranial nerves. This is accompanied by CSF abnormalities (pleocytosis, increased protein, and intrathecal specific antibody production). Patients respond to antibiotic therapy with stabilization of deterioration or with improvement although deficits often do not clear completely.

TABLE 39–3. Neurologic Lyme Disease Syndromes

I. Early local infection	• Premeningitis seeding (culture-positive CSF without pleocytosis)
II. Early disseminated infection	• Meningitis, meningoencephalitis • Cranial nerve palsy • Acute radiculoneuritis • Unusual symptoms: confusional states, transient ischemic attacks, cerebellar ataxia, intracranial hypertension (children/adolescents)
III. Late-stage infection	• Encephalopathy • Chronic polyradiculoneuropathy • Encephalomyelitis, meningoencephalomyelitis • Unusual syndromes: vascular syndromes, myositis, psychiatric manifestations

The diagnosis of Lyme disease ultimately rests on clinical grounds although it is ideally supported by epidemiologic and laboratory evidence (Table 39–4). Serologic testing is used to confirm exposure (detection of antibodies to *B. burgdorferi*) although a positive serology does not document active infection or Lyme disease. At the current time, a two-stage test is used: borderline or positive screening by ELISA confirmed by Western immunoblot. Seronegative infections can occur in patients who receive early but inadequate antibiotic therapy. The best-documented studies suggest that this occurs in approximately 7% of Lyme disease cases. Current ELISAs use a whole-cell sonicate, containing over one hundred organism-specific and nonspecific antigens. A strong response to nonspecific (shared) antigens can lead to a false positive ELISA. Western immunoblot looks at the antigen specificity of the response. The assay has been standardized with regard to what constitutes a positive IgM or IgG immunoblot. Positive IgM immunoblots must show at least two out of three specified bands (p23,p39,p41); a positive IgG immunoblot must show at least five out of ten specified bands (p18, p23, p28, p30, p39, p41, p45, p58, p66, p93). Unfortunately, there are problems with the current ELISA and immunoblot tests (Table 39–5). Serology assays should be improved shortly when recombinant and chimeric protein-based assay tests are marketed.

Cerebrospinal fluid studies are generally critical when diagnosing neurologic Lyme disease and documenting CNS involvement. A series of specific and nonspecific tests is available (see Table 39–4). A CSF culture is almost never positive, with the exception of occasional meningitis cases. A culture requires the use of specific media and typically takes weeks. Current PCR assays show low sensitivity (lower than 40%) when applied to the CSF of neurologic Lyme disease patients. This probably reflects the very low numbers of free spirochetes in CSF since these organisms are highly tissuetropic. Studying concentrated CSF increases the yield of PCR. Intrathecal *B. burgdorferi* antibody production, indicating preferential synthesis of specific antibodies in serum as compared with CSF, is the most useful test to document CSF infection. There are rare false positive reactions, however. Other CSF tests are nonspecific but can show abnormalities (particularly mononuclear pleocytosis) consistent with Lyme disease (see Table 39–4).

Treatment of neurologic Lyme disease generally involves intravenous ceftriaxone given for several weeks (Table 39–6). In cases of pure PNS involvement, oral doxycycline, which gives good tissue penetration, can probably be substituted for parenteral therapy. Ultimately, the most effective treatment for any infection is prevention. Two Lyme disease vaccines have been tested in large studies involving over 20,000 people and seem effective. They are both based on a single recombinant protein, outer surface protein (OspA). Immunoprophylaxis provides short-term protection against Lyme disease. The vaccines do not provide long-lasting immunity, however, and it appears that periodic revaccination will be necessary.

Headache is the most common symptom of neurologic Lyme disease. As indicated by Brinck (1993), it can be the presenting feature of Lyme disease. This was true in the first case. Headache is common at all stages of infection although it tends to be more prominent during early disease than late disease. It is estimated that over half of all patients with Lyme disease experience headaches (Table 39–7).

As reported by Steere, headache is present in up to 64% of patients with the EM skin lesion. Nadelman (1996) reported on 79 culture-documented cases

TABLE 39–4. Diagnosis of Neurologic Lyme Disease

Epidemiologic Clues	Laboratory Clues	Clinical Clues

• Exposure to endemic region
• Evidence of tick bite
   Type of tick, vector infection rate,
   duration of the attachment,
   tick engorgement
	• Blood
	   B. burgdorferi antibodies, nonspecific
	     tests (ESR, liver enzymes, cryoglobulins, VDRL,
	     anticardiolipin-Ab, IgM, hypergammaglobulinemia),
	     tests to exclude other diagnoses
	
	• CSF studies
	   Specific (intrathecal *B. burgdorferi* antibodies,
	     PCR, experimental antigen culture, immune complexes)
	   Nonspecific (cell count, protein, glucose, VDRL, cytology,
	     oligoclonal bands, IgG, myelin basic protein)
	
	• Ancillary studies
	   Neuroimaging (MRI, SPECT), neurophysiologic (EMG, NCV),
	     neuropsychologic testing, EKG, angiography
		• Flu-like syndrome
		
		• Extraneural features
		   Joint involvement, jaw pain,
		   myalgias, fatigue, cardiac and
		   ocular features
		
		• Characteristic neurologic
		   syndrome
		• Physical examination
		   Facial weakness, radicular signs,
		   polyneuropathy, arthritis,
		   Baker's cyst, cardiac and ocular
		   abnormalities

and noted headache in 42%. In some of these patients, the headache reflects CNS invasion that may be accompanied by normal CSF (premeningitis phase) or a CSF pleocytosis (occult meningitis). Invasion of the central nervous system is more likely when the headache is accompanied by a stiff neck or photophobia. Headache is also typically a feature of the early flu-like syndrome with seroconversion. The headache of early Lyme disease is generally bifrontal or occipital and is intermittent (or occasionally persistent) with periodic exacerbations. It often improves spontaneously and also improves with antibiotics. Scelsa (1995) reported on 49 patients hospitalized with Lyme disease of recent onset (within 4 months of infection), who did not have encephalitis or meningitis. Their headache pattern could mimic both tension-type headaches and migraine-like headache. In 80% of patients who were treated, the headache responded to antibiotics.

As noted by both Reik and Pachner, headache is the most common symptom of Lyme meningitis. It usually starts gradually rather than explosively, varies in intensity, and is bilateral in the frontal or occipital region. The headache worsens with physical activity. It can be intermittent or persistent. Most often, it is dull in quality and will improve somewhat with analgesics. Headache can be extremely mild in Lyme meningitis. Its intensity does not seem to correlate very closely with the degree of pleocyto-

sis. Some patients are almost headache free despite significant CSF pleocytosis. Other clues to Lyme meningitis are accompanying systemic symptoms (prominent fatigue, arthralgias, myalgias), extraneural features (EM, palpitations, tender joints, conjunctivitis), and suggestive signs (unilateral or bilateral facial nerve palsy, radicular involvement).

Headache is also common in the acute painful radiculoneuritis and facial nerve palsy syndromes of

TABLE 39–5. Current Problems in Lyme Disease Serology Assays

General	• Positive serology does not indicate
	  active infection
	• Seronegative cases
	• Negative until several weeks into
	  infection
	• Interlaboratory variability
	• Intralaboratory variability

ELISA	• No standardized assay antigen target,
	  reagents, positivity criteria
	• False positives due to nonspecific
	  antigen reactivity
	    —B-cell hyperreactivity
	    —autoantibodies
	    —other infections

Immunoblot	• No standardized assay antigen target,
	  reagents
	• Specific bands not counted
	• May be positive despite negative
	  screening ELISA

TABLE 39–6. Treatment for Lyme Disease

Infection Stage	Duration	Standard	Alternative
Early local infection	2 to 4 weeks	Doxycycline 100 mg b.i.d. PO (up to 200 mg b.i.d.) Amoxicillin 500–1000 mg t.i.d. PO	Cefuroxime axetil 500 mg b.i.d.
Early disseminated infection (mild, no CNS involvement)	2 to 4 weeks	Doxycycline 100 mg b.i.d. PO (up to 200 mg b.i.d.)	Ceftriaxone 2 g q.d. IV
Early disseminated infection (severe or CNS involvement), late-stage infection	2 to 6 weeks	Ceftriaxone 2 g q.d. IV	Cefotaxime 2 g t.i.d. IV Penicillin 4 million units q4–6h IV Doxycycline 200 mg b.i.d. PO

early dissemination. The characteristics are similar to the headache of Lyme meningitis. Lyme disease is a rare cause of secondary trigeminal neuralgia. In these cases, the CSF pleocytosis, response to antibiotics, and associated features of the systemic infection help to identify Lyme disease as the cause of this cranial neuropathy.

Temporomandibular joint arthritis is one of the early musculoskeletal manifestations of Lyme disease. This contrasts with other arthritides where TMJ inflammation is a late phenomenon. As noted by Moscatello (1991), patients may have jaw pain, preauricular pain, bitemporal headache, or pain during chewing.

As reported by Belman (1993), in children with neurologic Lyme disease, the most frequent clinical manifestation is also headache (71%). Usually, it is intermittent, with a frontal or occipital predominance, and it is generally associated with other systemic features (arthritis, myalgia, facial nerve palsy). In one series headache was the major neurologic feature in 30% of the children. Intracranial hypertension syndrome is an unusual age-specific (children, adolescents) disorder associated with the early dissemination stage. Patients present with significant headache and a normal neurologic examination except for bilateral choked disks. They are not obese, and CSF is generally abnormal. There may be a high protein concentration, pleocytosis, or intrathecal *B. burgdorferi* antibody production. This syndrome may be immune complex mediated since high levels of *B. burgdorferi*-specific complexes have been found in CSF without detectable organism.

TABLE 39–7. Headache and Lyme Disease

Headache associated with extraneural Lyme disease	• EM-associated headaches • Headache of the flu-like syndrome with seroconversion • Temporomandibular pain
Headache associated with neurologic Lyme disease	• Lyme meningitis headache • Cranial nerve palsy headache 　—Facial nerve palsy 　—Trigeminal neuralgia • Painful radiculoneuritis headache • Headache associated with intracranial hypertension syndrome • Chronic headache associated with encephalopathy • Encephalomyelitis with headache • Persistent infection with recurrent meningitis and headache
Headache associated with post-treatment Lyme disease	• Primary headache precipitated by Lyme disease • Headache of postinfectious chronic fatigue/fibromyalgia syndrome • Headache associated with infection due to other tick-borne pathogens • Headache associated with re-infection • Headache associated with persistent infection (rare)

In the neurologic syndromes of late-stage infection, headache may be an accompanying feature but cognitive deficits or objective signs of neurologic parenchymal damage predominate. The characteristics of the headache are similar to those of a chronic tension-type headache.

As reported by Lawrence (1995), in very rare circumstances, antibiotic therapy may not permanently eradicate CNS infection. This may reflect a defective response. The clinical course is characterized by recurrent bouts of meningitis with symptomatic improvement with antibiotic therapy. During these relapses, headache is common.

Finally, as reported by Gaudino (1997), headache may also be a problem in patients who are treated, yet have persistent post-treatment complaints sufficient to be diagnosed with a chronic Lyme disease/post-Lyme-disease syndrome. In view of the multiple possible explanations for this syndrome (see Table 39–2), headache in these patients could reflect a pre-existing headache disorder, a postinfection problem, persistent *B. burgdorferi* infection, or infection by other pathogens, among other possibilities.

Selected Readings

Belman A, Ier M, Coyle PK, et al. Neurological manifestations in children with North American Lyme disease. Neurology 1993;43:2609–14.

Brinck T, Hansen K, Olesen J. Headache resembling tension-headache as the single manifestation of Lyme neuroborreliosis. Cephalalgia 1993;13:207–9.

Gaudino E, Coyle PK, Krupp L. Post-Lyme syndrome and chronic fatigue syndrome. Neuropsychiatric similarities and differences. Arch Neurol 1997;54:1372–6.

Lawrence C, Lipton RB, Lowy FD, et al. Seronegative chronic relapsing neuroborreliosis. Eur Neurol 1995;35:113–7.

Moscatello A, Worden D, Nadelman R, et al. Otolaryngologic aspects of Lyme disease. Laryngoscope 1991;101:592–5.

Nadelman R, Nowakowski J, Forseter G, et al. The clinical spectrum of early Lyme disease borreliosis in patients with culture-confirmed erythema migrans. Am J Med 1996; 100:502–8.

Pachner A, Steere A. The triad of neurologic manifestations of Lyme disease: meningitis, cranial neuritis, and radiculoneuritis. Neurology 1985;35:47–53.

Reik L, Steere A, Bartenhagen N, et al. Neurologic abnormalities of Lyme disease. Medicine 1979;58:281–94.

Scelsa S, Lipton R, Sander H, et al. Headache characteristics in hospitalized patients with Lyme disease. Headache 1995; 35:125–30.

Steere A, Bartenhagen N, Craft J, et al. The early clinical manifestations of Lyme disease. Ann Intern Med 1983;99:76–82.

Editorial Comments

Cases of headache in patients with a systemic symptomology usually allow clinicians to begin a search for a specific underlying disorder, sometimes of infectious origin. In Lyme disease, headache is the most common neurologic symptom, as the authors point out in their comprehensive discussion of this disorder in the context of the two cases they present in this chapter. In endemic areas, the diagnosis is invariably considered but it also must be considered in other areas and clinical settings, and a high index of suspicion of the diagnosis is needed. Lyme disease is treatable and curable, so it is necessary for physicians seeing a multitude of headache disorders to know about this disease. In many ways, we are all aided by the discussion in this excellent chapter.

CHAPTER 40

THE WOMAN WITH FACIAL PAIN OF UNDETERMINED ORIGIN

STEVEN B. GRAFF-RADFORD, DDS

Case History

A 59-year-old, right-handed woman presented with continuous face, neck, left jaw, and postauricular pain. The quality described was a severe, throbbing, sharp, stabbing pain with a shooting sensation in the postauricular region. Light touch in the postauricular region was unbearable. The pain could suddenly and spontaneously worsen, with the exacerbated pain lasting anywhere from a few seconds to 20 minutes. These episodes occurred many times during the day and interfered with the patient's sleep. There were no specific autonomic changes or associated nausea, vomiting, and sensitivity to light or noise. Aggravating factors included touching the area lightly. Alleviating factors included acetaminophen.

The pain began 3 months prior to this evaluation. While moving a neighbor's trash can from her driveway she was hit in the face as the trash can flipped over unexpectedly. The injuries sustained included lacerations to the left nasal bridge as well as to the area inferior to the right eye over the zygoma. A plastic surgeon immediately repaired the lacerations. No fractures were identified. Pain in the neck and the lacerated area started immediately following the trauma. As the days progressed, a severe pain developed in her teeth, ear, and postauricular region. She felt that this was like a tooth abscess experienced approximately 5 or 6 years before. A general

dentist was consulted, who referred the patient to an oral surgeon. Further radiographs revealed no local pathology.

Current medications at the time of evaluation included acetaminophen, two to three every 4 hours, and omeprazole, 20 mg one per day. The patient's past medical history was positive for chickenpox and mumps, and possibly measles. Operations included a hysterectomy, appendectomy, and tonsillectomy. Allergies to aspirin were reported. A review of the patient's systems was positive for a hiatal hernia and some gastric sensitivity.

The patient is single, works as a sales representative, and likes her work. Her father died of old age and her mother, aged 97, recently had a stroke. Symptoms similar to the chief complaint were not present in any family member.

When asked about her mood, she described feeling irritable. Further questioning revealed a decrease in motivation and concentration but no suicidal ideation. Complaints regarding the laceration included feeling unattractive. The lacerations could not be seen unless there was close examination. There was litigation pending.

Examination

The patient's blood pressure was 130/80. Her heart rate was 54 beats per minute and regular.

A screening examination was conducted of cranial nerves II to XII. Abnormalities were noted in the fifth and seventh cranial nerves. A marked sensory loss in the V1, V2, and V3 distributions to both light touch and pinprick was evident. There was marked hyperalgesia and allodynia in the V1 distribution as well as in the C2 through C4 distributions. She was unable to seal her mouth when blowing up her cheeks. Reflexes were 1+ and symmetrical. Her coordination was normal. A Romberg's test was negative.

A stomatognathic examination revealed a normally functioning temporomandibular joint with an interincisal opening of 50 mm and 1 mm of passive stretch. Protrusion was 12 mm and left and right laterotrusion 10 mm, respectively. Temporomandibular joint noise was absent. Marked lateral and dorsal capsular tenderness was present on the left temporomandibular joint. Mucosal ridging on the tongue indicated a clenching habit. She had bridges in the upper right, upper left, and lower left quadrants. Occlusal contacts were normal.

An upper quarter and cervical spine examination revealed a symmetrical head position and unelevated shoulders. The anterior head position was 6 cm from a tangent to the thoracic spine which was normal. The transverse process of the atlas was nontender and nonrotated. The functions of the occiput on the atlas and the atlas on the axis were normal. Flexion was normal. Extension was slightly limited. Lateral flexion was limited to the right and painful on the left. Rotation was limited both left and right and painful on the left.

A myofascial examination revealed marked tenderness in the left splenius capitis region and the left trapezius in the neck which produced marked pain referral into the left facial area and reproduced her pain in part. She had an active trigger point in the left trapezius which referred and partially reproduced her neck pain. At the time of examination, the degree of pain was 4 out of 10. Touching the postauricular region markedly exacerbated the pain.

Questions about This Case

- What is the relevance of asking about autonomic changes and migraine-associated symptoms?
- What, if any, is the relevance of trigger points in this case?
- What diagnostic tests would you order?
- How would you manage her pain?
- What is the prognosis for this patient?

Case Discussion

The differential diagnosis was:
1. Rule out sympathetically maintained traumatic trigeminal neuralgia
2. Rule out sympathetically independent traumatic trigeminal neuralgia
3. Myofascial pain

Autonomic changes and migraine-associated symptoms (nausea, vomiting, photo- and phonophobia) are reviewed in all facial pain patients to rule out cluster headache and migraine presenting in the face. A common examination finding in facial migraine is tenderness in the carotid region radiating pain to the face. This has prompted Raskin to call this carotidynia. Magnetic resonance imaging (MRI) of the brain was ordered because the pain followed a trauma to the head and the symptoms indicated a broader pain distribution than one would expect. The associated sensory and motor changes were also a concern. Particular emphasis on the posterior cranial fossa and the upper cervical segments was requested. The MRI was reported within normal limits.

The second test ordered was a diagnostic sympathetic nerve block (stellate ganglion block). If patients show good response to this block, doing repeated blocks (up to 6) may be helpful. These are mostly effective in the first 3 to 6 months following the nerve trauma. Graff-Radford and Bittar reported that repeated somatic blocks have not proved effective in patients with traumatic trigeminal neuralgia. This patient had a profound response to the sympathetic nerve block (complete relief of pain for 12 hours). She noted pain relief that outlasted the duration of anesthesia. Usually the first block is done with a short-acting anesthetic, and if effective, subsequent blocks are done with a longer-acting anesthetic agent such as bupivacaine. It is suggested when a myofascial component is present, it should be re-evaluated after the sympathetic nerve block. Often the tenderness and referral will decrease. In these cases it may be tenderness secondary to hyperalgesia and not myofascial pain. If the pain referral persists, a more aggressive approach using physical therapies should be entertained. In this case, upper back and neck pain continued and prompted an orthopedic evaluation to rule out fractures. Once cleared, a home exercise-program was initiated, specifically addressing posture and range of motion. Within a few weeks the myofascial pain had improved. The medication chosen was nortriptyline. The recommended dosage was 10 mg at bedtime to be increased by 10 mg every 4 days. A maximum of 100 mg is usually recommended, although some patients require higher doses. Studies of facial pain by Solberg and Graff-Radford suggest an average dose of 80 mg as being beneficial in 80% of cases. In this case the facial pain resolved rapidly and within a month the patient was not having facial pain. She received three stellate ganglion blocks in total. After 2 months she complained of weight gain. At this time she was having intermittent upper back pain and occasional shooting pain in the occipital region. The nortriptyline was tapered off and gabapentin initiated in combination with an anti-inflammatory. The gabapentin was started at 300 mg and increased by 300 mg every 2 days to a maximum of 1800 mg in three doses. It may be necessary to increase the medication to as much as 3000 mg per day. Usually, if there has not been a response at 1800 mg, a further increase is not beneficial. An excellent response was seen with the gabapentin and after 3 months the drug was withdrawn and the patient remains pain free. Intermittent upper back pain continues. When it occurs, exercises are used to control the discomfort.

Behavioral testing including the MMPI (Minnesota Multiphasic Personality Inventory) was performed along with a standard evaluation by a pain center psychologist. Essentially all testing was within normal limits. She did display some anxiety and was provided three sessions with the psychologist to learn relaxation skills.

Management Strategies

There are various ways to manage traumatic trigeminal neuralgia and often a combination therapy is required. The management strategies will be summarized under topical applications, procedures, pharmacology, and behavioral therapy.

Topical Applications

The use of topical therapies has not been well studied. There is some evidence that capsaicin applied regularly will result in desensitization and pain relief. The recommended dose is five times per day for 5 days then three times per day for 3 weeks. If the patient cannot withstand the burning produced by the application, the addition of a topical local anesthetic, either 5% lidocaine or a lidocaine/prilocaine preparation is useful. Clonidine can be applied to the hyperalgesic region by placing a proprietary cutaneous delivery patch on the skin where it is most tender. Alternatively the use of a 4% gel can be compounded and delivered over a larger area. For local intraoral application a neurosensory stent has been conceived (Figure 40–1). Once this device is manufactured, the patient is instructed to apply the prescribed gel to the lingual surface. The device may also work to protect the region from persistent input.

Procedures

A neural blockade is very effective in differentiating sympathetically maintained pain from sympathetically independent pain. It may also be effective in controlling sympathetically maintained pain if used regularly. It is recommended that up to six blocks be received, repeated at about a week apart, provided that a cumulative effect is seen. If no significant response occurs after the third block, further intervention is withheld. In the head and neck, the sympathetic block is achieved by doing a stellate ganglion block. Although sphenopalatine ganglion blocks (topical) have been described as useful, the author feels they are not as effective as stellate ganglion blocks. Phentolamine infusion is another procedure described as useful in obtaining a chemical sympathetic block, but again the author feels that phentolamine infusion is not as useful as the stellate ganglion block.

A lidocaine infusion may be used therapeutically as well as to determine if mexiletine could be useful.

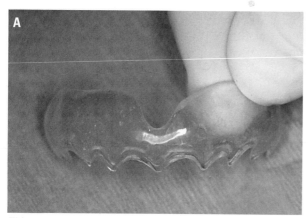
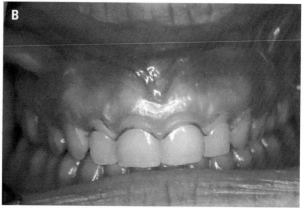

FIGURE 40–1. *A*, Acrylic stent for delivering medication to a painful site. *B*, Acrylic stent shown in place.

Patients with neuropathic pain receive 200 mg of lidocaine intravenously over 1 hour. The effect is measured using visual analog pain scales (VAS). It is useful to monitor the pain change using a diary or VAS for at least 24 hours post procedure. It is not uncommon for sympathetically maintained pain to decrease for periods that outlast the expected duration of the local anesthetic .

Neural stimulation of the trigeminal ganglion has been attempted with varying results. The author has been involved with 7 intractable facial pain patients who received ganglion stimulators. Initially, pain relief was achieved in 6 subjects and after 1 year, little residual benefit was achieved. The primary problem was drift of the electrode, ultimately due to hardware failure. This treatment did not work.

Intrathecal opioid pumps are also used in intractable cases. There is little published on the use of these devices for head and neck pain. Prior to considering this procedure a very careful work-up, including intrathecal trials, should be attempted. If patients do not respond to oral opioids, they are unlikely to respond to opioids delivered through other routes.

Pharmacology

It is well documented that tricyclic antidepressants are effective in many pain problems. Solberg and Graff-Radford have studied the response of amitriptyline in traumatic neuralgia. It is noted that the effective range is 10 to 150 mg per day usually taken in a single dose at bedtime. Table 40–1 summarizes the dosage range of tricyclic antidepressants. It is the author's opinion that nortriptyline is the choice drug because it has fewer anticholinergic side effects.

Membrane stabilizers are medications that include anticonvulsants, lidocaine derivatives, and some muscle relaxants. They have been typically used to treat intermittent sharp electric pains but are useful as individual agents, or in combination with the antidepressants in traumatic trigeminal neuralgia. Table 40–2 summarizes the common medications in this group and their doses.

Blood levels are available for some antidepressants and membrane stabilizers. The blood level may indicate a low level if there is a poor clinical outcome. In these situations, increasing the drug is beneficial. It is not uncommon to have patients on high doses with low blood levels. Usually this is also accompanied by minimal side effects. Further, the blood levels are useful if combination therapies are used to avoid toxicity. Special care should be taken when combining a tricyclic antidepressant with a selective serotonin reuptake inhibitor (SSRI). This is secondary to the build-up and added effects seen due to the slow cytochrome P-450 metabolism. There is very little effect seen with the SSRI as an individual therapy in traumatic trigeminal neuralgia.

Behavioral Strategies

Prior to beginning therapy it is essential to perform a behavioral assessment with appropriate testing.

TABLE 40–1. Common Antidepressants Used to Treat Trigeminal Neuralgia

Generic Name	Dosage (mg/d)
Trazodone	50–300
Amitriptyline	10–150
Desipramine	10–150
Nortriptyline	10–150
Doxepin	10–150
Imipramine	10–150

TABLE 40–2. Common Medications Used to Treat Traumatic Trigeminal Neuralgia

Generic Name	Dosage (mg/d)
Baclofen	10–80
Carbamazepine	100–1200
Phenytoin	100–400
Divalproex sodium	125–2000
Clonazepam	0.5–8
Pimozide	2–12
Gabapentin	300–3000

Common psychometric tests used at our center, include the Minnesota Multiphasic Personality Inventory (MMPI), Multidimensional Pain Inventory (MPI), Beck Anxiety and Beck Depression Inventories. Additional tests may be given to target specific problem areas, e.g., Ways of Coping Scale to determine the patient's coping strategies. Following the behavioral evaluation, management is directed at the factors which may affect treatment and determine the most appropriate interventions. Consideration should be given to the following factors: (1) behavioral or operant; (2) emotional; (3) characterologic; (4) cognitive; (5) side effects; (6) medication use; and (7) compliance. Therapy should intervene at two levels. First, the physical medicine techniques or pharmacology may be changed, and secondly, behavioral techniques may be incorporated, such as cognitive and behavioral management techniques, relaxation, biofeedback, and psychotherapeutic and psychopharmacologic interventions.

Case Summary

- This patient had sympathetically maintained traumatic trigeminal neuralgia.
- There was secondary myofascial pain which responded to physical medicine procedures.
- Therapeutic options include topical applications, nerve blocks, medications, and behavioral therapies.
- Traumatic trigeminal neuralgia can be sympathetically maintained or independent.
- The prognosis for traumatic trigeminal neuralgia is usually an 80% pain reduction. Medication is required for at least a year and some patients require extended treatment.

Overview of Traumatic Trigeminal Neuralgia

The basic pain quality associated with peripheral somatic nerves is a sharp electric or bright sensation which follows the affected nerves' dermatomal distribution. In the orofacial region the peripheral nerve disorders can be subdivided into (1) neuritis, (2) neuroma, and (3) neuralgias. The discussion here will be limited to traumatic trigeminal neuralgia (Table 40–3).

Traumatic neuralgia is defined as a continuous pain following complete or partial damage to a peripheral nerve. The pain is described as a continuous, burning numbness, and often as a pulling pain. The trauma is usually quite obvious, e.g., after facial trauma, root canal therapy or wisdom tooth removal, or after the placement of dental implants but may occur with minor traumas such as crown preparation. The discomfort can be self-limiting, depending on nerve regeneration. Campbell has described persistent pain following root canal therapy and apicoectomy in approximately 5% of patients. This may be attributed to the nerve damage and central sensitization or peripheral neural changes. Elies studied patients after mandibular dental implants and reported 17% developed persistent sensory

TABLE 40–3. Criteria for Traumatic Trigeminal Neuralgia

- History of trauma
- Continuous pain
- Associated hyperalgesia and allodynia
- Temperature change
- Block effect (sympathetic versus somatic)

change or pain. Other clinical characteristics of traumatic trigeminal neuralgia include associated hyperalgesia and allodynia, and a local temperature change. Thermographic studies reveal abnormal thermograms in all patients, some being hot in the pain distribution and some cold. None are normal. Graff-Radford et al. have described a hypothesis for these temperature changes that may be helpful in choosing treatment or understanding the mechanism producing the pain. Finally, traumatic neuralgia can be further divided by seeing the response to nerve blocks. If a sympathetic nerve block (stellate ganglion block) versus somatic (sensory) nerve block is effective, the traumatic neuralgia is defined as sympathetically maintained versus sympathetically independent.

Although thermography is somewhat speculative, it is an interesting finding that all thermograms are asymmetrical with the affected side being hot or cold. We assume that the mechanisms for hyperalgesia and allodynia are different for hot and cold thermogram presentations. We have hypothesized that hot thermograms due to injury or trauma would either indicate neurogenic inflammation or tissue inflammation produced by the release of substance P and calcitonin gene-related peptide (CGRP) both of which produce profound vasodilation. Cold thermal emissions may suggest a decrease in blood flow due to peripheral vasoconstriction. This is perhaps secondary to catecholamines binding onto new adrenergic receptors that have sprouted on vessels around the site of the trauma. These new receptors are bound by circulating catcholamines or by norepinephrine secreted by sympathetic nervous system activity. Other patients without obvious sympathetic overactivity (local somatic block stops the pain) may have sprouting of neuropeptide Y receptors on their vessels that will bind neuropeptide Y and circulating catecholamines, and then will show a cold thermogram.

If different mechanisms cause diverse temperature changes, one could hypothesize that different treatments could be developed to affect these mechanisms. Perhaps delivering capsaicin (a substance P depleter) may limit hot hyperalgesia and clonidine (a centrally acting alpha adrenergic stimulant) cold hyperalgesia.

Female patients in their 40s predominate in traumatic neuralgia. The reason for this is undetermined. It is clearly not a psychologic issue. Graff-Radford and Solberg have described MMPIs in this group and essentially the profiles are normal and similar to other same sex and duration head-pain patients. While sympathetically maintained pain occurs less frequently than sympathetically independent pain, it is the more complex problem to diagnose and manage. It is hoped that the many unnecessary treatments traumatic neuralgia patients receive may be limited by describing this problem.

Selected Readings

Campbell JN, Meyer RA, Davis KD, Raja SN. Sympathetically mediated pain a unifying hypothesis. In: Willis WD, editor. Hyperalgesia and allodynia. New York: Raven Press; 1992. p. 141–9.

Campbell Rl, Parks KW, Dodds RN. Chronic facial pain associated with endodontic neuropathy. Oral Surg Oral Med Oral Pathol 1990;69:287–90

Canavan D, Graff-Radford SB, Gratt BM. Traumatic dysesthesia of the trigeminal nerve. J Orofacial Pain 1994;8:391–6.

Ellies LG. Altered sensation following mandibular implant surgery: a retrospective study. J Prosthet Dent 1992;68:664–7.

Ellies LG, Hawker PB. The prevalence of altered sensation associated with implant surgery. Int J Oral Maxillofac Implants 1993;8:674–9.

Graff-Radford SB. Orofacial pain—an overview. J Back Musculoskeletal Rehabilitation 1996;6:113–33.

Graff-Radford SB, Ketalar M-C, Gratt BM, Solberg WK. Thermographic assessment of neuropathic facial pain: a pilot study. J Orofacial Pain 1995;9:138–46.

Graff-Radford SB, Solberg WK. Is atypical odontalgia a psychological problem? Oral Surg Oral Med Oral Pathol 1993;75: 579–82.

Gratt BM, Graff-Radford SB, Shetty V, et al. A six year clinical assessment of electronic facial thermography. J Dento Maxillo Facial Radiology 1996;25:247–55.

Lovshin LL. Vascular neck pain—a common syndrome seldom recognized: analysis of 100 consecutive cases. Cleve Clin Q 1960;27:5–13.

Okeson J, et al. Differential diagnosis and management considerations of neuralgias, nerve trunk pain, and deafferentation pain. In: Okesan J, editor. Orofacial pain: guidelines for assessment diagnosis and management. Chicago: Quintessence Books; 1996. p. 73–88.

Orofacial pain of neurogenous origin. In: Pertes RA, Gross SC, editors. Temporomandibular disorders and orofacial pain. Chicago: Quintessence Books; 1995. p. 329–42.

Raskin NH, Prusiner S. Carotidynia. Neurology 1977;27: 43–6.

Solberg WK, Graff-Radford SB. Orodental considerations of facial pain. Semin Neurol 1988;8:318–23.

Editorial Comments

Facial pain of undetermined origin can be extremely vexatious for the clinician and the patient in arriving at a correct diagnosis. There are so many causes and mechanisms for facial pain that at times clinicians faced with such patients are overwhelmed as to the diagnostic approach and management if the etiology is uncertain. Dr. Graff-Radford's case leads us through the maelstrom and shows us that one particular subtype, sympathetically maintained post-traumatic neuralgia, can be accurately diagnosed and managed in the majority of patients. Using evidence from his own studies, in large part, and his considerable experience, he teaches us a lot with this case, which should help us manage similar cases.

CHAPTER 41

THE WOMAN WITH RIGHT UPPER FACIAL PAIN

STEWART J. TEPPER, MD

Case History

A 72-year-old, right-handed woman presented with severe right upper face pain. The pain was described as an "electric shock-like sensation" in the first division of the trigeminal nerve in her eye, forehead, and right temple.

The pain was triggered by touching her eyebrow or combing her hair in the wrong direction. She also noticed that she could trigger brief, second-long attacks by jumping during aerobics, by walking in a breeze, or by other seemingly trivial activities of daily living.

She noted that between the pains she had a burning heaviness on that side of the head, so she was not entirely asymptomatic between the episodes.

None of the attacks lasted longer than a few seconds. All of the attacks were described as sudden, intense, sharp, superficially located, stabbing or burning in quality, and severe in intensity.

Her past medical history was significant for a right carotid endarterectomy for right transient monocular blindness 2 years before. She also had a history of migrainous aura with and without migraine headache, with vertigo and scintillating scotomata. She had Meniere's disease and hypertension. She had a right parotid tumor removed in 1943 and a malignant melanoma resection without evidence of recurrence.

Her neurologic examination was entirely normal except for the scars from the various surgeries. A magnetic resonance imaging (MRI) of the brain, without and with contrast, showed two small periventricular white matter lesions, which were nonspecific.

She had a complete resolution of her pain with 200 mg four times a day of carbamazepine. Two years later, she weaned herself off the carbamazepine, but within 6 months, she had a relapse requiring reinstitution of 200 mg of carbamazepine, twice daily. She has remained on this for 3 years and finds that she needs it.

Questions about This Case

- What is her diagnosis?
- What would be different if her age was 25?
- What features might be cause for concern?
- What work-up is appropriate?
- Which medical therapies may be considered in this disorder?
- Which surgical remedies may be considered for this disorder?

Case Discussion

This clinical presentation is certainly a classic case of trigeminal neuralgia. The International Headache Society (IHS) classification of 1988 lists the following criteria for diagnosing trigeminal neuralgia:

A. Paroxysmal attacks of facial or frontal pain which last a few seconds to less than two minutes

B. Pain has at least four of the following characteristics:

1. Distribution along one or more divisions of the trigeminal nerve

2. Sudden, intense, sharp, superficial, stabbing, or burning in quality
3. Pain intensity severe
4. Precipitation from trigger areas, or by certain daily activities such as eating, talking, washing the face, or cleaning the teeth
5. Between paroxysms the patient is entirely asymptomatic

C. No neurologic deficit

D. Attacks are stereotyped in the individual patient.

E. Exclusion of other causes of facial pain by history, physical examination, and special investigations when necessary

The patient's age is helpful in suggesting that this is "idiopathic" trigeminal neuralgia. In her age group, secondary causes include structural lesions involving the brain stem. Many are vascular such as stroke, aneurysm, and vascular compression of the trigeminal nerve. Other structural causes include syringobulbia, arachnoiditis, and basilar impression. Finally, neoplastic causes may include acoustic neuroma, epidermoid, meningioma, schwannoma, and cholesteatoma.

Her symptoms between paroxysms and her known cerebrovascular disease were cause for concern. However, her normal MRI excluded most potential structural and neoplastic causes for her symptoms. Stroke was a consideration, but her examination was normal, and the MRI failed to reveal a brain stem stroke. There are links epidemiologically between trigeminal neuralgia and hypertension and atherosclerosis.

In younger patients, the diagnosis is more likely to be secondary, and multiple sclerosis is the most frequent cause. Many neurologists would say that trigeminal neuralgia in a 25-year-old woman is multiple sclerosis (MS) until proven otherwise. In studies published since 1970, the frequency of secondary trigeminal neuralgia in MS patients ranged from 2.4 to 7.2%. Also, patients with multiple sclerosis often have neuralgic pain on both sides of the face during the course of their disease.

So, causes for concern over a secondary etiology would include younger age and bilateral facial pain. Pain outside the distribution of the trigeminal nerve would be worrisome. Of course, if the patient does not meet IHS criteria, that, too, should be a red flag.

Many specialists feel that an imaging study is necessary in the work-up of trigeminal neuralgia, even when the patient meets all criteria. In a study by Abbott and Killefer, 5 out of 57 patients had tumors, 3 out of 5 had no worrisome features, and 1 out of 5 responded to typical trigeminal neuralgia medication! An MRI is the best study with which to visualize the posterior fossa.

Medical treatment for trigeminal neuralgia involves the use of antiseizure drugs or baclofen. Carbamazepine is generally felt to be the first line of treatment. Although this patient used short-acting carbamazepine, many neurologists are recommending the use of extended-release preparations to avoid dosing three or four times a day.

Studies from 1968 to 1981 suggest a 70 to 80% response rate to carbamazepine. Zakrzewska recommends a careful, slow, low initiation of treatment with 100 mg per day, increasing by 100 mg every 3 days until there is symptomatic relief.

Carbamazepine can cause nausea, diplopia, sedation, and dizziness. Since it activates the cytochrome P-450 system, it autoinduces its own metabolism, and blood levels can fall after weeks of use. It may, therefore, be necessary to increase the dose again later in treatment.

Carbamazepine can cause idiosyncratic bone marrow aplasia in any or all cell lines. It can cause severe skin reactions, liver dysfunction, and the syndrome of inappropriate antidiuretic hormone secretion. Most neurologists monitor the blood at baseline and intermittently during therapy for complete blood count, differential, platelet count, electrolytes, and liver function tests.

Other antiseizure drugs can work in trigeminal neuralgia. Phenytoin can be used, either alone in patients who do not tolerate carbamazepine or adjunctively with carbamazepine.

Gabapentin is being studied currently, and its superior side-effect profile makes it very attractive. As with all of the antineuralgic drugs, it can be used alone or in combination.

There have been some limited studies on the use of divalproex sodium alone and in combination. This form is available in the U.S. and is composed of half valproate sodium and half valproic acid. Once again, lower doses of this drug are preferable, due to gastrointestinal side effects, and once again, blood monitoring is necessary. Divalproex sodium has less risk for hepatic toxicity when administered in mono-therapy rather than in copharmacy.

A few studies suggest that the benzodiazepine clonazepam can be effective in trigeminal neuralgia. Its use is severely constrained by the side effects of drowsiness, depression, induction of liver enzymes, and habituation.

Finally, baclofen is a unique antispasticity drug with inhibitory effects on neuronal action that may account for its antineuralgic activity. Several studies suggest efficacy in trigeminal neuralgia, and doses are from 15 to 60 mg per day. It can cause drowsiness, and it must be tapered off at withdrawal to avoid seizures.

Surgical remedies can be divided into peripheral interventions and central techniques. The peripheral trigeminal nerve can be disabled or destroyed by a variety of techniques including alcohol injection, freezing with cryosurgery, or radiofrequency thermocoagulation. The nerve itself can be cut with neurectomy. There is no comparative randomized study to clearly suggest that one operation is the best. In all peripheral surgeries, pain relief may be delayed for days, and symptoms usually recur within months. In all techniques, sensory loss occurs, and rarely anesthesia dolorosa.

The advantage of peripheral nerve approaches is that they are simple, give quick relief, and can be repeated easily. Alcohol injection carries with it the greatest risk for adverse events, and thermocoagulation requires expensive surgical devices. Zakrzewska notes that peripheral surgical interventions can be performed by oral and maxillofacial surgeons, as well as by neurosurgeons.

Centrally, surgery can be performed at the gasserian ganglion or in the posterior fossa. In the gasserian ganglion, the root can be thermocoagulated, injected with glycerol or alcohol, microcompressed, or cut. All these procedures cause loss of sensation and a decreased or absent ipsilateral corneal reflex. Risks include transient weakness of the muscles of mastication and the usual rare neurosurgical complications (e.g., meningitis, hemorrhage, other cranial neuropathies, etc.). Radiofrequency thermocoagulation of the gasserian ganglion remains the most frequently performed surgical procedure for trigeminal neuralgia. Recurrence tends to occur after years, rather than months.

Neurosurgical posterior fossa microvascular decompression has been championed in the U.S. by Jannetta, and is therfore referred to as the Jannetta procedure. This is a major neurosurgical procedure involving craniectomy. The trigeminal nerve is exposed, and if vessels are compressing it, they are separated and a Gelfoam-type material placed between the nerve and the compressing structure. If there is no compressing structure, sometimes a partial nerve-root resection is undertaken. Recurrence can occur and is felt to be due to irreversible lesioning of the trigeminal nerve by the compressive structure, with surgery too late to be curative. Burchiel et al. have described a recurrence rate of 2.0 to 3.5% per year.

Since the procedure is major and the outcome not perfect, careful medical consideration should be brought to bear before embarking on this route. Some surgeons feel that the operation should be done early to prevent permanent lesions and to decrease the likelihood of recurrence. Burchiel et al. have noted that when symptoms recur, the use of medication can often obviate the need for a second craniectomy.

Of course, the therapy must be individualized. In the case presented, the patient was easily managed with carbamazepine at a low dose in a convenient twice-daily regimen. The more severe and refractory the neuralgic pain, the more likely is the need for surgical intervention. Unfortunately, often the older the patient, the greater is the risk involved in central neurosurgical procedures.

Management Strategies

- It is very important to make sure that the diagnosis is primary trigeminal neuralgia and not secondary trigeminal neuralgia. In general, it is necessary to obtain an MRI to adequately visualize the posterior fossa.
- If there are reasons to suspect a vascular cause, magnetic resonance angiography (MRA) or conventional angiography may be necessary.
- Medical management usually involves the use of anti-seizure drugs, and carbamazepine remains the drug of first choice. The use of most anti-seizure drugs requires familiarity with side effects

and blood monitoring. The exception to the rule is gabapentin, and studies are underway to evaluate its efficacy in trigeminal neuralgia.

- If antiseizure drugs are not tolerated, baclofen should be used.
- When the neuralgia is inadequately controlled by drugs, surgical options should be considered next.
- Surgery can be peripheral or central, either at the gasserian ganglion or in the posterior fossa via craniectomy and the Jannetta procedure.
- Peripheral surgeries are, in general, cheaper, less invasive, and can be performed by oral surgeons. But, symptoms recur more quickly, within months. Peripheral surgeries include cryosurgery, radiofrequency thermocoagulation, and neurectomy.
- Radiofrequency thermocoagulation of the gasserian ganglion is the most commonly performed surgical technique for trigeminal neuralgia. Recurrence occurs after years.
- The Jannetta procedure, a posterior fossa craniectomy with microvascular decompression of the trigeminal nerve, also yields a high success rate, with recurrence after years. Often the recurrence can be treated with medication, as opposed to more surgery. On the other hand, it is the most invasive of all the options for trigeminal neuralgia, so it is theoretically a higher risk, higher gain situation.

Case Summary

- This patient has idiopathic trigeminal neuralgia or tic douloureux according to International Headache Society criteria.
- Her age, normal examination, normal MRI, and response to medication add certainty to the diagnosis.
- Her response to carbamazepine is heartening, and she will probably require no other treatment.
- Had her neuralgia been recalcitrant, gabapentin or phenytoin would have been reasonable antiseizure drug alternatives or adjuncts. Baclofen remains a useful choice, as well.
- If drug management fails, surgical procedures should be considered, ranging from simple peripheral cryosurgery to the nerve, to radiofrequency thermocoagulation of the gasserian ganglion, to the Jannetta procedure—a posterior fossa craniec-

tomy to achieve a microvascular decompression. These increasingly invasive procedures often yield better results with longer time to recurrence, but there is no consensus regarding the optimal surgical treatment and no definitive cross-surgery randomized study to guide individualized therapy.

Overview of Trigeminal Neuralgia

The International Headache Society classification describes trigeminal neuralgia as a "painful unilateral affliction of the face, characterized by brief electric shock-like (lancinating) pains limited to the distribution of the trigeminal nerve. Pain is commonly evoked by trivial stimuli including washing, shaving, smoking, talking, and brushing the teeth, but may also occur spontaneously. The pain is abrupt in onset and termination and may remit for varying periods." The location is almost always unilateral, and there can be trigger areas on the face or in the mouth.

On clinical examination, if the examination is not completely normal, there may be trigeminal sensory loss, and often the patient is unaware of the deficit.

Observation of a patient during an attack is useful as the patient will show a characteristic facial contortion which may be accompanied by other movements such as an arm or hand movement. The "tic" of "tic douloureux" is the reproducible behavioral movement that accompanies the pain.

It is worth remembering that the severity of trigeminal neuralgia pain is extreme and can lead a patient into depression and suicide. This accounts for the "douloureux" of "tic douloureux."

The prevalence of trigeminal neuralgia has been estimated by Zakrzewska as 4.7 per 1 million men and 7.2 per 1 million women. Kurland estimated that there were four new cases per 100,000 people per year at the Mayo Clinic in 1958. Rothman and Monson estimated a women to men ratio of 1.17:1 in 1973.

White and Sweet noted that 29% of trigeminal neuralgia patients experienced onset in the sixth decade and 28% in the seventh decade. Decreases in the rate of onset were observed at the two extremes with 18% presenting in the fifth decade, 6% in the fourth decade, and 12% in the eighth decade.

Onset is earlier in multiple sclerosis (MS)-induced secondary trigeminal neuralgia, and this can be used to alert the practitioner to the possibility of a secondary cause. Also, as noted, MS is often the situation in which the pain is on both sides or is atypical.

The differential diagnosis of primary trigeminal neuralgia can be divided into those primary headache disorders which can be confused with trigeminal neuralgia, and the secondary causes for trigeminal neuralgia.

The disorders that can sometimes be confused with trigeminal neuralgia include:

- Cluster headache. The duration of the headache is longer at 15 to 180 minutes, and the dysautonomic findings (e.g., conjunctival injection, nasal congestion, rhinorrhea, and Horner's syndrome) are also characteristic.
- Glossopharyngeal neuralgia. This is a stabbing neuralgic pain in the glossopharyngeal distribution of the tongue, pharynx, and angle of the jaw, but it can overlap the ear and can be triggered by similar triggers, i.e., talking and swallowing. Anatomic distribution is the best differentiation.
- Postherpetic neuralgia. The preceding zoster, of course, helps with the diagnosis, and the pain is often more achy or searing and less lightning-like. The location is often not trigeminal.
- Hemifacial spasm. This is a motor disorder and not painful. The tic of the face in trigeminal neuralgia is not an involuntary movement disorder. It can be controlled and is secondary to the pain.
- Idiopathic stabbing headache ("ice-pick pain"). Although the ice-pick pains are jabs and jolts, they are less painful than trigeminal neuralgia and are frequently single jabs. Occasionally they may occur in volleys, but, unlike trigeminal neuralgia, idiopathic stabbing headache usually responds to indomethacin.
- SUNCT (short-lasting unilateral neuralgiform headache with conjunctival injection and tearing). Although short lasting, the other features are unmistakable.
- Migraine. It lasts 4 to 72 hours and thus is not similar to trigeminal neuralgia.
- "Atypical facial pain." This is not trigeminal neuralgia, and it does not meet the IHS criteria for any other benign recurring headache disorder. The IHS classification official term is "facial pain not fulfilling criteria" and it is "not associated with physical signs or a demonstrable organic cause." It usually does not respond to medication, and it "persists for most or all of the day."

The secondary causes for trigeminal neuralgia include:

- Dental/temporomandibular joint causes
- Sinusitis
- Autoimmune disease—giant cell arteritis
- Eye disease—iritis, neuritis, glaucoma
- Vascular causes—stroke, aneurysm, vascular compression of the trigeminal nerve
- Neoplasm—acoustic neuroma, epidermoid, schwannoma, cholesteatoma
- Structural causes—syringobulbia, arachnoiditis, basilar impression

A work-up would include, at the least, an MRI to evaluate the posterior fossa. Angiography or an MRA may be considered if a vascular cause is suspected. Autoimmune serologies with a sedimentation rate are necessary when an autoimmune disease or giant cell arteritis is suspected. Referral to specialists in dentistry, oral surgery, otolaryngology, and ophthalmology may be indicated when a particular organ system is implicated.

The cause of trigeminal neuralgia is unknown. The most recent theory is that of Rappaport and Devor from 1994, which suggests that it may begin with an injury to the trigeminal ganglion or nerve root, and that this translates into a self-sustaining, self-generating area in the trigeminal ganglion which fires autorhythmically.

Another theory suggests a similarity between hemifacial spasm of the seventh nerve and trigeminal neuralgia in the fifth nerve. An injury to the nerve would result in ephaptic transmission with retrograde paroxysmal discharges.

The nature of the injury could be a demyelinating process, with impaired or altered transmission, or inadequate autoregulation or inhibition.

As noted, medical treatments begin with carbamazepine and/or gabapentin, with baclofen also being useful. Additional antiseizure drugs can be used such as phenytoin, clonazepam, or divalproex sodium.

Surgical treatments can involve peripheral techniques such as cryosurgery, alcohol injection, or radiofrequency thermocoagulation of the trigeminal nerve. Gasserian ganglion surgery is more invasive, but radiofrequency thermocoagulation remains the most commonly performed surgery. The Jannetta procedure is a posterior fossa craniectomy which allows for a microvascular decompression.

Symptoms may recur after procedures at all three levels, but they tend to occur with less frequency and at a longer time after the procedure with increasingly invasive techniques. Surgical therapy has not been satisfactorily randomized for study, and the decision on surgery must be individualized.

Selected Readings

Abbott M, Killefer FA. Symptomatic trigeminal neuralgia. Bull Los Angeles Neurol Soc 1970;35:1.

Brisman R. Trigeminal neuralgia and multiple sclerosis. Arch Neurol 1987;44:379–81.

Burchiel KJ, Clarke H, Haglund M, Loeser JD. Long term efficacy of microvascular decompression in trigeminal neuralgia. J Neurosurg 1988;69:35–8.

Fromm GH, editor. The medical and surgical management of trigeminal neuralgia. New York: Futura; 1987.

Fromm GH, Terrence CF, Chattha AS. Baclofen in the treatment of trigeminal neuralgia: double-blind study and long-term follow-up. Ann Neurol 1984;15:240–4.

Headache Classification Committee of the International Headache Society. Classification and diagnostic criteria for headache disorders, cranial neuralgias and facial pain. Cephalalgia 1988;8 Suppl 7:1–96.

Jason TS, Rasmussen P, Reske-Nelson E. Association of trigeminal neuralgia with multiple sclerosis: clinical and pathological features. Acta Neurol Scand 1982;65:182–9.

Kiluk KI, Knighton RS, Newman JD. The treatment of trigeminal neuralgia and other facial pain with carbamazepine. Mich Med 1968;67:1066–9.

Kurland LT. Descriptive epidemiology of selected neurologic and myopathic disorders with particular reference to a survey in Rochester, Minnesota. J Chron Dis 1958;8:378–418.

Rappaport ZH, Devor M. Trigeminal neuralgia: the role of self-sustaining discharge in the trigeminal ganglion. Pain 1994; 56:127–38.

Rothman KJ, Monson RR. Epidemiology of trigeminal neuralgia. J Chron Dis 1973;26:1–12.

Rovit RL, Murali R, Jannetta PJ, editors. Trigeminal neuralgia. Baltimore: Williams and Wilkins; 1990.

Sillampaa M. Carbamazepine. Pharmacology and clinical use. Acta Neurol Scand 1981;64 Suppl 88:115–9.

Smirne S, Scarlato G. Clonazepam in cranial neuralgias. Med J Aust 1977;1:93–4.

White JC, Sweet WH. Pain and the neurosurgeon. A 40-year experience. Springfield (II): Charles C. Thomas; 1969.

Zakrzewska JM. Trigeminal neuralgia. London: WB Saunders Company; 1995.

Zakrzewska JM, Patsalos PN. Drugs used in the management of trigeminal neuralgia. Oral Surg Oral Med Oral Pathol 1992; 74:439–50.

Zakrzewska JM, Thomas DGT. Patients' assessment of outcomes after three surgical procedures for the management of trigeminal neuralgia. Acta Neurochir 1993;122:225–30.

Editorial Comments

Dr. Tepper carefully reviews the IHS diagnostic criteria for trigeminal neuralgia and takes us through brief descriptions of the disorders that can be confused with it.

The diagnosis of trigeminal neuralgia is usually straightforward when patients present with classic symptoms. If there is any variance, however, further investigation and diagnostic considerations are indicated. In fact Dr. Tepper recommends, in general, neuroimaging of the posterior fossa in typical cases. Given the low incidence of trigeminal neuralgia, as well as the numerous secondary etiologies, such a recommendation seems sensible. This is especially so before destructive or invasive surgical intervention is contemplated. Many therapies are available, as is the case for most idiopathic pain disorders. Carbamazepine still remains the clinican's and patients' most valuable ally.

CHAPTER 42

THE PATIENT WITH NECK PAIN AND HEADACHE

NIKOLAI BOGDUK, MD, PhD, DSc

Case History

This patient was a 21-year-old nurse when her headaches started. She reported that the headaches were precipitated by a period of work during which she assisted in a radiology department and had to wear lead aprons for some 4 to 5 hours per day, 4 days a week for about 1 month. She developed severe neck pain and headache, associated with a decreased range of movement of her neck. She was relieved of work for 2 weeks, but upon resuming work she had to stop after 10 days because the pain had become worse. She presented some 2 years after the onset of her pain.

On presentation, her pain was felt high in the right posterior cervical region and radiated into the right occipital region and orbit, and sometimes to the right shoulder, right arm, and forearm. The symptoms were mainly on the right but sometimes passed to the left. The quality of the pain was dull and aching. It was present daily and aggravated by lifting, turning her head, sudden movements of the head, getting into awkward positions, and by looking down. The pain was relieved somewhat by application of heat and by lying down. Irregularly, the pain was associated with tingling over the right periorbital region and cheek.

She reported an episode some 3 months prior to presenting in which she was craning forward and felt a "clunk" in the back of her neck, which was followed by spasm of her neck muscles and very severe pain which obliged her to take to her bed. The next morning she felt that her neck was still "out of place" and was very painful. This persisted for some days until, when she was picking up something from her lap, she lifted her head backward and again felt a "clunk," after which there was a dramatic relief of her pain.

She had no family history of illness. Her own medical history included appendicitis and conjunctivitis, both resolved. A systems review revealed no symptoms of concurrent illness. Neurologic examination revealed no sensory or motor deficits in the distribution of the cranial or spinal nerves. Specifically, there was no numbness or hyperesthesia in the distribution of the trigeminal nerve or C2 spinal nerve.

Questions about This Case

- What are your diagnostic considerations in this case?
- Why have her headaches continued?
- Do you wish to know more about this particular case; if so, what pertinent information would you like to know?
- How would you have investigated this patient's headaches, and what specific therapies would you suggest?
- What long-term management strategies would you suggest for her case?

Case Discussion

Several features in this case implicate the neck as the source of pain. Headache is the predominant complaint, but the patient also complains of neck pain. The orbital region is involved but the pain spreads from the posterior upper neck to the orbit, rather than arising in the orbit. Neck movements aggravate the pain, as do activities of daily living that involve moving or loading the neck, such as lifting.

The headache suffered by this patient lacks the periodicity and associated features of migraine. It lacks any vascular features. The relationship to neck movements and activities denies a diagnosis of chronic tension-type headache. The unilateral distribution of the headache and the lack of systemic illness or neurologic signs, and the lack of progression exclude intracranial diseases.

Prior to presenting, she had seen a variety of health professionals, each of whom inferred that the neck was involved, although none offered a specific diagnosis. Nevertheless, therapy was applied empirically to the neck. Treatment by a chiropractor did not help; manipulative therapy by three different physiotherapists gave the patient some intermittent relief, as did acupuncture; but nonsteroidal anti-inflammatory drugs afforded no particular benefit. The challenges in a case like this are whether the headache stems from the neck, and if so, from where exactly.

One of the manipulative therapists who saw the patient reported signs of abnormal joints at C2-3 and C3-4, consisting of abnormal quality of movement and abnormal end-feel, with reproduction of the patient's pain upon passive intersegmental motion. An orthopedic surgeon requested plain radiographs of her neck. These showed slight (grade 0.5) spondylolisthesis at C2-3 and C3-4, but this grade of translation is within the normal limits of motion at these levels.

Medical imaging is notoriously useless in determining a diagnosis of cervical headache. Tumors, infections, and inflammatory diseases of the cervical spine are rare causes of headache. In the vast majority of patients there is nothing that might possibly be evident on radiographs of the neck that either implicates or refutes a diagnosis of cervical headache. Spondylosis is not a cause of headache, because the same spondylotic changes are evident in the same proportion of patients as in asymptomatic individuals of the same age.

Manipulative therapists believe that they can pinpoint abnormal and symptomatic joints in the neck by careful manual examination. This has been validated in the case of one manipulative therapist but the results of that study cannot be generalized. It has not been shown that manipulative therapists at large are either reliable or valid in their claims of diagnostic acumen. Serendipitously, the manipulative therapist in the present case proved to be correct.

Diagnostic blocks are the only available, valid means of pinpointing a source of neck pain or cervical headache. Various joints and ligaments in the neck, that might be the source of the pain, are simply not palpable, but they are accessible to needles. Under radiographic control, needles can be used to anesthetize selected joints, ligaments, or nerves, in order to test if that structure is the source of the patient's pain, or in the case of nerves, if that nerve mediates the patient's pain.

At the request of her orthopedic surgeon, she underwent a diagnostic block of her right C2-3 zygapophysial joint. Upon injection of contrast medium into that joint her pain was aggravated, but upon injection of local anesthetic and corticosteroid, her pain was promptly relieved. This provided prima facie evidence that the C2-3 zygapophysial joint was the source of her headache, and this preliminary diagnosis was subsequently explored.

The C2-3 zygapophysial joint is innervated by the third occipital nerve. A right third occipital nerve block, using 0.5% bupivacaine, promptly and completely relieved her of her headache for several hours. Subsequently an intra-articular injection of 0.8 mL of a mixture of 1 mL 0.5% bupivacaine and 1 mL (5.7 mg) of betamethasone provided complete relief of her headache for some 12 weeks. A repeat injection of 0.5 mL of betamethasone alone resulted in a further period of 12 weeks of relief, on each of two subsequent occasions.

Although grateful for the quality of relief that these injections afforded, the patient wanted to obtain longer-lasting relief. She had been informed of the prospect of percutaneous radiofrequency neurotomy, and she wanted to pursue this.

A prognostic block of her right third occipital nerve was performed and, again, completely relieved her headache. On the basis of this response and her consistent response to third occipital nerve blocks and to intra-articular steroids, she was scheduled to undergo percutaneous radiofrequency neurotomy of her right third occipital nerve.

This was performed and she obtained complete relief of her headache. The relief lasted for some 9 months, but she suffered two side effects, each predicted from the prognostic blocks. She had numbness in the cutaneous territory of the third occipital nerve, which was not a problem, but she also had ataxia. This gave her trouble walking down stairs, but she could cope if she held the banister and looked straight ahead instead of at her feet. The ataxia and the numbness, however, resolved as her headache returned.

As the relief of her headache waned, she asked if she could have the neurotomy repeated. Told that if she had a repeat operation the ataxia would recur, and asked if she wanted to suffer that side effect again, she responded, "Are you kidding? I would swap these headaches for unsteadiness any day."

Ataxia is a regular side effect of third occipital neurotomy and occurs temporarily when that nerve is blocked with local anesthetics. It arises because of interference with tonic neck reflexes, ostensibly because of block of conduction in proprioceptive afferents from muscles innervated by the third occipital nerve.

Ten months after the initial neurotomy, she underwent a repeat neurotomy and regained complete pain relief. Eleven months later the pain recurred, and she underwent another repeat neurotomy. This afforded her complete relief again, this time lasting some 12 months.

Almost as regularly as clockwork she has enjoyed complete relief every year since, with pain recurring at about 12 months, only to be relieved by a repeat neurotomy. On February 22, 1997, she celebrated the seventh year of relief from her headaches.

During this period her life was rehabilitated. After having been unemployed and disabled for some 3 years, the pain relief allowed her first to complete a university degree, and maintain part-time employment. Upon graduating she was able to assume full-time employment, which she has maintained since.

The only interruption has been the 1 day a year that she requires to have a repeat neurotomy, and 5 days' leave for recuperation. The one side effect that she has developed is addiction to the pain relief she has obtained. She cannot bear going back to the way she was, if radiofrequency neurotomy was no longer to be available.

Management Strategies

- Patients with suspected cervical headache require a precision diagnosis.
- A diagnosis might be established using the skills of a well-trained manual therapist, but the validity and reliability of such skills in the community at large has not been established.
- Manual therapy might be tried, but there is little guarantee that it will work at all or, if it does seem to work, that it will have any profound or lasting effect.
- For many sources of cervical headache, diagnostic blocks are available for precision diagnosis. The putatively painful joint or its nerve supply can be selectively anesthetized under radiographic control. Complete relief of pain pinpoints the offending structure.
- Oral drug therapy is of no proven benefit for cervical headache and has not even attracted anecdotal support.
- Intra-articular steroids are potentially of benefit for some patients, but most patients do not obtain lasting relief. Pain recurs within 1 to 2 weeks in more than 80% of patients.
- The only treatment known to have any lasting effect on cervical headache is radiofrequency neurotomy, but this procedure has not been proved in a controlled trial.

Case Summary

- This patient suffered cervical headache which was pain referred from her right C2-3 zygapophysial joint to her occiput and orbit.
- The pain was repeatedly and consistently relieved by local anesthetic blocks of her third occipital nerve or by intra-articular injections of a corticosteroid.
- This pain relief, however, was only temporary, lasting hours with local anesthetic and only weeks with steroids.

- Percutaneous radiofrequency third-occipital neurotomy abolished her headache for periods of up to 1 year and beyond.
- Despite side effects of numbness and ataxia, she craved and insisted on relief from her pain.
- As the effects of the operation wore off, so did her side effects.
- Repeat neurotomy has reinstated her relief regularly for 7 years.
- Relief of her pain has restored her life.

Overview of Cervical Headache

Diseases or injuries of the upper cervical spine can cause local pain and pain referred into the head. The referred pain is perceived in the occiput and may extend through the parietal region and into the frontal and orbital regions.

The anatomic basis of cervical headache appears to be convergence between cervical and trigeminal afferents in the trigeminocervical nucleus, which consists of the pars caudalis of the spinal nucleus of the trigeminal nerve and the dorsal horns of the first three cervical spinal cord segments. Exactly where the referred pain is felt depends on which nerves converge in this nucleus. Convergence between cervical joint afferents and the first division of the trigeminal nerve will result in referral to the frontal region and orbit. Convergence between joint afferents and fibers of the C2 spinal nerve will result in referral to the occiput.

Although the specific neuroanatomy has not been demonstrated, several clinical experiments in normal volunteers have demonstrated the capacity of the neck to refer pain into the head.

Campbell and Parsons and Feinstein et al. showed that stimulating the upper posterior neck muscles could produce headache in normal volunteers. Dwyer et al. show the same for the C2-3 zygapophysial joint, and Dreyfuss et al. for the atlanto-occipital and lateral atlantoaxial joints.

In patients with headache, Ehni and Benner reported temporary relief of pain following periarticular blocks of the lateral atlantoaxial joints, and McCormick reported relief following intra-articular blocks of these joints. Bogduk and Marsland reported relief following blocks of the C2-3 zygapophysial

joints, later confirmed by Lord et al. using double-blind, controlled blocks.

Lord et al. established that in patients with chronic headache following whiplash, the headache could be traced to the C2-3 joint in some 50% of cases. Joints below C2-3 are uncommonly the source of headache, if at all.

Jull et al. reported that an expert manual therapist was capable of accurately diagnosing cervical zygapophysial joint pain. The diagnostic features of a symptomatic joint were abnormal quality of movement, abnormal end-feel and reproduction of pain upon passive movement of the joint. These findings, however, have not been followed by subsequent studies to show that any other manual therapist is equally accurate.

Nevertheless, using Jull as the diagnostic instrument, Treleavan et al. found that many cases of so-called postconcussional headache could be traced to the C1-2 or C2-3 joints.

Ironically, cervical headache is one of the best defined types of headaches, yet the least respected. The definition of cervical headache and its diagnostic criteria are far more explicit and objective than those for tension-type headache, yet the latter entity is honoured far more than cervical headache.

The definition of cervicogenic headache proposed by the North American Cervicogenic Headache Society is that the headache is referred pain that stems from a structure innervated by one or other of the cervical spinal nerves. This definition expressly differentiates cervical headache from another type of headache, some of whose clinical features might be shared. But the diagnosis of cervical headache rests not on recognizing clinical features; it rests solely on demonstrating a cervical source of pain, by whatever means, provided that those means are valid. At present, controlled diagnostic blocks are the only valid means.

Opposition to the concept of cervical headache seems to stem largely from lack of familiarity with the concept, or lack of ability or reluctance to apply or obtain the necessary diagnostic procedures. Because the diagnosis cannot be established by conventional clinical examination, neurologists and others are not equipped or trained to make the diagnosis. For this reason, the entity has been embraced far more strongly by anesthesiologists in pain medicine, and by radiologists who have at their disposal the needle skills and imaging facilities required to pursue the diagnosis.

Although the earlier literature relied on uncontrolled diagnostic blocks of cervical joints or cervical nerves in the pursuit of cervical headache, controlled blocks are now mandatory. Controlled blocks guard against false-positive responses due to placebo effects. Controls are required in each and every case.

Placebo controls pose ethical and logistic problems. In most countries, impromptu, single-blind, placebo injections are unethical without informed consent. Therefore, if placebos are to be used, a series of three diagnostic blocks is required to make a diagnosis of cervical headache. The first block must be with an anesthetic agent in order to first establish that the target joint is, indeed, painful. Unless that is shown, it would be a waste of time and resources to complete the series on a joint that is not symptomatic. The second block cannot routinely be the placebo, for an observant patient would know that the second block was always the dummy. In order to maintain blinding and the element of chance, the second block must be either a placebo or an active agent. To complete the series, the agent not used on the second occasion is administered as the third block. A positive response would be one in which the patient obtains complete relief of their headache whenever a local anesthetic was used, but no relief when normal saline was used.

A more practical form of control is a comparative local anesthetic block. This circumvents the ethical and logistic problems of placebo-controlled blocks. On separate occasions the diagnostic block is performed using different local anesthetic agents. A positive response is deemed to have occurred if on each occasion the patient obtains complete relief of their pain but short-lasting relief when a short-acting agent is used, and long-lasting relief when a long-acting agent is used.

Lord et al. have shown that these criteria are robust against placebo-challenge; they are highly specific, but lack optimal sensitivity. Some patients who obtain complete relief but inordinately prolonged relief with lignocaine defy the diagnostic criteria of comparative blocks, but nonetheless do not respond to placebo. Such patients may fail to be included as positive if the diagnostic criteria for comparative blocks are rigidly applied.

Diagnostic blocks of many upper cervical structure are not difficult to perform. Therefore, in principle, few possible sources of cervical headache can escape pursuit. What is required is the willingness to entertain these sources, and the skills and technical resources to pursue them. Blocks can be performed of the atlanto-occipital, lateral atlantoaxial, and zygapophysial joints, as well as the C2 and C3 spinal nerves. Only the median atlantoaxial joint is inaccessible for blocks.

What remains unknown is the extent epidemiologically to which cervical headaches stem from the atlanto-occipital, atlantoaxial, C2-3 zygapophysial joints and other cervical structures that are responsible for headaches. To date, the only index is that the C2-3 joint is a very common source of headache after whiplash.

The pathology of cervical headache is unknown. Presumably it arises as a result of some form of injury to one or other cervical structure. Frustratingly, contemporary medical imaging cannot resolve such injuries even though they may be present. Postmortem studies have shown that injuries to the atlantoaxial, atlanto-occipital, and cervical zygapophysial joints, evident on dissection, are invisible on radiographs of the specimen, even on retrospective review.

In the case described in this chapter, 1 mm CT scans were taken perpendicular to the surface of the C2-3 and other zygapophysial joints. The joints at C2-3 were extremely narrowed, to less than 1 mm, implying virtually no articular cartilage. This feature was not evident at lower joints and intuitively must be abnormal for a 21-year-old woman. However, there are no data against which this intuition might be tested. Not only do we not know what the CT appearance is of painful zygapophysial joints, we do not even know what their normal appearance is at different ages. Until that normative data is at hand, CT scanning cannot be used to investigate the cause of zygapophysial joint pain.

Treatment of cervical headache remains at the frontier of medical research. No conventional therapy is known to work. There are no data on the usefulness of arthritis drugs, and no compelling data on physical therapy or manipulative therapy. No one has yet conducted a trial of any therapy for patients with proven cervical headache.

Intra-articular steroids might be countenanced as an upmarket medical intervention, but the study carried out by Barnsley et al. showed that few patients respond, and that steroids confer no benefit over local anesthetic alone.

Radiofrequency neurotomy remains an unproven treatment, and applicable only for cervical headache stemming from the C2-3 zygapophysial joint. Lord et al. found that radiofrequency neurotomy works for zygapophysial joint pain at levels below C2-3 for the treatment of neck pain, but they encountered technical difficulties when treating pain from C2-3 which limited application of the procedure. Whereas some patients responded outstandingly, as in the present case, others responded dismally. The flaw did not lie in the diagnosis; it lay in the operative technique. If the third occipital nerve is effectively coagulated, and remains coagulated, the patients reliably obtain relief. In essence, if they go numb, they lose their pain; but if the nerve is missed, and they do not go numb, their pain remains.

Current research is focused on perfecting the technique for third occipital neurotomy. For joints other than C2-3, some form of definitive therapy still needs to be conceived, let alone evaluated.

Selected Readings

Barnsley L, Lord S, Bogduk N. Comparative local anesthetic blocks in the diagnosis of cervical zygapophysial joints pain. Pain 1993;55:99–106.

Barnsley L, Lord SM, Wallis BJ, Bogduk N. Lack of effect of intraarticular corticosteroids for chronic pain in the cervical zygapophyseal joints. N Engl J Med 1994;330:1047–50.

Bogduk N, Marsland A. On the concept of third occipital headache. J Neurol Neurosurg Psychiatry 1986;49:775–80.

Bogduk N. Anatomy and physiology of headache. Biomed Pharmacother 1995;49:435–45.

Campbell DG, Parsons CM. Referred head pain and its concomitants. J Nerv Ment Dis 1944;99:544–51.

Dreyfuss P, Michaelsen M, Fletcher D. Atlanto-occipital and lateral atlanto-axial joint pain patterns. Spine 1994;19:1125–31.

Dwyer A, Aprill C, Bogduk N. Cervical zygapophysial joint pain patterns I: a study in normal volunteers. Spine 1990; 15:453–7.

Ehni G, Benner B. Occipital neuralgia and the C1-2 arthrosis syndrome. J Neurosurg 1984;61:961–5.

Feinstein B, Langton JBK, Jameson RM, Schiller F. Experiments on referred pain from deep somatic tissues. J Bone Joint Surg 1954;36A:981–97.

Jull G, Bogduk N, Marsland A. The accuracy of manual diagnosis for cervical zygapophysial joint pain syndromes. Med J Aust 1988;148:233–6.

Lord S, Barnsley L, Wallis B, Bogduk N. Third occipital headache: a prevalence study. J Neurol Neurosurg Psychiatry 1994;57:1187–90.

Lord SM, Barnsley L, Bogduk N. The utility of comparative local anaesthetic blocks versus placebo-controlled blocks for the diagnosis of cervical zygapophysial joint pain. Clin J Pain 1995;11:208–13.

Lord SM, Barnsley L, Bogduk N. Percutaneous radiofrequency neurotomy in the treatment of cervical zygapophysial joint pain: a caution. Neurosurgery 1995;36:732–9.

Lord S, Barnsley L, Wallis BJ, et al. Percutaneous radiofrequency neurotomy for chronic cervical zygapophysial joint pain. N Engl J Med 1996;335:1721–6.

McCormick CC. Arthrography of the atlanto-axial (C1-C2) joints: technique and results. J Intervent Radiol 1987;2:9–13.

Treleaven J, Jull G, Atkinson L. Cervical musculoskeletal dysfunction in post-concussional headache. Cephalalgia 1994; 14:273–9.

Editorial Comments

The relationship of headache to neck disorders and neck pain has long been a source of debate, with wide and varied views put forth by many individuals. Dr. Bogduk presents an important case, with a diagnosis and management strategy supported by his considerable knowledge and experience with similar cases. The concept of convergence of cervical and trigeminal pathways makes intuitive sense, both anatomically and clinically. Diagnostic and therapeutic blocks can be harder to accept, except in Dr. Bogduk's hands. There is much for the reader to learn from this case, whether you agree with the diagnosis and treatment or not. The fact that diagnosis of cervicogenic headache depends not on a recognizable pattern in the patients' histories but on the results of a nerve block makes the concept hard to accept. Even if one does not accept the entity of cervicogenic headache, that diagnostic possibility should be considered and investigated in cases such as these.

CHAPTER 43

HEADACHE AND FACIAL PAIN IN AN ELDERLY MAN

HARVEY J. BLUMENTHAL, MD

Case History

A 79-year-old man was admitted to hospital for chest pain which was found to result from myocardial infarction. There was a long history of vascular disease, and he had undergone successful coronary artery bypass surgery in the past. Upon this admission, he was treated with heparin and warfarin. He had a past history of bladder cancer and the patient was actually in his urologist's office when the chest pain developed and he was sent to the emergency department. I was consulted because of severe left periorbital pain which developed 5 days after hospitalization, pain which was unlike anything the patient had ever experienced. He awakened at 3 AM the morning of the consultation with severe left periorbital pain. He was given acetaminophen with codeine without relief and the medication caused mild nausea. When I first saw him at 7 PM, the pain had subsided considerably and he was feeling better than he had all day but his left cheek was mildly painful. He had never experienced anything like this before.

Four months earlier, the patient became confused while driving and found himself on the wrong road. He was able to drive home. Two months later, he experienced blurred vision while driving, and then he did not recall driving off the road and into a culvert, which damaged his car. He was able to drive home, and when he arrived home, he saw that the car was damaged but could not remember how. A

neighbor called his home and told the patient's wife that her husband had been driving erratically and had driven off the road into the culvert. The patient had no memory of this one-car accident.

A physician suspected a light stroke. A brain scan was done 2 months before I was consulted and was normal.

For the previous 3 months, the patient had suffered mild fluctuating pain in the left cheek lasting only a brief moment. This brief paroxysmal pain might not occur for 2 or 3 weeks and then reoccur.

The patient had normal vital signs. He was alert, intelligent, fluent, and extremely talkative. He was hard of hearing. His carotid pulses were strong and equal, and I heard no carotid or subclavian bruits or bruit over his orbits. There was no tenderness of the temples or cheek. Sensation over his face was normal. Visual fields, pupils, and optic fundi were normal. There was no facial asymmetry. His cardiologist had suspected left ptosis earlier that evening but I could not appreciate it, and when I called this to the patient's attention, he told me that the pain had been so severe he was merely closing his left eye when examined earlier. There was no down-drift or tremor of his outstretched arms and he had excellent grip and proximal muscle power. Tests of cerebellar coordination were performed smoothly with arms and legs. Stretch reflexes were normal but he had Babinski's sign on the right and not on the left. The sensory examination yielded normal responses.

Computed tomography brain scan and carotid Doppler tests were normal. Sedimentation rate was 59 mm per hour, and temporal arteritis was considered. The pain improved spontaneously and the patient was dismissed 2 days later, taking warfarin but not prednisone.

Questions about This Case

- Formulate a differential diagnosis for the cause of this patient's headache.
- How might the headache condition be related to his other medical and neurologic problems?
- What additional diagnostic tests would you consider?

Case Discussion

Within a week after discharge, at home, the facial pains recurred, and a dentist was consulted. A left maxillary premolar apical abscess was diagnosed and the patient was treated with antibiotics. The dentist was fearful of performing any procedures because the patient was taking warfarin. The pain improved, and 2 months later the tooth fell out spontaneously. The patient has had no headache or facial pain since. He did well at home until 1 year later when he experienced a spontaneous convulsion and had two subsequent seizures in the next 3 days. He was treated by his home-town physician with phenytoin. A magnetic resonance imaging brain scan proved normal.

Dental Disease Presenting with
Headache and Facial Pain

The patient's chief headache complaint was acute left periorbital pain, and although this was the reason I was consulted, the patient's headache and neurologic condition were more complex than a simple headache problem. Four months earlier, he became confused while driving. Two months later, he experienced blurred vision, wrecked his car, and did not remember the accident. An experienced cardiologist suspected a stroke.

Three months before the acute headache presentation, the patient developed infrequent brief parox-

ysmal jabs of mild pain in his left cheek, finally culminating in the acute left orbital and left cheek pain the day I was consulted. All of this was superimposed upon the acute myocardial infarction 5 days before the acute left orbital and facial pain.

This complex problem of multisystem involvement, particularly in the elderly, is a common challenge for the clinician. And in this case there were multiple neurologic elements which may or may not have been related: the acute left-sided headache, the paroxysmal left facial pain, and the two episodes of reversible confusion.

The acute left frontal headache accompanied by right Babinski's sign 5 days after the myocardial infarction raises the question of cardiogenic cerebral embolism. The patient was under treatment with heparin, and a therapeutic level of anticoagulation had been achieved with partial thromboplastin time of 50.7 seconds. While heparin reduces the risk for cardiogenic embolism, it does not eliminate the risk completely. Headache associated with stroke is discussed in Chapter 29.

A second diagnostic consideration in a 79-year-old man with new headache must be temporal arteritis. Giant cell arteritis can also cause mental confusion and blurred vision, which the patient complained of at the time of his accident 2 months before presenting with the acute left periorbital headache. Blurring of vision occasionally precedes the sudden blindness which can result from temporal arteritis. One of the great tragedies in medicine is for the patient to have a treatable condition which is overlooked until too late. In the case of temporal arteritis, 50% of patients are at risk of irreversible blindness, but this outcome is preventable in most instances by early diagnosis and treatment with corticosteroids.

The patient had bladder cancer and, in fact, was in his urologist's office for routine follow-up when he developed the chest pain which sent him to the emergency department. Cancer metastatic to the head may cause localized headache, and the left facial pain immediately focuses our attention on the trigeminal nerve. Most often posterior fossa tumors are responsible, but metastasis to Meckel's cave may invest the trigeminal ganglion and cause facial pain. Metastatic disease to the base of the skull or orbital apex can cause orbital pain and blurred vision. Visceral cancer may result in a hypercoagulable state and stroke is the second most common neurologic complication of cancer after metastasis. Nonbacterial thrombotic endocarditis (NBTE) or marantic endocarditis is a common cause of embolic stroke in cancer patients. Rarely, lung cancer may compress or infiltrate the vagus nerve near the trachea and cause referred facial pain. Intracranial neoplasms presenting with headache are discussed in Chapter 27.

The paroxysmal left facial pains which began 3 months before the acute left periorbital headache call tic douloureux to mind. This condition is common in the elderly and may fluctuate and remit spontaneously. Once again, our attention is directed to the trigeminal ganglion to rule out any structural compression or irritation. Tic douloureux is discussed in detail in Chapter 41.

Although I did not observe ptosis, the cardiologist thought the patient did have left ptosis, and the combination of facial pain and ptosis make carotid artery dissection a diagnostic consideration.

The combination of ipsilateral ptosis and facial pain may also result from cranial mononeuropathy multiplex. Infiltrations at the base of the skull by malignancy, granulomatous infiltrations, or tuberculosis, or fungal infections may cause this syndrome.

New facial pain or orbital headache may be the presenting symptom of purulent sinusitis. Engorged and swollen nasal mucosa, purulent turbinates, and significant nasal discharge are usually present. Sphenoid sinusitis especially is a condition which must be diagnosed early, and endoscopic drainage and antibiotic treatment are urgent because of the frequent spread of infection to nearby structures. If the treatment of acute sphenoid sinusitis is delayed, there is 100% serious morbidity such as cortical vein or cavernous sinus thrombosis, meningitis, or retro-orbital abscess.

Acute periorbital pain may result from the expansion of a supraclinoid aneurysm which can compress the ophthalmic branch of the trigeminal nerve as it enters the orbit through the superior orbital fissure.

I missed the diagnosis in this case because I did not consider that pain referred through the maxillary division of the trigeminal nerve might result from dental disease. Solberg and Graff-Radford make a very strong statement which I shall remember when I next see a similar case: "So versatile are dental pains that it has been a rule of thumb to consider all pains about the mouth and face to be of dental origin until proved otherwise."

Sensory innervation of the teeth is strictly unilateral and inflammation of the dental pulp causes a deep orofacial pain, less easily localized by the patient than superficial pain from the gingiva. Typically, dental pain is a sharp, deep pain often evoked by an external stimulus and subsides within a few seconds. Hot or cold liquids, food, and air are common stimuli, but the patient did not volunteer such symptoms and I failed to ask. Inflammation, usually infection of the dental pulp, may cause a throbbing pain or dull, deep aching pain. Pain caused by pulpitis is less often affected by chewing than by thermal changes. In difficult cases a local dental anesthetic will block the peripheral dental pain, whereas the more central pain of tic douloureux would not be helped.

Dental disease may cause referred pain, secondary muscle spasm, and autonomic symptoms which may further confuse the clinician. Dental pain may be referred between the upper and lower dental arches on the same side, but do not give any anatomic explanation. Anesthetic blockade of the secondary site will be equivocal adding to the diagnostic confusion while anesthesia of the offending tooth will abolish pain at both sites. Myocardial pain may be referred to the teeth; psychogenic tooth pain must also be considered.

There is considerable literature on atypical odontalgia (see Solberg and Graff-Radford for the many dental references). This condition is poorly understood and the diagnosis is made with persistent pain localized to apparently normal teeth and may be a localized form of atypical facial neuralgia. Antidepressants have been helpful in some cases.

When considering dental disease as a cause of facial pain, specific questions regarding thermal provocation, local tenderness to a gloved digital palpation of the gum area, or gently tapping the tooth may lead to the correct diagnosis. Dental consultation may be helpful in difficult cases of facial pain.

Case Summary

In conclusion, this 79-year-old man's case was complicated by neurologic symptoms which remain unexplained and were almost certainly unrelated to the dental abscess which caused the headache and facial pain. The lesson to be remembered is that in complicated cases, especially in the elderly, there may be more than one simultaneous pathophysiologic process which can cause headache or neurologic complications unrelated to the headache problem.

The author gratefully acknowledges and thanks Bruce Stewart, DDS, for reviewing the dental aspects of this chapter.

Selected Readings

Barker FG, Jannetta PJ, Bissonette DJ, et al. The long term outcome of microvascular decompression for trigeminal neuralgia. N Engl J Med 1996;334:1077–83.

Blumenthal HJ. Temporal arteritis, a medical emergency. J Ark Med Soc 1978;75:201–5.

Bongers KM, Willigers HMM, Koehler PJ. Referred facial pain from lung carcinoma. Neurology 1992;42:1841–2.

Cheng TMW, Cascino TL, Onofrio BM. Comprehensive study of diagnosis and treatment of trigeminal neuralgia secondary to tumors. Neurology 1993;43:2298–302.

Forsyth PA, Posner JB. Headaches in patients with brain tumors. Neurology 1993;43:1678–83.

Jorgensen HS, Jespersen HF, Nakayama H, et al. Headache in stroke. Neurology 1994;44:1793–7.

Lew D, Southwice FS, Montgomery WW. Sphenoid sinusitis. Lancet 1983;309:1149–54.

Raps EC, Rogers JD, Galetta SL, et al. The clinical spectrum of unruptured intracranial aneurysms. Arch Neurol 1993;50:265–8.

Silbert PL, Mokri B, Schievink WI. Headache and neck pain in spontaneous internal carotid and vertebral artery dissections. Neurology 1995;45:1517–22.

Slivka A, Philbrook B. Clinical and angiographic features of thunderclap headache. Headache 1995;35:1–6.

Solberg WK, Graff-Radford SB. Orodental considerations in facial pain. Semin Neurol 1988;8:318–23.

Editorial Comments

We all learn a great deal from the limited number of cases that we either fail to diagnose or in which our specialty orientation leads us down the wrong path. Dr. Blumenthal clearly illustrates the lessons that can be learned from such cases. We commend Dr. Blumenthal for sharing a "missed diagnosis" with us. We all have them. Pain knows no boundaries, and we all can be grateful for the advice and help of neurologists, dental specialists, and cardiologists. Read this case carefully; it "teaches" us a lot.

CHAPTER 44

THE OENOPHILE WITH THE DISAPPEARING MIGRAINE

ROBERT F. NELSON, MD, FRCPC

Case History

This patient is a healthy, athletic 40-year-old wine connoisseur (oenophile) who has suffered from migraine headaches dating back to childhood, when he was also very susceptible to motion sickness. The headaches became quite severe in his twenties, when he noted that the headache might be precipitated by red sandwich meat, pizza, and red wine. There was never any prelude or aura, and the pain began as a throbbing in the right occipital region that spread forward to the right eye. The eye might tear but he had never noted drooping of the eyelid or alteration of vision. When he was a teenager, the headaches were usually accompanied by nausea and vomiting. As he grew older, vomiting rarely occurred and he had not vomited in recent years. He usually had to lie down in a darkened room and found that acetaminophen with codeine or ibuprofen reduced the intensity of the pain only slightly. Of a number of triggers, red wine was the most potent and he found that even half a glass of red wine invariably induced a headache within an hour and often sooner. He found that particular wines with a high tannin, oak, or sulfur content were most noxious and certain Bordeaux, Riojas, and ports would trigger a headache almost immediately. This lead him to curtail his hobby, although he continued to collect rare wines. In the past few years, his migraine attacks occurred once or twice a month, often precipitated by abrupt changes in the weather or let-down periods after emotional stress.

His family history is positive for migraine. His mother suffered from severe migraine, also precipitated by red wine. His father suffers from Meniere's disease, but not headache, and his paternal uncle suffers from migraine. His maternal grandmother has continued to suffer from migraine through to her nineties, but her headaches improved after she was prescribed medication for hypertension.

On a very hot day one August, the patient and a friend trekked for 4 hours up a low mountain and after reaching the top they lifted some heavy rocks to make a cairn. On straining to lift a particularly heavy rock, the patient developed a burning itchy sensation in his right eye and felt light-headed. After a few minutes he noted a tingling on the right side of his lips that spread to the adjacent cheek area. After a further few minutes his left hand developed a crawling tingling sensation and this spread proximally. His left toes went numb and this numbness also spread up the left leg. By the end of 5 minutes his whole left side, from the neck down, felt numb. This was not followed by any headache but he felt faint and profoundly tired. After a further 5 minutes, the symptoms gradually cleared completely and he headed down the mountain. At no time did he have any weakness or loss of function of his limbs. However, as he trekked downhill he experienced the same sequence of events twice again, always starting in the right upper lip and appearing within minutes in the left limbs.

From August through to the following June he experienced many of these stereotyped attacks. By June they were occurring several times a day, often occurring in a flurry, where he might experience three or four attacks in a few hours, each lasting only a few minutes. On a few occasions, however, the numbness or buzzing sensation in his right lip and left hand persisted for 20 to 30 minutes. He describes the attacks in detail as follows. First, the right upper lip becomes "tingly" and this spreads to involve the right side of the nose, and the nostril stings as if he is about to sneeze. Then numbness spreads to the adjacent cheek area, and then the lower lip and the inside of the mouth on the right become numb. The right eye develops a burning, itchy feeling but there is no tearing. Then after a few seconds, the left fingers and hand become numb. The patient does not think that any one digit becomes numb first, but rather the fingers and whole hand become numb simultaneously and then the left arm and foot are affected, with the whole march occurring over 5 minutes. Eventually his torso is involved and everything is numb from the neck down. The foot feels tingly as if it were "asleep," but when he touches it he can feel the contact and does not appear to have lost touch sensation. He may feel "spacey," which he compares to the "runner's high" he used to get as an athlete. He sometimes feels dizzy and he senses that his hearing is diminished. There may be a vague left frontal discomfort that he says is very different from the old migraine. Pain is not a prominent feature, nor is there nausea. Most of the attacks have been associated with heavy physical activity and he noted that occasionally attacks have been triggered by bending down when picking up a heavy object, particularly when he keeps his neck hyperextended while still in the bending position, as when lifting weights.

The patient was seen by several physicians who carried out electroencephalography (EEG) and magnetic resonance imaging (MRI) which were normal, and the attacks were interpreted as an evolution of his migraine. Eventually he was prescribed the β-adrenergic receptor blocker nadolol. This seemed to reduce the frequency of the attacks for a time but after several

months they again became more frequent. He himself believed that they were quite distinct from his previously experienced migraine attacks. Indeed, during the year since the acute event, he has never experienced another episode of what he had previously considered to be migraine attacks. Furthermore, he tested himself by consuming four glasses of Côtes de Rhône and two glasses of Rioja. He developed a sensation of nasal stuffiness and flushing, which he had, in the past, interpreted as a warning that he was going to get a migraine. However, on this occasion no other symptoms occurred.

When seen some 9 months after the event on the mountain, the patient was noted to be an exceptionally fit, athletic-appearing man. His blood pressure was normal and no bruits were heard over the head or neck. The only abnormal finding was a slight vertical skew deviation with diplopia when the patient looked up, due to reduced elevation of the right eye. There was no ptosis or pupillary asymmetry. A brief attack was witnessed in which he complained of a numb tingling of the right upper lip that spread in a few seconds to the right cheek area and, within 30 seconds, to his left hand but did not proceed further and lasted only about 2 minutes. During this time there was no change in pulse rate or blood pressure and no alteration of consciousness.

Magnetic resonance imaging scans did not demonstrate any structural changes in the hemispheres or in the brain stem. Magnetic resonance angiography (MRA), however, revealed a narrowed intracranial right vertebral artery, which appeared to end in the posterior inferior cerebellar artery (PICA) without connecting to the basilar artery. Traditional cerebral angiography demonstrated more clearly the abnormality in the vertebral-basilar territory. The vertebral artery itself showed abnormalities in the intracranial portion with areas of dilation and narrowing of the lumen consistent with a resolving dissection. The left vertebral artery was entirely normal and supplied the basilar artery and the remaining branches, including the left PICA, which were well visualized. No abnormalities were seen in the cervical carotid arteries or their intracranial branches. The circle of Willis was intact.

After the angiography the patient had many daily attacks of ipsilateral face and contralateral limb numbness and he was then started on warfarin sodium and aspirin. He was also prescribed gabapentin at a dose of 300 mg, three times a day. Within a week his attacks lessened and he was then free of all attacks over the next 3 months, by which time it was decided to stop the anticoagulants. In the month subsequent to stopping the warfarin sodium, he remained attack free while taking only gabapentin. One evening he decided to put himself to the test by consuming three-quarters of a bottle of his best Bordeaux. He experienced facial flushing but did not develop any symptoms of migraine that evening. The following morning he awoke with a feeling of nasal stuffiness and was certain he was going to develop a migraine. He went back to sleep for another 2 hours and then awoke refreshed and headache free. On another occasion, he consumed several glasses of port. He has had none of his transient sensory episodes and has had no headache. Needless to say, he is delighted that he no longer suffers from migraine and apparently can resume enjoyment of his old hobby, which he had had to put aside for almost 20 years. Repeat MRI and MRA have been done and show no change in the configuration of the vessels and no evidence of brainstem infarction.

Questions about This Case

- What is the nature of the sensory attacks?
- How does one explain an apparent sensory march in the brain stem?
- Can spreading depression occur in the brain stem?
- Why are the sensory attacks no longer occurring?
- Why does he no longer suffer from migraine?

Case Discussion

This man's sensory attacks seem to follow a pattern consistent with a localization in the brainstem. As every medical student knows, any neurologic syndrome that involves one side of the face and the opposite limbs is presumed to have its basis in the brain stem. The ventral spinothalamic tract in the lateral medulla is arranged with the face fibers medial and adjacent to the arm fibers, which are slightly more lateral, whereas trunk and lower limb fibers are arranged still more laterally. The blood supply consists of small arterial branches of the posterior inferior cerebellar artery that penetrate the lateral medulla from the surface. Thus, the face fibers being situated most deeply would be the most susceptible to ischemia. The anatomical localization seems quite clear. However, the problem of pathogenesis is more difficult.

Transient neurologic phenomena are usually either of electrical or vascular origin. The time frame of the attacks would suggest an anatomical progression or march. Since this man had suffered from migraine headaches in the past, one might have wondered whether the march was akin to that seen in migrainous aura where there is spreading depression over the visual cortex. There the rate of depression has been calculated to proceed at a rate of 3 mm per minute. Sensory pathways in the brain stem are very compact and the area occupied by sensory fibres in the spinothalamic tract and the adjacent trigeminal sensory fibers is quite minute. Consequently, a march of depression could appear to be much more rapid. However, spreading depression is presumably a neuronal phenomenon and is not known to occur in bundles of axons. Nevertheless, the time frame seems similar to other marches ascribed to migraine. Andermann reports a woman with migraine (and epilepsy), who described a tingling in the upper and lower lips and tongue that spread over 10 minutes to involve the hand and lasted an hour. The only difference from our case is that it involved the ipsilateral face and hand and presumably arose from cortical structures.

Another explanation must be found for this man's clinical picture. The analogy to amaurosis fugax is more applicable. Patients who experience amaurosis fugax describe a progression of their visual deficit, which presumably indicates an extension of the area of the retina that becomes ischemic as emboli pass through the retinal circulation (curtain sign). Perhaps what this man describes is due to ischemia that is initially localized in the sensory fibers serving the face area and as the ischemic area spreads, sensory fibers coming from the contralateral hand become ischemic, the leg fibres being involved only during a few attacks. As noted, the face fibers would be most susceptible to reduced perfusion through the small penetrating branches of the PICA and might explain why his attacks always start in the face. The nature of these attacks then would seem to be most probably due to decreased perfusion through a precarious blood supply via the PICA and the abnormal right vertebral artery. The supply is particularly precarious in that there is no obvious collateral flow from the opposite vertebral or basilar arteries.

Dissection of cervicocranial vessels is now becoming recognized with increasing frequency, in part due to the ease with which the diagnosis can be established with newer imaging techniques. The underlying cause for most dissections remains obscure, although many have a history of trauma. Even in these cases, it may be presumed that there is an underlying defect in the vessel wall. Occasionally patients are known or are found to have fibromuscular dysplasia.

Dissection of the carotid arteries has been reported in patients suffering from migraine, but the association may well be fortuitous. However, a recent study reported migraine in 40% of a series of 50 patients with dissection versus a 24% occurrence of migraine in controls suggesting a greater than chance connection. It has been suggested that recurrent attacks of migraine in which there is much vasospasm may render the vessel wall susceptible to dissection. In experimental studies, ergotamine may play a role in thickening the arteries. This patient had never taken ergotamine or methysergide.

In this man's case, the onset of the dissection presumably occurred when he did some heavy lifting. Whether or not his many attacks of migraine in some way predisposed the particular vessel to dissection is unclear. It is of interest that the previous migraine pain was perceived on the same side as that of the dissection. It may well be that a congenital anomaly, a failure of the terminal vertebral artery to connect on that side with the basilar artery, may have predisposed him to dissection; but could it also have in some way determined the side of the migraine?

Dissection may also present with head pain. Indeed pain may be the only manifestation of dissection of either the carotid or vertebral arteries. We have recently encountered a nonmigrainous young serviceman whose only evidence of dissection of a vertebral artery was continuing intense pain behind the mastoid with no neurologic deficit. In the case recounted here, the patient had had migraine all his life until he suffered what was presumably an event that caused brainstem ischemia. The subsequent attacks are difficult to ascribe to a specific diagnostic category. Are they migraine equivalents? Are they transient ischemic attacks (TIAs), due to emboli or transient reduced perfusion? Are they epileptic phenomena? The actual event and subsequent events are most unusual. Two aspects are particularly interesting: the time frame in which they occur and the apparent anatomical localization of their origin.

The time frame in which the events occur is most suggestive of some sort of "march," as has been discussed already. "Marches" are seen in epilepsy and migraine and possibly in ischemia. The timing of the march of a visual aura in migraine presumably corresponds to the timing of the spread of depression of cortical activity over the visual cortex and usually spans about 20 minutes. The march of an epileptic seizure, either sensory or motor, is presumed to follow the anatomic distribution of cortical representation of peripheral somatic structures but the timing generally is very rapid, the whole process being accomplished in a matter of seconds. The development of a neurological deficit in an acute transient ischemic attack lasts minutes according to the territory rendered ischemic. Amaurosis fugax, which is essentially a TIA localized to the retina, usually occurs over a few minutes. If the attacks are due to some sort of spreading depression, their brief duration would certainly suggest a very small area to be covered as one might expect in the tightly packed brain stem, compared to the relatively extensive cortical gyri to be covered in a process proceeding over the visual cortex or the postrolandic area.

There is a suggestion that the spreading depression is related to hypoxia in that methods that augment oxygenation may abolish the symptoms. Wolff found that whereas 10% carbon dioxide inhalation abolished the aura temporarily, adding 90% oxygen abolished both the aura and the subsequent development of headache. Presumably the hypercapnic hyperoxic state alters the cortical spreading depression. Perhaps then the spreading sensory symptoms in this patient arise in the brain stem from a state of localized ischemic hypoxia.

However, even if the localization can be established, a physiological problem remains in hypothesizing a "march" or at least a spreading depression in the brain stem. Generally a march involves activity in neuronal cell bodies or their immediate dendritic networks. The brainstem structures generally involved in producing a Wallenberg's syndrome are neuronal pathways or axons.

Why have the presumed TIAs stopped? Is this because the warfarin sodium prevented clot formation, thus removing a source for emboli ? Why did the migraine attacks stop ? It would be fascinating to hypothesize that they stopped because of some change in the migraine generator. Recently neurologists have sought the migraine generator with as much enthusiasm as Ponce de Leon sought the fountain of youth. On the basis of observations of patients who had stimulating electrodes inserted into the periaqueductal grey matter in an effort to control pain, Raskin hypothesized that there might be a migraine generator in the brain stem. Work with positron emission tomography (PET) scanning on migraineurs by Weiller and Diener and others have shown that there may well be a center in the brain stem that sets off and maintains the sequential events of the migraine episode. Their studies show that an area in the mid-dorsal pons remains activated even after the clinical symptoms of the migraine attack have been terminated by sumatriptan, which presumably acts peripherally to block the migraine process. Perhaps in this patient, the migraine generator has been rendered inactive, at least for the present, so that even a previously effective stimulus such as red wine fails to start the process. Space does not permit discussion of the interesting association between wine and headache, why it only happens with certain wines and to certain people and even to them only at certain times. This patient had many ideas on this topic and we can learn a great deal from thoughtful and observant patients. This is the stuff neurologic armchair philosophers muse over with a glass of port, but sober neurophysiologists in the laboratory may soon be able to answer some of these questions and our patients will benefit immensely.

Management Strategies

Management depends almost entirely on the presumed diagnosis. Initially it was thought that this man, having had typical migraine attacks all his life,

was now developing a more complex migraine presentation. Consequently the treatment recommended was a medication commonly prescribed for the prophylaxis of migraine, i.e., nadolol at an initial dose of 40 mg per day. When the attacks continued to be very frequent the dose was doubled.

It later became apparent that the patient's attacks were not typical of migraine, not even of "basilar artery migraine," and further investigation was indicated. It is a good general rule that when there is a change in migraine pattern, the patient be carefully re-evaluated and other nonmigraine processes be considered. The second diagnosis considered was transient cerebral ischemic attacks from an as-yet-undiscovered source. Aspirin was then prescribed. When this did not reduce the frequency of the attacks, it was clear that much more extensive investigation was needed such as an MRI. This lead to the discovery of the anomalous posterior circulation and the performing of an angiogram that demonstrated a dissection. Even though it is presumed that the dissection had actually taken place some 9 months previous to the discovery of the dissection, anticoagulants were prescribed. Since there was still some doubt about the actual cause of the symptoms, and on the basis that there might still be some sort of neuronal activity underlying the attacks, gabapentin was precribed simultaneously, although the justification for its use at this time might be questioned. At the time of writing, the patient was very loath to give up the one medication that seemed to bring relief at last. It will be of interest to see if the attacks return when eventually the gabapentin is also stopped.

Case Summary

A 40-year-old man with lifelong unilateral migraine, readily precipitated by red wine, suffered a dissection of the ipsilateral vertebral artery. Thereafter he suffered frequently recurring attacks of brainstem sensory symptoms but the migraine attacks no longer occurred, even when he drank red wine, an invariable precipitant prior to his dissection. The attacks were reduced by nadolol, aspirin, and warfarin sodium, but only after the addition of gabapentin was he free of both sensory attacks and migraine. This freedom continued when all medications other than gabapentin were withdrawn.

It may be that migraine predisposed the particular artery to dissection but the reason for the cessation of migraine attacks after the dissection can only be surmised. What would be most intriguing is the possibility that the dissection and subsequent brainstem ischemia in some way altered the hypothesized pontine migraine generator.

Selected Readings

Andermann F. Clinical features of migrain-epilepsy. In: Andermann F, Lugaresi E, editors. Migraine and epilepsy. Boston: Butterworth; 1987. p. 17–8.

D'Anglejan-Chatillon J, Ribiero V, Mas JL, et al. Migraine, a risk factor for dissection of cervical arteries. Headache 1989; 29:560–1.

Guillon B, Biousse V, Massiou H, Bousser MG. Orbital pain as an isolated sign of internal carotid artery dissection. A diagnostic pitfall. Cephalalgia 1998;18:222–4.

Raskin NH, Hosubuchi Y, Lamb S. Headache may arise from perturbation of the brain. Headache 1987;27:416–20.

Sinclair W. Dissecting aneurysm of the middle cerebral artery associated with migraine syndrome. Am J Pathol 1953; 29:1083.

Torda C, Wolff HG. Experimental studies on headache: transient thickening of walls of cranial arteries in relation to certain phenomena of migraine headache and action of ergotamine tartrate on thickened walls. J Arch Neurol Psychiatry 1945; 53:329.

Weiller C, May A, Limmroth V, et al. Brain stem activation in spontaneous human migraine attacks. Nat Med 1995;1: 658–60.

Editorial Comments

The pathophysiology of migraine is increasingly being defined in more precise neurobiologic terms and concepts, yet remains complex and somewhat enigmatic. Cases such as this one by Dr. Nelson raise many questions about the basic nature of migraine and its genesis. What turns the putative "generator" on, and importantly, what turns it off? Does it really exist? There is a lot of room for speculation and reflection on these matters, a process that has served neurologists particularly well while waiting for definitive answers, which we all hope will come sooner rather than later.

CHAPTER 45

THE PATIENT WITH AN UNUSUAL FAMILIAL HEADACHE DISORDER

KATAYOUN VAHEDI, MD

MARIE-GERMAINE BOUSSER, MD

Case History

This patient is a 37-year-old, right-handed woman who has had migraine with aura since the age of 25 years. Her attacks always begin with a bitemporal severe throbbing headache followed 5 minutes later by bilateral blurred vision with scintillating white spots of 15 minutes' duration. She then feels numbness on the right side of her face and her tongue spreading over a few minutes to her right hand, and has some difficulty in moving her right arm because of weakness and numbness. Her gait is slightly disturbed. Neurologic symptoms last about 20 minutes. During her attacks she is hypersensitive to light and sound, she is nauseated, and has to be in bed in complete darkness. She usually does not take any medication and awakens headache free in a few hours. The frequency of the attacks is around two per month. She occasionally reports emotional stress as a triggering factor. Recently she has had three severe attacks during which the usual aura symptoms lasted 3 hours while the headache lasted 2 days. During the very last attack, in addition to the long-lasting aura symptoms, she felt extremely tired and had confusion, with memory disturbances and gait ataxia lasting for 3 days.

She has smoked 20 cigarettes per day since the age of 18 years and has no other vascular risk factor. Her general and neurologic examinations are normal as well as her blood pressure (120/85).

Her 39-year-old sister had experienced attacks of migraine with typical visual aura since the age of 12 years. On occasions, she suffers attacks characterized by the same visual symptoms (scintillating scotoma) lasting 30 minutes, but without any headache. She has recently experienced an episode of sudden pure right hemiplegia lasting for 3 weeks in the absence of headache or visual disturbances. She has no vascular risk factors.

Their mother died at the age of 60 years of a so-called "vascular dementia." She had had an episode of acute left hemiplegia with dysarthria when she was 45 years old and a second episode with a right hemiplegia at the age of 52 years. She then worsened gradually over the years, became progressively demented, unable to walk, bedridden, tetraplegic, and pseudobulbar. She died suddenly 15 years after her first stroke. She had never experienced migraine and had no vascular risk factors whatsoever. She had a cranial magnetic resonance imaging (MRI) scan showing a diffuse leukoencephalopathy with multiple areas of subcortical infarcts (Figure 45–1).

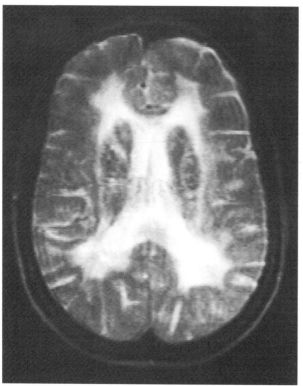

FIGURE 45–1. Magnetic resonance T2-weighted image of the mother of the patient showing diffuse and confluent leukoencephalopathy with multiple areas of subcortical infarcts.

Questions about This Case

- What are your diagnostic considerations? Why is this migraine not "just a migraine?"
- What other information is important in this case?
- Do you wish to have more information regarding the neurovascular investigations that have been performed on the mother and the sister of this patient?
- Would you perform neuroimaging investigations in this case? If so, would you perform a computed tomography (CT) scan or MRI?
- Would you perform other investigations?
- What treatment do you suggest?

Case Discussion

In this patient, the clinical characteristics of migraine correspond to those defined by the International Headache Society's (IHS) classification for migraine with aura. Indeed, she has fully reversible successive aura symptoms (visual, sensory, and motor) that develop gradually over more than 4 minutes and last usually fewer than 30 minutes. In migraine with aura, sensory or motor symptoms may be bilateral, or more frequently unilateral as in this patient, in some cases always involving the same side of the body. These aura symptoms are associated with a bilateral headache which starts shortly before the neurologic symptoms, as seen in some patients with migraine with aura, and which has two of the clinical characteristics of migraine, i.e., the headache is severe and throbbing. Furthermore, the patient is nauseated, she cannot tolerate light and sound, and she is unable to pursue any normal physical or intellectual activity. She has to stay in bed in complete darkness. The headache is relieved by sleep, as reported by many migrainous patients.

If we consider in more detail the IHS criteria for different subtypes of migraine with aura, the three recent migraine attacks in this patient have the clinical characteristics of migraine with prolonged aura, since the neurologic symptoms lasted more than 60 minutes and fewer than 7 days. Otherwise, they were identical to her previous migraine attacks in all other aspects. As regards the very last attack, the best corresponding diagnosis would be basilar migraine because of the associated gait ataxia and the decrease in the level of consciousness which indicate that the aura symptoms probably originated from the brain stem.

The general and neurologic examination of this patient is normal, as should be the case in migraine.

It is tempting to conclude that this patient simply has "migraine with aura." This migraine is somewhat unusual in that most patients who experience attacks of migraine with aura also have attacks without aura. Furthermore, this patient has three varieties of aura, consisting of typical aura, prolonged aura, and basilar aura, and her last attack was particularly severe in its duration (3 days) and associated symptoms (confusion, memory disturbances, and ataxia) so that a differential diagnosis would be a reversible ischemia in the basilar territory. Though unusual, these features are nevertheless still compatible with migraine with aura. This migraine with aura is familial since her sister has typical attacks of migraine with visual aura. Such a familial pattern—though not considered as a diagnostic criteria in the IHS classification—has long been recognized as an important characteristic of migraine. This story is thus compatible with a familial migraine with aura, except for one aspect that should immediately raise suspicion, and that is the striking family history of strokes in young women which have occurred in the absence of vascular risk factors. Stroke in young women is rare and although migraine has been shown to be a risk factor—with a relative risk of 3—for ischemic stroke in this group, the occurrence of a stroke should always prompt investigations to try to find the etiology. In the present case, the suspicion is raised that there is in the family a disorder that is responsible for both migraine and stroke.

Besides her migraine, the sister of the patient suffered a hemiplegia of acute onset, which was clearly distinct from an attack of migraine. This hemiplegia was said to be "pure," which means that there were no other signs such as dysphasia, sensory disturbances, or visual field defect. This pattern immediately points to a small infarct (lacuna) either in the pons, or more frequently, in the internal capsule. Such small, deep infarcts are extremely rare in young subjects, particularly in the absence of arterial hypertension. The patient probably underwent investigations but we do not know what etiology of stroke, if any, was discovered.

The mother of this patient did not suffer from migraine but had a typical history of a small artery disease of the brain with recurrent lacunar strokes (left hemiplegia with dysarthria, right hemiplegia), pseudobulbar palsy, dementia, and MRI signs of leukoencephalopathy and small, deep infarcts. Again, the striking features here are the young age at onset and the absence of hypertension. It would be extremely useful to know more about the neurovascular investigations performed in this case such as duplex scanning, a transcranial Doppler examination, magnetic resonance (MR) angiography, or echocardiography.

Thus, this patient has, firstly, a personal history of migraine with typical aura, migraine with prolonged aura, and basilar migraine, and secondly, a family history of migraine with aura and ischemic stroke in her sister, and subcortical infarcts, vascular dementia with pseudo-bulbar palsy, and leukoencephalopathy in her mother. This immediately points to a familial vascular disease involving the small arteries of the brain, which has been responsible for subcortical infarcts in two family members and dementia in the mother, and possibly having migraine as its clinical presentation. In that hypothesis, migraine would be symptomatic and not idiopathic.

None of the three family members had hypertension which is the major risk factor for lipohyalinosis of small vessels. So we can rule out Binswanger's disease, which is also responsible for small, deep infarcts and vascular dementia but is related to hypertension. In addition, migraine and familial inheritance are not reported to be features of Binswanger's disease.

Antiphospholipid syndrome may cause ischemic stroke, dementia, and migraine. In addition, families with antiphospholipid syndrome have been reported as having an autosomal dominant pattern of inheritance. Although there is no history of venous thrombotic events or miscarriage in this patient and in her family, anticardiolipin and antiphospholipid antibodies should be checked in this patient.

A mitochondrial vasculopathy such as **m**itochondrial **m**yopathy, **e**ncephalopathy, **l**actic **a**cidosis, and stroke-like episodes (MELAS) is also a possible etiology for both migraine and ischemic stroke. It is, however, unlikely in the absence of clinical signs of a mitochondrial disease in any of the three family members, such as myopathy, ophthalmoplegia, retinitis, hypoacousis, cataract, seizures, or diabetes mellitus. A muscle biopsy searching for ragged red fibers and a full mitochondrial work-up do not seem necessary in this case unless no other cause is found.

A recently identified genetic nonatherosclerotic and nonamyloid arteriopathy, **c**erebral **a**utosomal **d**ominant **a**rteriopathy with **s**ubcortical **i**nfarcts and **l**eukoencephalopathy (CADASIL), may be strongly suspected in this case. CADASIL involves predominantly the small arteries of the brain and is responsible for recurrent small, deep infarcts, beginning in midadulthood and leading progressively or step by step to subcortical dementia with pseudobulbar palsy. In the final stage of the disease, a diffuse and symmetrical periventricular leukoencephalopathy with multiple areas of small subcortical infarcts is always demonstrated by MRI, as in the case of the mother of this patient. Migraine with aura is a frequent symptom in CADASIL and it usually precedes the first ischemic strokes by a mean of 15 to 20 years. Symptoms of migraine in CADASIL correspond to those defined by the IHS criteria for migraine with aura. However, attacks of migraine with prolonged aura and attacks of acute-onset aura without headache are particularly frequent, as in the two sisters reported here. The personal and family history of the patient is thus very illustrative of CADASIL. Therefore, in response to the first question about this case, we can say that on this occasion, migraine is not "just a migraine," despite the fact that the clinical IHS diagnostic criteria for migraine are satisfied. It is a "symptomatic migraine" related to a familial cerebral artery disease. This emphasizes the crucial importance of the family history, and in the present case, it is of the utmost importance to draw a full genealogical tree. CADASIL has an autosomal dominant pattern of inheritance which means that nonaffected subjects have no risk for their offspring whereas 50% of the children of affected subjects will also be affected.

Thus, in response to the second question about this case, more information about the rest of the family is crucial, both for diagnosis and for future management.

The diagnosis of migraine remains essentially clinical and very rarely requires ancillary investigations. However, in the present case, the unusual features of some of the attacks (3 days' duration) and the family history of stroke were sufficient to prompt investigations. Indeed, because of the last episode of migraine with prolonged aura which had unusual associated neurologic symptoms, this patient had been referred to a neurologist, who asked for a cranial MRI, considering the diagnosis of ischemic stroke as an alternative diagnosis to migraine. The results of this MRI are shown in Figure 45–2. You can see multiple areas of symmetrical, periventricular white-matter abnormalities, particularly on T2-weighted images. Meanwhile, the neurologist in charge of the patient's sister sent us the MRI of her patient (Figure 45–3), which showed very comparable white-matter abnormalities, and also the results of the neurovascular investigations which were negative.

Magnetic resonance imaging white-matter abnormalities in CADASIL consist of leukoencephalopathy on T2-weighted images and small subcortical areas of hyposignal suggestive of small, deep infarcts on T1-weighted images. Magnetic resonance imaging white-matter abnormalities (leukoencephalopathy) in CADASIL precede by many years (10 to 20) the first symptoms of ischemic stroke. These abnormalities are found in young CADASIL patients suffering from migraine with aura as the sole clinical manifestation of the disease. In this regard, it is interesting to discuss the relationship between white-matter abnormalities and migraine, since previous controlled studies have emphasized the high frequency of white-matter abnormalities (of unknown pathophysiology and significance) in migrainous patients (varying from 12 to 46%). Compared to a CT scan, there is no doubt that MRI, particularly on T2-weighted images, is the method of investigation of choice for the detection of cerebral white-matter abnormalities. The finding of a leukoencephalopathy in these two sisters would constitute a strong argument toward the diagnosis of CADASIL. On the other hand, the absence of any MRI white-matter abnormalities would constitute a strong argument against the diagnosis of CADASIL, since the MRI penetrance of this condition is near complete after the age of 35 years, which means that all individuals older than 35 and having inherited the mutated gene would have at least some subtle areas of periventricular leukoencephalopathy on MRI.

Since the alterations of the vascular smooth-muscle cells that are characteristic of the disease are not limited to the central nervous system, ultrastructural study performed on vessel walls of arteries in other organs and tissues easily available, such as the skin, would be a very useful diagnostic tool.

With the very recent identification of the underlying genetic defect that causes CADASIL, genetic testing with the use of molecular techniques can now confirm the diagnosis in patients such as those reported here. However, this raises major ethical and psychologic issues since CADASIL is a late-onset disease with a severe prognosis and for which there is no effective treatment. Therefore, it is of great importance to refer the patient before any genetic testing takes place to an experienced neurogeneticist for appropriate genetic counseling.

There has been so far no therapeutic trial comparing the efficacy of different antimigraine drugs in

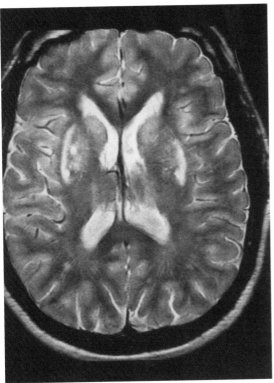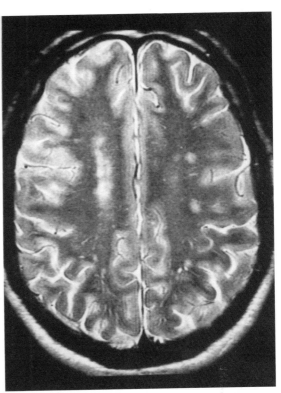

FIGURE 45–2. Magnetic resonance T2-weighted image of the patient showing diffuse white-matter abnormalities. Sections are at the level of the basal ganglia (*left*) and just above the lateral ventricles (*right*).

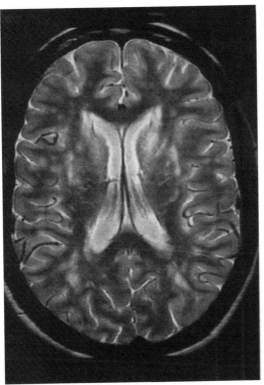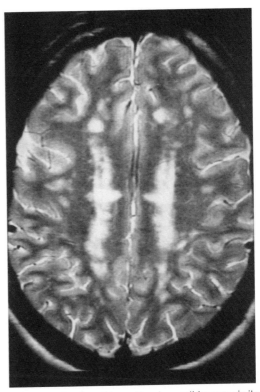

FIGURE 45–3. Magnetic resonance T2-weighted image of the sister of the patient showing white-matter abnormalities very similar to those in the patient's MRI. Sections are at the level of the basal ganglia (*left*) and just above the lateral ventricles (*right*).

CADASIL patients who suffer from migraine. This is obviously because it is a newly defined condition. One could just treat CADASIL-related migraine as any migraine but because of the underlying arteriopathy, the high risk of ischemic stroke, and the high frequency of attacks of migraine with prolonged aura, it seems reasonable to avoid all vasoconstrictive drugs. Thus, as far as acute treatment is concerned, ergot derivatives and triptans should preferably be avoided, whereas aspirin and nonsteroidal anti-inflammatory drugs would be the acute treatments of choice. As regards prophylactic treatment, beta-blockers, which can occasionally prolong the aura, should be used with caution and methysergide would be contraindicated. Given the risk of ischemic stroke, a more logical approach is to use aspirin which has been shown to have a preventive effect both in migraine and in cerebral infarction, although there are no data specifically devoted to CADASIL patients.

The long-term management of either symptomatic or asymptomatic CADASIL patients is not yet defined. The natural history of this condition leads to the recurrence of ischemic strokes, to increasing leukoencephalopathy on MRI, and to the constitution of a progressive dementia sometimes preceded by severe mood disturbances. No treatment has so far been prospectively studied in this disease. Most patients are on aspirin for the reasons mentioned above. It is hoped that the recent identification of the gene will help us understand the pathophysiology of this condition and to develop effective treatments.

Management Strategies

- When seeking diagnosis, take into consideration the family history of subcortical stroke, vascular dementia, and diffuse leukoencephalopathy in the absence of any known vascular risk factor. Try to make a genealogical tree to support the hypothesis of a genetic disorder. Search particularly in the older generations for a history of strokes leading to dementia with pseudobulbar palsy.
- Try to have all the information available about the neurovascular investigations that have been performed on the patient's sister and on her mother, who had suffered ischemic strokes.

- An MRI is indicated for this patient as well as for her 39-year-old sister. If a leukoencephalopathy shows on T2-weighted images (as in Figures 45–2 and 45–3), we can conclude that there is a familial arteriopathy, having as its major phenotypes ischemic subcortical strokes, dementia, migraine, and leukoencephalopathy. CADASIL will then be the first diagnosis to be proposed. This would be reinforced if the sister's MRI already shows small, deep infarcts on T1-weighted images.
- A skin biopsy for the ultrastructural study of vessel walls is of great help in demonstrating alterations of the vascular smooth-muscle cells with characteristic granular deposits in their basal membrane.
- Genetic testing using the techniques of molecular biology, when available, will confirm the diagnosis of CADASIL. However, it would be necessary to refer this patient to a specialist for appropriate genetic counseling before any genetic testing was performed.
- What we can propose to this patient as therapeutic strategies for her migraine is very limited, since the underlying mechanisms of migraine in CADASIL are not yet understood. However, we can suggest that she avoids ergot compounds and triptans because of the underlying arteriopathy and the high risk of ischemic strokes. It would also be preferable to avoid beta-blockers because of the previous episodes of migraine with prolonged aura. Otherwise, there are as yet no long-term therapeutic strategies for CADASIL patients except for the control of other vascular risk factors if they are present (which was not the case in the present family).

Case Summary

- This patient does have symptomatic migraine with aura associated with MRI white-matter abnormalities, due to a newly defined genetic arteriopathy, CADASIL .
- In a patient with attacks of migraine, the early diagnosis of CADASIL, before the onset of ischemic strokes or dementia, is seldom realized because of the usually typical features of migraine in CADASIL. What may help the diagnostic procedure is the presence of MRI white-matter

abnormalities. But in cases of typical migraine, it is not recommended to undertake such investigative procedures. So the major point that has to be taken into consideration in the diagnostic procedure is the family history of subcortical infarcts and dementia particularly when associated with a diffuse leukoencephalopathy in the absence of any major vascular risk factors.

- This case would be extremely rare, compared to the many migraine-with-aura patients that you see in your practice, but the correct diagnosis of CADASIL is of importance because of the radical difference in prognosis: migraine is a benign disease, whereas CADASIL is a severe condition. It is also important to recognize CADASIL for the understanding of its natural history, the correct estimation of its prevalence, appropriate genetic counseling, and the organization of future therapeutic trials.

Overview of CADASIL

Cerebral autosomal dominant arteriopathy with subcortical infarcts and leukoencephalopathy is a newly defined nonatherosclerotic and nonamyloid arteriopathy, involving mainly the small arteries penetrating the white matter and basal ganglia of the brain. Pathologic studies reveal a diffuse myelin loss of the hemispheric white matter and multiple, small, deep infarcts. Microscopic examination shows marked alterations of arteries, consisting of a concentric thickening of the vessel walls, mainly due to an extensive nonamyloid eosinophilic material in the media and sometimes to a reduplication of the internal elastic lamina. Ultrastructural study of the arteries shows destruction of the vascular smooth-muscle cells and the presence of characteristic granular osmiophilic material of unknown nature within their basal membrane (Figure 45–4). These vessel alterations are found not only in the brain arteries but in a systemic manner in all tissues. However, the clinical expression of the disease seems to be limited to the central nervous system.

The main manifestations of CADASIL are recurrent subcortical infarcts involving primarily the periventricular white matter, the basal ganglia, the

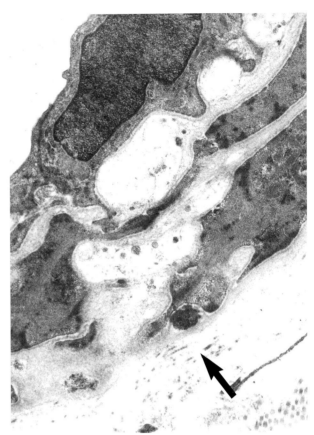

FIGURE 45–4. An ultrastructural study of a skin small artery in CADASIL demonstrating characteristic granular deposits in the basal membrane of a vascular smooth muscle cell (*arrow*) (courtesy of Dr. MM Ruchoux, CHRU Lille, France).

thalamus, the pons, and the dentate nucleus. The recurrence of ischemic events leads progressively to the constitution of a multi-infarct dementia with pseudobulbar palsy. The mean age of onset of infarcts is 49 years, ranging from 27 to 65. The mean age of demented CADASIL patients is 60 years and the mean age at death is 68. In 10% of cases, dementia occurs in a progressive manner without any previous episode of ischemic stroke. However, in these patients as well as in other demented CADASIL patients, MRI shows a diffuse and symmetrical periventricular leukoencephalopathy and multiple areas of subcortical infarcts (Figure 45–1). Interestingly, MRI white-matter abnormalities constitute the earliest manifestation of this arteriopathy, preceding by a mean of 10 to 20 years the first ischemic events.

Migraine is one of the most frequent clinical manifestations of CADASIL. It has been reported in 20 to 30% of CADASIL patients. It consists mainly of attacks of migraine with aura, either typical or atypical. Atypical migraine consists of attacks of migraine with prolonged aura, basilar migraine, hemiplegic migraine, or attacks of acute-onset aura without headache. The mean age of onset of migraine with aura is 30 years, ranging from 6 to 48. In some patients, migraine with aura may begin very early in life, even in childhood; age of onset as early as 5 or 6 years has been reported. There is no gender preponderance in migraine with aura among CADASIL patients. However, the mean age of onset of migraine with aura in CADASIL is significantly lower in women compared to men. In comparison with migraine as an entity, there are no specific triggering factors in migraine attacks in CADASIL. Their frequency and severity are extremely variable from one individual to another and over one individual's life. Interestingly, there is a preponderance of migraine in some CADASIL families, whereas in others migraine is rare or even absent. This variable expression of migraine in a given CADASIL family and between unrelated CADASIL families is not yet understood. What differentiates migraine in CADASIL from migraine as defined by the IHS is the presence of striking MRI white-matter abnormalities usually in young patients without major vascular risk factors. The relationships between these white-matter abnormalities and migraine are not yet understood.

Severe mood disturbances, either depressive or manic episodes, are reported in 20% of CADASIL patients and may be the first presenting symptoms of this arteriopathy. Seizures and confusion have rarely been reported. There are no clinical manifestations involving the peripheral nervous system or the muscular system, and no infarcts involving tissues other than the brain.

CADASIL has an autosomal dominant mode of inheritance with near complete penetrance. In the absence of any known biochemical defect, the genetic abnormality has first been mapped, by genetic linkage analysis, on chromosome 19p. Subsequently, different point mutations in the Notch3 gene have been demonstrated in CADASIL patients. The function of Notch3 is still unknown.

What we know is that in Drosophila, Notch gene encodes a glycosylated transmembrane receptor involved in development. Further research is ongoing to try to understand the mechanisms that lead Notch3 mutations to induce alterations of the vessel walls, destruction of vascular smooth muscle cells, constitution of small deep cerebral infarcts, leukoencephalopathy, dementia, and migraine in some patients. Progress in understanding the pathophysiology of CADASIL will hopefully lead to the development of new therapeutic approaches.

Selected Readings

Babikian V, Ropper AH. Binswanger's disease: a review. Stroke 1987;18:2–12.

Baudrimont M, Dubas F, Joutel A, et al. Autosomal dominant leukoencephalopathy and subcortical ischemic stroke. A clinicopathological study. Stroke 1993;24:122–5.

Chabriat H, Tournier-Lasserve E, Vahedi K, et al. Autosomal dominant migraine with MRI white-matter abnormalities mapping to the CADASIL locus. Neurology 1995;45:1086–91.

Chabriat H, Vahedi K, Iba Zizen MT, et al. Clinical spectrum of CADASIL: a study of 7 families. Lancet 1995;346:934–9.

Headache Classification Committee of the International Headache Society. Classification and diagnostic criteria for headache disorders, cranial neuralgias and facial pain. Cephalalgia 1988;8(Suppl 7):19–28.

Hutchinson M, O'Riordan J, Javed M, et al. Familial hemiplegic migraine and autosomal dominant arteriopathy with leukoencephalopathy (CADASIL). Ann Neurol 1995;38:817–24.

Joutel A, Corpechot C, Ducros A, et al. Notch3 mutations in CADASIL, a hereditary adult-onset condition causing stroke and dementia. Nature 1996;383:707–10.

Koo B, Becker L, Chuang S, et al. Mitochondrial encephalomyopathy, lactic acidosis, stroke-like episodes (MELAS): clinical, radiological, pathological, and genetic observations. Ann Neurol 1993;34: 25–32.

Levine SR, Deegan MJ, Futrell N, Welch KMA. Cerebrovascular and neurologic disease associated with antiphospholipid antibodies: 48 cases. Neurology 1990;40:1181–9.

Ruchoux MM, Guerouaou D, Vandenhaute B, et al. Systemic vascular smooth muscle cell impairment in cerebral autosomal dominant arteriopathy with subcortical infarcts and leukoencephalopathy. Acta Neuropathol 1995;89:500–12.

Tournier-Lasserve E, Joutel A, Melki J, et al. Cerebral autosomal dominant arteriopathy with subcortical infarcts and leukoencephalopathy maps on chromosome 19q12. Nat Genet 1993;3:256–9.

Vérin M, Rolland Y, Landgraf F, et al. New phenotype of the cerebral autosomal dominant arteriopathy mapped to chromosome 19: migraine as the prominent clinical feature. J Neurol Neurosurg Psychiatry 1995;59:579–85.

Editorial Comments

Much can be learned from the thorough study of rare neurologic disorders and, in particular, when migraine and stroke are components. CADASIL is such a disorder, and Drs. Vahedi and Bousser give us an in-depth and erudite review of this disorder, as well as its genetic basis. This is exciting since we all can learn from such cases. Importantly, there are some significant management differences, in terms of the use of vasoconstrictors and genetic counseling, between CADASIL and other migraine disorders. Calcium channel antagonists, such as verapamil, may be helpful therapeutic agents, especially if the patient has frequent visual auras. Further knowledge about this disorder and about familial hemiplegic migraine should help us unravel the migraine mystery and serve our patients better in the future.

CHAPTER 46

AN INTERESTING RESOLUTION OF AN UNUSUAL HEADACHE

PETER J. GOADSBY, MD, PhD, DSc, FRACP, FRCP

Case History

A 58-year-old man was sent for review. He had a 5-year history of short-lasting headaches. He reported that he had been having between 3 and 4 to a maximum of 50 to 60 attacks a day of right supraorbital and retro-orbital pain. These attacks lasted 5 to 30 seconds with no trigger factors and no aura symptoms. There was no nausea, photophobia, or phonophobia but his wife volunteered, and he confirmed, tearing of the eyes without redness or nasal congestion. The pain was unaffected by movement. He had never had a significant break from the attacks over the 5 years. There was no effect of wind, swallowing or chewing, and no temporomandibular joint tenderness or clicking. He was on no medications.

His past history was largely unremarkable. There was no significant family history. He was a nonsmoker who drank alcohol occasionally, and this did not trigger attacks.

On examination he was well and in no distress. The fundi were normal and the visual fields full. The eye movements were normal and full and the pupils equal and normal. There was no trigeminal sensory loss, temporal artery tenderness, or facial asymmetry. The jaw opened normally. In the limbs, tone and power were equal and normal and the reflexes symmetrical with down-going toes. Gait and coordination were normal. The general examination was normal with a normal blood pressure.

A diagnosis was made and therapy commenced. At review he was completely pain free. He has remained so at least 6 months later.

Questions about This Case

- Are there any other points from the history that could be clarified?
- What, if any, tests would you do?
- What is the provisional diagnosis?
- What treatment would you advise?

Comments on the Questions

1. History taking is a very individual matter and this case is no exception. One could come to a reasonable differential diagnosis with the history as it is. Perhaps the possibility, albeit remote, of giant cell arteritis could have been explored more.
2. The range of tests will always reflect a compromise between how confident one is, how confident the patient is with what you say, and the realities of the medicolegal climate in which one practices. Certainly, a test for electrolytes, a blood count, ESR, and brain imaging seem reasonable as a minimum.
3. The differential diagnosis is relatively limited by the very short-lasting nature of the attacks. I have included some diagnoses in the list which are really not there but interesting to discuss. One possible list would include:
   - SUNCT (short-lasting neuralgiform headache with conjunctival injection and tearing)
   - Paroxysmal hemicrania
   - Chronic cluster headache
   - Chronic sinusitis
   - Giant cell arteritis
   - Trigeminal neuralgia

It is most unusual to have autonomic features in trigeminal neuralgia and, coupled with the longish attacks (30 seconds) and the lack of any trigger, it is hard to sustain that diagnosis. The other diagnoses are possible; although giant cell arteritis would be very unusual in this age group, it is dangerous to overlook it.

4. Treatment to a certain extent will depend on the diagnosis. The treatment of the secondary problems, such as giant cell arteritis and sinusitis, is reasonably established. He had been treated with carbamazepine, valproate, and baclofen with the provisional diagnosis of trigeminal neuralgia but these were unhelpful.

Results of Investigations

The patient had normal electrolytes, blood glucose, and blood count. The ESR was not raised and he had had a temporal artery biopsy before initial review. He had had a normal magnetic resonance imaging (MRI) of the brain and no sinus disease.

Case Outcome

I initially thought that this was the history of SUNCT without the C, with the differential diagnosis being chronic paroxysmal hemicrania. He was treated with indomethacin 50 mg t.i.d. for a few weeks but this made no difference and was stopped. He saw his dentist who did some work on the right side of an ill-fitting denture and he has been completely well since that time.

Case Discussion

Initially, I had wondered whether this man had SUNCT without the C or a paroxysmal hemicrania. As it turned out, he had ill-fitting dentures. It is worthwhile to discuss SUNCT in this case because the patient presented with the same clinical picture and it is possible that he had SUNCT which went into spontaneous remission, in addition to the more simple explanation that it was fixed entirely by the dental work. The differential diagnosis, after secondary headache has been eliminated, for this type of presentation would include chronic paroxysmal hemicrania and cluster headache, which are discussed elsewhere in this volume.

Most patients diagnosed with SUNCT are males. The paroxysms of pain are very short-lasting, being usually between 15 seconds and 2 minutes. Patients may have up to 30 episodes an hour although more usually would have 5 to 6 per hour. The occurrence of bouts also may vary and a frequency as low as once or twice in 1 to 4 weeks has been seen in a male patient who, at other times, had up to 20 attacks a day. In another reported case, the patient had almost continuous attacks for up to 3 hours. The conjunctival injection seen with SUNCT is often the most prominent of the autonomic features, and tearing also may be obvious. Although these and other autonomic stigmata, such as sweating of the forehead or rhinorrhea, may be seen in many short-lasting headache syndromes, the injection and tearing are an order of magnitude more obvious in SUNCT. Most cases have some associated precipitating factors which may be movements of the neck.

There have been a few reported secondary or associated SUNCT syndromes. The first reported secondary SUNCT syndrome was due to a homolateral cerebellopontine angle arteriovenous malformation diagnosed on MRI. It is notable that two other secondary SUNCT syndromes have both been posterior fossa arteriovenous malformations so that cranial MRI is justified in these patients. The various short-lasting headaches, including their treatments, have recently been reviewed in detail.

Selected Readings

Goadsby PJ, Lipton RB. A review of paroxysmal hemicranias, SUNCT syndrome, and other short-lasting headaches with autonomic features, including new cases. Brain 1997;120: 193–209.

Editorial Comments

Rare and unusual short-lasting headaches are interesting and diagnostically important because of often effective, specific therapeutic interventions. Therefore, such cases are even more amazing when their causation is found to be not related to the disorders described. Dr. Goadsby presents such a case and indicates that the patient's headaches resolved when "ill-fitting dentures" were repaired! It is so easy to overlook dental causes of facial and head pain. Remember the possibility of dental disease in any patient with an atypical presentation of head or facial pain. This case also provides a good overview of SUNCT. Time will tell whether Dr. Goadsby's patient remains headache free; let us hope such is the case.

CHAPTER 47

Two Women with Headache Associated with Loud Noise

William Pryse-Phillips, MD, FRCP, FRCPC

Anna M. Wong, MD

Introduction

The value of the medical adage that "common things occur commonly" is diluted by the observation that some things considered to be rare may also occur quite often—if one looks for them. The syndrome described here is generally considered to be both rare and benign; our observations, however, confirm the opinion of the researcher who described it most recently that it is not unusual (though seldom the basis for complaint). We present here both a benign case and one of a patient in whom this syndrome occurred within the context of a mitochondrial encephalopathy.

Case 1 History

A 72-year-old woman presented to her family physician with the complaint of being woken up by a sudden loud noise and headache. This had happened on several occasions over the past 2 months and she was concerned that she had a brain tumor. After these sudden awakenings, she described herself as being fearful with breathlessness, diaphoresis, and a pounding heartbeat.

The attacks occurred soon after falling asleep. The origin of the explosive noise was uncertain, but she was sure that the noise was coming from within her head. She did not recall any involuntary move-

ments. When asked to describe the "headache," she admitted, on reflection, that there was no actual pain involved. She had no problems after the panicky feeling settled and was able to sleep on through the remainder of the night. No sequelae were noted in the morning.

She was quite distressed by these events but had been afraid to tell her husband about them; he had not noticed any unusual events occurring during his wife's sleep. Her past history was unremarkable except for well-controlled hypertension. She had had mild sporadic headaches throughout her adult life with no recent change in pattern. There was no family history of migraine or seizure disorder. A functional inquiry was unremarkable. She was a nonsmoker and rarely drank alcohol. Her general examination was normal with a normal blood pressure and regular heart rate; her neurologic examination was completely normal. She was reassured and over the next few months the events ceased.

Case 2 History

A 52-year-old woman presented to the emergency room and was admitted to the psychiatry ward in a confusional state. Her past medical and neurologic histories revealed nothing other than a recent history of an anxiety state treated with benzodiazepines. A clinical examination of her nervous system and support systems revealed no abnormalities. On the fourth day of hospitalization, the patient suffered two generalized tonic-clonic seizures, despite the recent prescription of valproate sodium. A neurologic examination revealed no localizing nor lateralizing findings, and no anticonvulsant therapy was prescribed. After standard treatment for anxiety, the patient was discharged.

Three months later, she returned to the emergency room with the complaint that she was woken up by a loud explosion-like sound within her head, accompanied by the feeling as though it were bursting. This could occur up to three times during the night, at any time, and was followed by acute anxiety and a clouded state during which she appeared to her husband as being confused. She was reassured, clomipramine was prescribed, and she was discharged, only to return four times over the next 10 days with recurrent symptoms, now occurring by day as well as by night. At the last presentation she was admitted to the psychiatric ward in a confusional state.

Her central nervous system (CNS) examination remained normal, but a computed tomography scan showed moderate bilateral calcification of the basal ganglia and patchy white-matter lucencies, also seen on a magnetic resonance imaging scan. The only abnormal investigation among those performed in a search for the cause of the abnormalities on the images was an elevation of resting serum lactate levels. A diagnosis of **m**itochondrial **e**ncephalopathy, **l**actic **a**cidosis, and **s**troke-like episodes (MELAS) was made, a conclusion later supported by the results of a muscle biopsy and genetic analysis.

Questions about These Cases

- What is the differential diagnosis of the cranial sensation?
- What other information/investigations would you seek?
- Is there any therapy you would recommend?
- What is the prognosis?

Case Discussion

The diagnosis in each case is "exploding head syndrome." This implies the occurrence of episodes of

sudden waking to a sudden bang or explosive noise within the head, occurring most typically soon after falling asleep. In this (usually benign) condition the noise lasts only a split second and has often gone away by the time the patient is fully aroused. Some patients describe a flash of light associated with the noise. The event usually leaves patients alarmed for several minutes afterwards and they usually seek help because they believe that they have suffered a brain hemorrhage or have a tumor. Most of them initially call the sensation a "headache" but on further questioning agree that there is no actual pain with these awakenings.

This little-known but probably common syndrome was described in 1988 by Pearce who reported 10 cases. Prior to this there had been sporadic mention in the literature of similar phenomena. Weir Mitchell was among the first to describe such "sensory shocks," reporting descriptions such as "as if struck," "a feeling of rending," and "a bolt driven through the head." In 1920, Armstrong-Jones invited his scientific colleagues to suggest an explanation for "snapping of the brain." In his letter, he described patients who complained of a sudden crash or noise "as if something had snapped or given way in my brain." He felt that such perceptions may have arisen from some labyrinthine disorder or spontaneous cerebral auditory imaging. Pearce, in a follow-up report to his initial description of the syndrome summarized the descriptions of an additional 40 patients, in response to the barrage of information that he received from colleagues describing their experiences (either personal or patient-based) after his initial report.

The syndrome affects all age groups between 11 and 80 years but the commonest age of presentation is after the age of 50 years. There is a slight preponderance of women.

Descriptions of the feeling vary, but the sensation is usually brief and quite loud and has been described variously as a loud bang like that produced by a shotgun or an explosion, a thunderclap, a loud metallic noise, the clash of cymbals, a door slamming, or a loud electric explosion. Other descriptions include a "noise as if my head will burst open," like a Christmas cracker bursting, or like a human voice uttering a vowel sound. Associated phenomena may include the sensation of cessation of breathing, an overactive mind, an aura of floating, concern or panic, confusion, sitting bolt upright, tinnitus on waking, a sense of falling, missed heartbeats, or a flash of light. Most people report the occurrences soon after they fall asleep. No patients hitherto reported have been found to have any pathology prior to the onset of the symptoms and none appeared to have developed problems later, despite some having had these symptoms for over 20 years. The natural history indicates that the condition is self-limiting, lasting a few weeks to months, although it may reappear in later years.

Numerous explanations have been suggested. Early hypotheses favored an exaggerated perception of, or response to, normal changes in the peripheral auditory apparatus. Pearce hypothesized that the syndrome is the auditory analogue of the nocturnal myoclonus that occurs during the transition from wakefulness to stage 1 sleep. Sachs and Svanborg performed polysomnographic recordings of five patients with this syndrome and considered that the attacks occurred during relaxed wakefulness. Two of their subjects had evidence of increasing alertness associated with the attacks. There was no indication of an epileptic etiology in any of their cases. Clomipramine was prescribed for three of their subjects, who experienced prompt symptomatic relief.

The brevity of the phenomenon, its timing (usually in or around stage 1 sleep), its occurrence (in our second patient) contemporaneously with the onset of generalized seizures, and its high prevalence, (as we have confirmed through an informal survey of colleagues) all lead us to agree with Pearce that it represents the sensory equivalent of the "sleep start" or "hypnic jerk." This is a sleep-wake transition parasomnia consisting of generalized single myoclonus-like bodily jerks on falling asleep, unaccompanied by changes on electroencephalography (EEG) but sometimes with a perception of falling or a sensory flash, followed by intense arousal.

Regarding its prognosis, the syndrome has hitherto always been reported as benign and self-limiting. Some patients report that these occurrences coincide with times of stress, fatigue, or depression, but otherwise no trigger factors have been noted. Reassuring the patient about the benign nature of these attacks is a major part of management and may alone decrease the severity of the symptom. If this is not the case, prescription of clomipramine may be of value.

Other entities to consider when a patient presents with this complaint are intracerebral hemorrhage, hypnagogic hallucinations, benign paroxysmal cranial neuralgias, and seizures. The repetitive occurrence of the symptom in healthy people who have no clinical deficit makes the diagnosis of intracerebral hemorrhage unlikely. Hypnagogic hallucinations are vivid auditory or visual perceptions incorporated into dream-like periods in the rapid eye movement (REM) sleep periods of narcoleptic patients and in the lightest stages of non-REM sleep in normal subjects. They are considered to represent the sleep/dream imagery of REM sleep occurring inappropriately and may be the sensory equivalent of hypnic jerks; if that is the case, then they are identical to the symptom in question. They usually comprise voices, animal noises, or music.

Benign paroxysmal cranial neuralgias (also known as "ice-pick pains," "needle-in-the-eye syndrome," or cephalgia fugax) are unaccompanied by any sounds and are painful; the exploding head syndrome is seldom so. Partial seizures originating in the temporal lobes may give rise to auditory hallucinations, but these are more commonly of formed, recognizable sound sequences which seldom occur without other symptoms or in the absence of some localized abnormality on the EEG or on brain imaging.

Selected Readings

Armstrong-Jones R. Snapping of the brain. Lancet 1920;2:720.

Oswald I. Sleeping and waking. New York: Elsevier; 1962.

Oswald I. Exploding head. Lancet 1988;2:625.

Pearce JMS. Exploding head syndrome. Lancet 1988;2:270.

Pearce JMS. Clinical features of the exploding head syndrome. J Neurol Neurosurg Psychiatry 1989;52:907–10.

Pryse-Phillips WEM. Companion to clinical neurology. Boston: Little, Brown; 1995.

Sachs C, Svanborg E. The exploding head syndrome: polysomnographic recordings and therapeutic suggestions. Sleep 1991;14:263–6.

Weir Mitchell S. Some disorders of sleep. Int J Med Sci 1890; 100:109–27.

Editorial Comments

Although we all deal regularly with common primary headache disorders, there are many rare and unusual cases of headache and head symptoms often seen in the office or clinic. Often these "rare disorders" turn out to be a variation of a more common headache condition. However, in these two cases presented by

Pryse-Phillips and Wong, the condition described is not frequently complained of by those who experience it. What is truly fascinating is the discussion of the putative mechanism of "exploding head syndrome." Its relationship to normal sleep mechanisms and other headache disorders is interesting and these cases should increase our awareness of this type of entity.

Chapter 48

The Woman with Occipital Headache and Acute Neurologic Deficits

Mark W. Green, MD

Stephan A. Mayer, MD

Case History

This 29-year-old woman initially developed migraine at the age of 19, when she experienced one episode of left-sided pulsatile headache associated with transient tingling paresthesia in the right arm and leg. Her headaches were typically unilateral and pulsatile in nature and were associated with photophobia and nausea. They were easily treated with ibuprofen and would occur just a few times a year.

The patient works as a nurse and also has what she calls "typical tension" headaches from time to time at the end of a hard day of work. She is otherwise healthy.

She was in her usual state of good health until the day she developed a strong occipital headache, which persisted for 2 days. On the third day at 7:30 AM the pain in her occiput acutely worsened, and she experienced numbness, which traveled from the right leg to the occiput to the right arm, followed by a claw-like contraction of the right hand. During this episode, which lasted 30 minutes, she also had right facial weakness and difficulty speaking. She was admitted to a local emergency room (ER). At that point her deficits had completely resolved and she was released.

The next day, she had a second episode, which began with a severe bilateral occipital headache fol-lowed shortly thereafter by numbness, which traveled up both legs, beginning in the feet, progressing to the thighs, then to both arms and then to the mouth. At this point she was completely unable to speak. Her parents took her to another ER, where she was treated with oxycodone and ibuprofen. After approximately 40 minutes, as these deficits resolved, she experienced severe photophobia and saw white spots. A computed tomography (CT) scan was obtained and was normal. She was released on pain medication.

One day later, she saw a neurologist who diagnosed complicated migraine and prescribed a suma-triptan injection. That evening, while driving home from the appointment, she experienced a third episode, which again began with a severe occipital headache, followed by numbness in the right leg, which traveled to the right arm. When she got home the symptoms persisted and she took a dose of sumatriptan. Her symptoms resolved immediately.

The next day, her neurologist ordered a magnetic resonance imaging (MRI) and magnetic resonance angiography of the brain, which were completely normal.

Finally, in the evening 3 days later, while at home, she experienced a fourth episode of severe occipital headache. At the onset of this attack she noticed diffi-culty holding the phone in her left hand. She then rapidly developed an acute agitated confusional state. She was taken to another local ER, where her temperature was 104°F. At that time she had a left hemiplegia. It was also noticed that as she tried to dress to go to the ER she had not put her clothes on the left side of her body, and a neurologic examination confirmed the presence of left hemispatial neglect.

A spinal tap was performed which showed a lymphocytic pleocytosis and elevated protein (Table 49–1). She was transferred to a tertiary care hospital for further management. On arrival at the intensive care unit she was agitated. A mental status examination showed her to be oriented but mildly encephalopathic, with delayed verbal responses, verbal perseveration, and emotional lability. Over the next few days, her mental status completely cleared and her left hemiparesis resolved. Two days after admission her condition was normal except for bilateral knee clonus and a mildly unsteady tandem gait. A second lumbar puncture (LP) showed slight improvement in the lymphocytic pleocytosis (Table 48–1). Her work-up at this time included electroencephalography, which showed mild bilateral slowing, another CT scan which was normal, and a brain single photon emission computed tomography (SPECT) scan which was normal. She was treated with acyclovir, antibiotics, and phenytoin and experienced no further episodes. She was discharged after 10 days with a normal examination and was off all medications.

Negative laboratory tests included cerebrospinal fluid (CSF) herpes simplex virus–polymerase chain reaction (HSV-PCR); CSF Lyme antibody; antinuclear antibodies (ANA); Coxsackie virus titers; echovirus titers; arboviral titers; viral rectal and throat cultures; CSF bacterial, fungal, and viral cultures; CSF immunoglobulin G (IgG) index; CSF cryptococcal antigen; CSF Venereal Disease Research Laboratory (VDRL); and CSF angiotensin converting enzyme (ACE) activity. Oligoclonal bands were positive in the CSF.

Five days after discharge from the hospital, she experienced a fifth stereotypical episode of occipital headache followed by numbness which ascended from the right leg to the occiput to the right arm followed by speech difficulty. She called her doctor and had evidence of anomic aphasia with semantic paraphasic errors on the telephone. This episode

again lasted 30 minutes. She was told to begin taking valproic acid but did not fill the prescription.

When driving home from her doctor's appointment, she experienced another severe attack, which began with occipital headache and numbness spreading from the right leg to the occiput to the right arm, followed rapidly by a confusional state and aphasia. She was again taken to the ER, where she was in an agitated delirium with aphasic speech and a right hemivisual deficit. Another lumbar puncture was performed which again showed lymphocytic pleocytosis (Table 48–1). She improved markedly over the next 24 hours and by the next day had a normal mental status with mild right hyperreflexia and difficulty with tandem gait. At this point, all serologic tests for viral meningitis were negative. She was treated with dexamethasone and loaded with valproic acid. On hospital day 1, she had a transcranial Doppler examination which showed evidence of accelerated flow consistent with spasm of the distal basilar artery (Table 48–2). This was repeated 2 days later and showed normalization of basilar flow, confirming the presumed diagnosis of complicated basilar artery migraine with secondary pleocytosis. An MRI of the brain was normal.

Thereafter, the dexamethasone was tapered off over a period of 10 days and she continued to take valproic acid with levels ranging from 75 to 120 mg per dL. She experienced no further episodes of complicated migraine. After 3 months, the valproic acid was tapered off and the patient has done well ever since with no further episodes of basilar migraine.

Questions about This Case

- What are your diagnostic considerations in this case?
- Do you think that sumatriptan was an appropriate treatment after the second attack of occipital headache and neurologic deficit?
- How would you have managed this patient's clinical course?

Points for discussion:

- This patient clinically had a history compatible with basilar migraine. The differential diagnosis would have included partial seizures or viral meningitis.
- Sumatriptan and other vasoconstricting agents are

TABLE 48–1. Lumbar Puncture Results

Date	WBC (cells/mm^3)	RBC (cells/mm^3)	Protein (mg/dL)	Glucose (mg/dL)	Differential Lymphocytes/Monocytes
Baseline	280	300	142	67	99/1
4 days later	135	15	65	70	95/5
9 days later	215	20	36	51	97/3
21 days later	50	0	47	72	97/3

WBC = white blood cell count; RBC = red blood cell count.

generally considered to be contraindicated in this condition but happened to be effective in this case.

- Pleocytosis has been described in association with complicated migraine and supports the hypothesis of a neurogenically mediated inflammatory response (trigeminovascular hypothesis) in the etiology of complicated migraine.
- The presence of distal basal artery constriction documented by transcranial Doppler is strongly confirmatory for the presumed diagnosis of basilar artery migraine.
- Valproic acid was associated with a dramatic cessation of symptoms in this case and may be effective for the treatment of complicated migraine. Other treatment possibilities might include calcium channel blockers.

Case Discussion

Diagnostic considerations in the case include a recurring encephalitis, a cerebral vasculitis such as extrinsic compression from rheumatoid inflammatory tissue, basilar artery dissection, or the syndrome of mitochondrial encephalopathy, lactic acidosis, and stroke-like episodes (MELAS). A lactic acid level was not obtained, and she might also have undergone a muscle biopsy looking for ragged red fibers, which are characteristic of a mitochondrial cytopathy, albeit nonspecific. Infarctions in MELAS do have a predilection for the posterior cerebral region but this patient has exhibited a benign course, unlikely to be the case in MELAS.

Sumatriptan is contraindicated in the treatment of basilar migraine but appeared to be effective in this case. It is contraindicated because of fear that it might further reduce cerebral perfusion in a situation felt likely to be associated with cerebral ischemia. Practically, it is contraindicated because the studies on this agent which led to FDA approval excluded any patients with basilar migraine. Therefore, it is untested in such patients. Sumatriptan is clearly a potent constrictor of human dural arteries but less so of cerebral and temporal arteries. Sumatriptan, as well as ergotamine, does appear to affect flow velocity on transcranial Doppler (TCD) studies in some migraineurs, particularly involving the middle cerebral and basilar arteries, although the majority of patients studied do not show any alteration in blood flow velocities. A theory still exists that arteriovenous anastomoses open in migraine and that sumatriptan and dihydroergotamine constrict these anastomoses. Should that be the case, these drugs could prove useful by improving perfusion.

Several convincing cases of migraine with CSF pleocytosis and elevations in CSF protein have been reported. Pleocytosis supports the trigeminovascular hypothesis that is described in detail elsewhere in this book. Most cases of migraine have not been associated with any abnormalities of the CSF but several cases of "hemiplegic" migraine have had similar CSF profiles to that of our patient. It is recognized that lumbar punctures are not routinely performed in patients with migraine with aura and therefore the actual incidence of these abnormalities is not known. Cerebrospinal fluid viral cultures and CSF Lyme titers in this patient were normal but that does not entirely exclude an infectious cause of the attacks. We also know that vasodilator polypeptides

TABLE 48–2. Basilar Artery Transcranial Doppler Examination Results

Date	Depth (mm)	Peak Velocity (cm/sec)	Mean Velocity (cm/sec)	Pulsatility Index
Baseline	104	105	70	0.82
2 days later	100	63	46	0.62

accumulate in the CSF of migraineurs and that there is an increase in capillary permeability. It is not difficult to imagine that a migraine headache could therefore simply reflect the neurogenic inflammation of a severe migraine attack.

The presence of distal basilar artery constriction may confirm the presumed hypothesis of basilar migraine. We know that this disorder can be associated with cerebral infarction, which is thought to be secondary to vasospasm, particularly since morphologic changes within these patient's vessels have not been identified. Cerebral angiography performed during attacks of basilar migraine is generally normal but at the height of an attack, constriction of the basilar artery has been seen. Unfortunately, studies of TCD features have not yielded consistent results. It appears that the intracranial mean flow velocities may be high in all cerebral arteries. It is also possible in this case that an unidentified cause of meningoencephalitis served as a nonspecific trigger for attacks of basilar migraine. Others (Barleson) have concluded that a syndrome of migrainous attacks with a mononuclear CSF pleocytosis suggests a benign syndrome that might not justify an invasive evaluation with cerebral angiography nor any therapeutic intervention. Furthermore, it has been suggested from the anecdotal experiences of several authors that migrainous patients may have an excessive complication rate from cerebral angiography.

The final point deals with how to manage this patient. Valproate appeared to have helped resolve these attacks. In similar cases, attacks are often infrequent, making a conclusion about the efficacy of any preventive agent difficult. Most patients with basilar migraine have their attacks widely spaced and are nonprogressive. Therefore, prophylaxis is often not suggested. In fact, all treatment recommendations for basilar migraine are based on anecdotal experiences, and no controlled studies really exist to guide us. Another reasonable treatment is with calcium channel blockers, noting that these agents reduce vasospasm since calcium regulates vascular smooth-muscle contraction. A few case reports suggest that propranolol may have precipitated attacks and some believe these agents are contraindicated. Other headache experts have recommended these agents for the prophylaxis of basilar migraine.

Management Strategies

- Rule out infectious causes of the encephalopathy, and treat for a meningoencephalitis if the diagnosis is uncertain. It is preferable to overtreat for an infectious etiology than to undertreat for migraine.
- Avoid treatment with 5-HT 1 agonists if the differential diagnosis includes hemiplegic or basilar migraine.
- Remember that a response or lack of response to an abortive antimigraine therapy cannot be used as evidence for the diagnosis of migraine.
- A neurology consultation is always appropriate in such a gravely ill patient.
- A transcranial Doppler can be a valuable study, if available, in a hospital setting if an attack might be observed.
- Should the diagnosis of basilar migraine be made, a decision about whether to use prophylactic agents will be dependent upon the frequency and severity of such attacks, but recognizing that there is no proven effective therapy.

Selected Readings

Barteson J, Swanson J, Whisnant J. A migrainous syndrome with cerebrospinal fluid pleocytosis. Neurology 1981;31:1257–62.

Day T, Knezevic W. Cerebrospinal-fluid abnormalities associated with migraine. (Med) Aust 1984;141:459–61.

Limmeroth V, May A, Auerbach P, et al. Changes in cerebral blood flow velocity after treatment with sumatriptan or placebo and implications for the pathophysiology of migraine. J Neurol Sci 1996;138:60–5.

Motta E, Rosciszewska D, Miller K. Hemiplegic migraine with CSF abnormalities. Headache 1995;35:368–70.

Schraeder P, Burns R. Hemiplegic migraine associated with an aseptic meningeal reaction. Arch Neurol 1980;37:377–9.

Editorial Comments

Unusual variations of migraine are not infrequent in clinical practice. However, this case by Drs. Green and Mayer raises numerous questions about diagnoses and appropriate management, as well as reminding clinicians that mononuclear pleocytosis in the CSF is seen in many headache disorders, including migraine. The authors conclude that this patient has basilar migraine possibly triggered by meningoencephalitis. Readers should draw their own conclusions.

APPENDIX: DIAGNOSTIC TABLE OF CONTENTS

PART II SECONDARY, RARE, AND UNUSUAL HEADACHE DISORDERS

Index

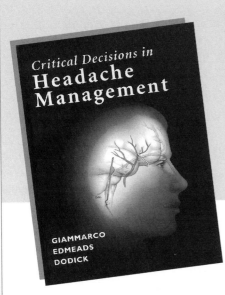
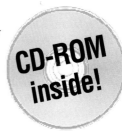
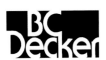

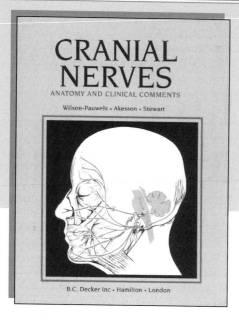
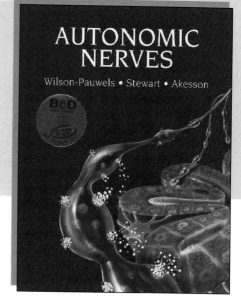
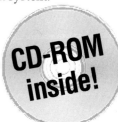

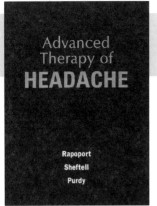
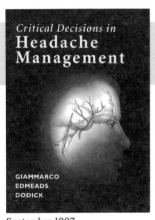

BUSINESS REPLY MAIL

FIRST-CLASS MAIL   PERMIT NO. 25   LEWISTON, NY

POSTAGE WILL BE PAID BY ADDRESSEE

B C DECKER INC
ATTN ORDER DEPARTMENT
P O BOX 785
LEWISTON NY 14092-9956

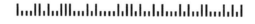

BUSINESS REPLY MAIL

FIRST-CLASS MAIL   PERMIT NO. 25   LEWISTON, NY

POSTAGE WILL BE PAID BY ADDRESSEE

B C DECKER INC
ATTN ORDER DEPARTMENT
P O BOX 785
LEWISTON NY 14092-9956